MRI: CENTRAL NERVOUS SYSTEM

· · · · · · · · · · · · · · · · · · ·

MRI: CENTRAL NERVOUS SYSTEM

edited by

WALTER KUCHARCZYK, MD, FRCP (C)

• •

CLINICAL DIRECTOR
TRI-HOSPITAL MAGNETIC RESONANCE CENTRE
TORONTO GENERAL HOSPITAL
ASSISTANT PROFESSOR OF RADIOLOGY
UNIVERSITY OF TORONTO
TORONTO, ONTARIO, CANADA

foreword by

DEREK C. HARWOOD-NASH, MB, ChB, FRCP

PAEDIATRIC NEURORADIOLOGIST, THE HOSPITAL FOR SICK CHILDREN
PROFESSOR OF RADIOLOGY, UNIVERSITY OF TORONTO
TORONTO, ONTARIO, CANADA

J.B. LIPPINCOTT   PHILADELPHIA
GOWER MEDICAL PUBLISHING   NEW YORK , LONDON

Distributed in USA and Canada by:
J.B. Lippincott Company
East Washington Square
Philadelphia, PA 19105
USA

Distributed in Southeast Asia, Hong Kong, India, and
Pakistan by:
Harper and Row (Asia) Pte Ltd.
37 Jalan Pemimpin 02–01
Singapore 2057

Distributed in UK and Continental Europe by:
Harper and Row Ltd.
Middlesex House
34–42 Cleveland Street
London W1P 5FB
UK

Distributed in Japan by:
Igaku Shoin Ltd.
Tokyo International
P.O. Box 5063
Tokyo
Japan

Distributed in Australia and New Zealand by:
Harper and Row (Australia) Pty Ltd.
P.O. Box 226
Artarmon, N.S.W. 2064
Australia

Library of Congress Cataloging–in–Publication Data
MRI: central nervous system/ edited by Walter
    Kucharczyk: foreword by Derek C. Harwood–Nash.
        p.   cm.
    Includes bibliographical references.
    ISBN 0–397–44670–5
    1. Central nervous system—Magnetic resonance
        imaging.
    I. Kucharczyk, Walter, 1955–
        (DNLM: 1. Central Nervous System Diseases—diagno-
sis. 2. Magnetic Resonance Imaging.   WL 141
M939)
RC349.M34M75   1990
616.8'047548—dc20
DNLM/DLC
for Library of Congress   89–13762
                                                CIP

British Library Cataloguing in Publication Data
Kucharczyk, Walter, *1955-*
    MRI: central nervuos system.
    1. Man. Central nervous system. Diagnosis. Magnetic
    resonance imaging
    I. Title
    616.8047575

    ISBN 0-397-44670-5

Copyright © 1990 by Gower Medical Publishing.
101 Fifth Avenue, New York, NY 10003

Printed in Hong Kong by Imago Publishing, LTD.

Editors: William B. Millard, Nancy Berliner
Illustrators: Alan Landau, Wendy Jackelow
Designers: Thomas Tedesco, Nava Anav, Glen Biren

10 9 8 7 6 5 4 3 2 1

FOREWORD

● ●

The development of the art and science of neuroradiology has always been based on three basic aspects: anatomic, technical, and clinical. Publications have become landmarks because of the satisfactory integration and exposition of these in equal proportion toward the intricacies of the normal and abnormal central nervous system.

To anatomy by Leonardo da Vinci and Vesalius, techniques of Dandy and Moniz, and clinical teachings of Cushing and Brain were first added pneumoencephalography, catheter angiography, and ultimately water-soluble myelography. A veritable explosion in physics and computer technology provided real-time ultrasound with Doppler, and now the major advances of computed tomography and magnetic resonance imaging.

It is necessary, therefore, to organize experience in such a way to display recognizable patterns. The patient and diagnostic images are only appearances; the pattern must be inferred. The analysis of these patterns provides an order, an order which is a synthesis derived from experience and thus makes experience comprehensible. The multiplication and addition of our knowledge intensifies the need to develop integrating principles. Numerous publications are extant which detail the many facets of MRI. What has been needed is a compact yet comprehensive treatise on MRI of the central nervous system for day-to-day clinical practice. This book is just that. It will become a landmark.

The initiative, enthusiasm, and talents of Dr. Walter Kucharczyk have produced this outstanding contribution toward the use of magnetic resonance imaging within the central nervous system. It is a concise and readable presentation of normal and abnormal anatomy, techniques, and the clinical concepts of neurologic disease. He and his co-authors have continued the tradition of significant contributions to medicine characteristic of the medical fraternity of the University of Toronto.

Noteworthy is this heritage of accurate anatomy, exquisite images, and the accent on clinical neuroradiology. Dr. Kucharczyk and his colleagues have combined the large and broad experience of pediatric, adult, and geriatric clinical MRI material from one of the largest, most diverse neuroscience departments in North America, with the assistance and experience of two colleagues at the University of California, San Francisco and the University of Manitoba.

Attractive to me, and I know to many others, will be the concise script with large print and well-defined topics in titled paragraphs. I particularly like the method of labeling anatomy and abnormalities at the margin of the images, together with a bold statement of the disease or entity in question above a succinct statement of the relevant observations. The references, containing a suitable blend of the essential historical and the necessary recent journal publications, have been chosen with care.

It is my privilege to be associated with Dr. Walter Kucharczyk, once a pupil and now my teacher, and all of the other authors. Their hard work and considerable clinical expertise are obvious. They have achieved what they set out to do. This is the essence of a valuable book.

Whether one is a clinician, anatomist, physicist or technician, student, intern, resident, or fellow, each of the three basic constituents (anatomy, technology, and clinical medicine) is most useful and readily understandable by all. Many copies will, I fear, receive the ultimate accolade for any good book, and that is to be permanently borrowed.

DEREK C. HARWOOD-NASH, MB, ChB, FRCP (C)

To Michael, Sasha, and Jennifer
FOR AMUSING THEIR MOTHER DURING THE PREPARATION OF THIS BOOK

To Dale
FOR BEING SO EASILY AMUSED

ACKNOWLEDGMENTS

I would like to extend my thanks and sincere gratitude to the many people who contributed their time, their effort, and their best cases to the production of this book. Drs. Keller, Kelly, Chuang, Bertram, Sutherland, Lee, Smith, and McClarty spent much of their free time searching for cases, and then writing, drawing and labeling their contributions. Surprisingly, they continued to do so despite my constant nagging either in person or on the phone. Drs. Harwood-Nash and Wortzman provided a constant source of encouragement and advice before and during this project. Mike and Betty Starr performed all the photography, usually on short notice because the prints were needed "now." Gina Sciortino was diligent, efficient, and even at times enthusiastic in typing the entire manuscript. Her future position in preparing manuscripts is forever assured. I am particularly grateful to Abe Krieger at Gower Medical Publishing for arranging this project and seeing it through to its completion. Finally, I thank my family, my mother and father for their encouragement, my wife Dale for her patience with me, and my children for never spilling anything on the prints.

PREFACE

The introduction of magnetic resonance imaging (MRI) into medical practice during the early 1980s created new opportunities for diagnosis. Based on proton density and the proton relaxation times T1 and T2, physical properties of tissue previously unexplored in clinical medicine, this technique produced spectacular images even with the earliest prototype instruments. Numerous reports attesting to the capabilities of MRI quickly accumulated and assured its place as a valuable diagnostic modality.

MRI's initial years in medicine exemplified a period of very rapid technical improvements, improvements so rapid that the quality of published material consistently lagged behind the technical level available in daily radiologic practice. More recently, the rate of these improvements has slowed and image quality has reached a relative plateau. This has enabled the collection and distillation of state-of-the-art images of a wide variety of disorders into this one concise publication. The figures in this book for the most part have all been obtained in an 18-month period on a 1.5 Tesla magnetic resonance system.

This book is directed to practicing radiologists, radiology residents, and physicians in related specialties such as neurology, neurosurgery, otolaryngology, and orthopedics, who are exposed to MRI of the brain, head and neck, and spine as part of their daily practice, whether they be experienced users or new in the field. The subject matter is comprehensive in scope; most topics receive some discussion, from classic manifestations of rare disorders to unusual manifestations of common disorders. In the interests of brevity, however, discussion of any one disorder is limited to the most salient and diagnostically important features.

The book contains five chapters: the brain, sella turcica and skull base, head and neck, orbit, and spine. Each chapter is organized into three sections, opening with a discussion and extensive illustrations of the normal anatomy, followed by a short section on MRI technique, and finally ending with an extensive collection of images depicting pathology.

The normal anatomy illustrations are displayed on opposing pages. The figures are laid out with a "scout" or "localizer" view that indicates the plane and position of section, and adjacent line diagrams indicate the structures of interest. MRI technique is discussed in terms as general as possible, recognizing that rapid changes are inevitable in this area. General objectives are emphasized rather than specific details. A technique table is provided in each chapter; these can be used as starting points and modified as necessary as new developments dictate. The pathologic material is extensively illustrated. The pathology figures are labeled directly, avoiding the use of various sizes and shapes of arrows. The abnormalities and diagnosis are readily apparent using this system without having to resort to long and complicated figure legends. The reading list accompanying each chapter is brief. The books and articles listed are representative of the literature on the various topics.

The format of the book allows quick and easy reference to most topics of interest in this area. At the same time, the concise nature of the book permits its complete reading in a relatively short period of time, either as a review or as a first exposure to the field.

WALTER KUCHARCZYK, MD, FRCP (C)

CONTRIBUTORS

• •

E.G. BERTRAM, PhD

Professor Emeritus
Department of Anatomy
University of Toronto
Toronto, Ontario, Canada

SYLVESTER H. CHUANG, MD, ChB, FRCP (C)

Department of Radiology
The Hospital for Sick Children
Toronto, Ontario, Canada

Associate Professor of Radiology
University of Toronto
Toronto, Ontario, Canada

WILLIAM M. KELLY, MD

Department of Radiology
David Grant Medical Center
Travis Air Force Base, California

Clinical Associate Professor of Radiology
University of California
San Francisco, California

M. ANNE KELLER, MD, FRCP (C)

Department of Radiology
Toronto General Hospital
Toronto, Ontario, Canada

Assistant Professor of Radiology
University of Toronto
Toronto, Ontario, Canada

WALTER KUCHARCZYK, MD, FRCP (C)

Clinical Director
Tri-Hospital Magnetic Resonance Centre
Toronto General Hospital
Toronto, Ontario, Canada

Assistant Professor of Radiology
University of Toronto
Toronto, Canada
Toronto, Ontario, Canada

KEVIN LEE, MD, FRACR

Department of Radiology
Toronto General Hospital
Toronto, Ontario, Canada

ROGER M.L. SMITH, MB, ChB, FRCS

Department of Radiology
Toronto General Hospital
Toronto, Ontario, Canada

BLAKE M. McCLARTY, MD, FRCP (C)

Department of Radiology
St. Boniface Hospital
Winnipeg, Manitoba, Canada

Assistant Professor of Radiology
University of Manitoba
Winnipeg, Manitoba, Canada

SCOTT SUTHERLAND, MD, FRCP (C)

Department of Radiology
University Hospital
Winnipeg, Manitoba, Canada

Assistant Professor of Radiology
University of Manitoba
Winnipeg, Manitoba, Canada

TABLE OF CONTENTS

chapter one

the brain

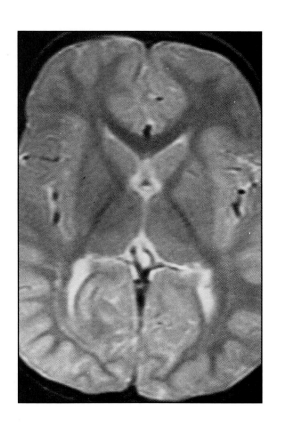

WALTER KUCHARCZYK   WILLIAM M. KELLY   SYLVESTER CHUANG

E. G. BERTRAM

INTRODUCTION

The diagnostic approach to patients with intracranial disorders has been markedly influenced by MRI's superb soft tissue contrast, multiplanar image acquisition, and freedom from beam-hardening artifact. Computed tomography, previously the only method of examining the brain parenchyma and skull base in detail, has been significantly displaced—but by no means replaced—by MRI. Although it has taken 3 to 4 years for physicians to become comfortable with MRI, many patients now come directly to MRI for diagnosis, bypassing CT. This is especially true for lesions in the middle and posterior fossae, and those adjacent to the vertex and skull base. Magnetic resonance imaging has become the diagnostic modality of choice for most congenital disorders, brain tumors, infections, white matter diseases and vascular malformations. Computed tomography, however, remains the preferred examination technique for acute trauma and suspected subarachnoid hemorrhage.

NORMAL ANATOMY
(Figs. 1.1 to 1.9)

THE CEREBRUM (TELENCEPHALON AND DIENCEPHALON)

TELENCEPHALON (CEREBRAL HEMISPHERE)
The **telencephalon** consists of the cortical **gray matter (cortex)**, the **medullary center (white matter)**, the **basal ganglia**, and the **lateral ventricles**. The cortex covers the surface of the cerebrum in a series of irregular convulutions, or gyri. The medullary center is a large area of consolidated nerve fibers coursing to and from the cortical gray matter. It is bounded peripherally by cortex and centrally by the lateral ventricle and corpus striatum. The individual fibers of the medullary center cannot be identified on MR images, but large groups of fibers form distinct tracts. For example, the projection fibers interposed between the caudate nuclei, lentiform nucleus, and thalamus form the internal capsule; and fibers interposed between the lentiform nucleus and claustrum form the external capsule.

The **internal capsule** consists of an anterior limb, genu, posterior limb, and retrolenticular and sublenticular parts. All the fibers originating from the motor cortex, and constituting the motor pathways (corticospinal and corticobulbar tracts), pass through the internal capsule toward the basal area of the brainstem. Large bundles of commissural fibers above the ventricles converge and cross medially to constitute the **corpus callosum** connecting the cerebral hemispheres. Easily identified portions are the splenium (posterior), body, genu, and rostrum (anterior), the last continuing inferiorly as the lamina terminalis (anterior wall of the third ventricle). Radiating commissural fibers from each occipital pole (forceps major) pass through the splenium; fibers from each frontal pole pass through the genu (forceps minor). The **anterior commissure**, a bundle of commissural fibers that crosses the midline within the lamina terminalis, connects the anterior portions of each temporal lobe.

The **basal ganglia** (gray matter) are located near the base of each cerebral hemisphere and consist of the **caudate nucleus**, the **lentiform nucleus**, the **claustrum**, and the **amygdaloid nucleus**. The large head of the caudate nucleus bulges into the frontal horn of the lateral ventricle. Its slender curved tail extends backward to curve around the dorsal surface of the thalamus in the floor of the body of the lateral ventricle, and then continues anteriorly to lie in the roof of the temporal horn of the lateral ventricle. The amygdaloid nucleus, situated in the ventral region of the uncus of the temporal lobe, blends with the tail of the caudate nucleus and forms part of the limbic system.

The lentiform nucleus is wedge-shaped, with the apical part (**globus pallidus**) of the wedge medial, and the **putamen** lateral. These are separated by an internal medullary lamina of nerve fibers. The head of the caudate nucleus and the putamen are continuous with one another beneath the anterior limb of the internal capsule. These three structures—the head of the caudate nucleus, the anterior limb of the internal capsule, and the putamen of lentiform nucleus—constitute the **corpus striatum**. The claustrum, a thin sheet of gray matter, is separated from the putamen by the **external capsule**, a thin layer of white matter. The **extreme capsule** separates the claustrum from the insular cortex.

The lateral ventricles contain the choroid plexus and cerebrospinal fluid (CSF). Each consists of a body from which three horns—frontal, occipital, and temporal—extend within their respective lobes. The body of the lateral ventricle is surrounded superiorly by the corpus callosum; laterally by the internal capsule; inferiorly by the thalamus and the structures that lie on its dorsolateral surface (tail of caudate nucleus and stria terminalis); and medially by the fornix.

The frontal horn is enclosed by the corpus callosum superiorly and anteriorly. The head of the caudate nucleus bulges into the inferolateral wall of the frontal horn and the septum pellucidum forms its medial wall, separating it from its counterpart on the opposite side. The interventricular **foramen of Monro** is located posterior to the septum and connects the lateral ventricle with the third ventricle.

The occipital horn is surrounded by the posterior medullary center. Two elevations on its medial wall are noteworthy: the bulb of the posterior horn, composed of the fibers of the forceps major, and the calcar avis, formed by the indentation of the calcarine sulcus.

The temporal horn is also surrounded by the medullary center. The tail of the caudate nucleus courses along its roof to the amygdaloid nucleus. The **hippocampus**, the anterior part of the limbic system, lies in the floor of this horn. The **fornix** originates from the hippocampus and courses within the ventricle from the undersurface of the thalamus, around its posterior aspect and onto the dorsomedial surface of the thalamus.

THE DIENCEPHALON

The **diencephalon** forms the central core of the cerebrum. It is almost completely surrounded by each cerebral hemisphere and is divided into two halves by the third ventricle. It consists of four regions: the **thalamus**, **epithalamus**, **subthalamus** and **hypothalamus**. Functionally, the thalamus and hypothalamus are the most important areas of the diencephalon.

The thalamus comprises approximately 80% of the diencephalon by volume. It lies between the interventricular foramen of Monro and the posterior commissure, extending laterally from the third ventricle to the posterior limb of the internal capsule. It consists of several nuclear areas that have connections for motor, general, or special sensory functions. On MR images these are not easily distinguished. Two paranuclear areas, the medial and lateral geniculate bodies, which function for hearing and vision, respectively, are located beneath the posterior overhanging area (**pulvinar**) of the thalamus.

The epithalamus is part of the superior surface of the diencephalon and consists of the pineal body, the habenular nuclei, and the stria medullaris thalami.

The hypothalamus, ventral to the medial thalamic area, forms the floor and lateral walls of the third ventricle up to the hypothalamic sulcus. It extends backward from the optic chiasm to the caudal border of the mamillary bodies. All the gross hypothalamic structures are visible on sagittal images, including the **infundibulum**, **tuber cinereum**, and **mamillary bodies**. The hypothalamus is divided into medial and lateral nuclear groups by anterior fibers of the fornix which end in the mamillary bodies. The hypothalamus governs the autonomic nervous system and is concerned with visceral, endocrine, and metabolic activity as well as with emotion, sleep, and temperature regulation.

The subthalamus is located ventral to the lateral thalamic nuclear area, between the hypothalamic area medially and the internal capsule laterally. It is a transitional zone composed of the subthalamic nucleus and many fiber tracts. All ascending sensory tracts and projection fibers from the cerebellum pass through the subthalamus en route to the ventral thalamic nuclei.

THE BRAINSTEM

The **brainstem**, consisting of the **midbrain**, **pons**, and **medulla oblongata**, is developed from the mesencephalon and rhombencephalon of the three primary brain vesicles. The brainstem contains white and gray matter. The white matter is composed of ascending (sensory) and descending (motor) tracts; the gray matter is composed of collections of nerve cells organized into the nuclei of the cranial nerves, and nuclei associated with coordinating motor activity (e.g., the red and olivary nuclei, reticular formation, and substantia nigra). The sensory and motor nerve fibers of cranial nerves III–XII enter or emerge from the ventral and lateral aspects of the brainstem; cranial nerve IV, however, emerges from the dorsal midbrain.

The midbrain is a short segment of the brainstem between the pons and diencephalon. From ventral to dorsal it is divided into the **cerebral peduncles**, **tegmentum**, and **tectum**. The **cerebral aqueduct** separates the tegmentum and tectum. The cerebral peduncle contains the basis pedunculi (the descending motor tract fibers including the corticospinal, corticobulbar, corticopontine, and corticoreticular tracts). The tegmentum consists of ascending sensory tracts and diffuse nuclear areas. The tectum is made up of the quadrigeminal plate. On the ventral surface, the cerebral peduncles are separated by the interpeduncular fossa. The optic tracts curve around each peduncle en route to the lateral geniculate bodies. On the dorsal surface, the colliculi are prominent landmarks. In the tegmentum of the midbrain, the central area of gray matter (around the aqueduct), and two distinct motor nuclei—the **red nucleus** and the **substantia nigra**—are easily identified. The tegmentum also contains the nuclei of cranial nerves III and IV, but these are not visible on MRI. Caudal to the red nucleus, the decussation of the brachium conjunctivum (superior cerebellar peduncles) is prominent on sagittal images.

The **pons** is a large structure caudal to the midbrain. It contains a prominent basal portion of descending motor tracts and nuclear areas, and a dorsal portion—the tegmentum—of diffuse areas of gray and white matter. The motor nuclei of cranial nerves V, VI, and VII, the sensory nuclei of cranial nerves V and VII, and the motor reticular nuclei are found in the tegmental pons as well as in the ascending sensory tracts. The smooth, flat dorsal surface of the pons forms the floor of the fourth ventricle. On the ventral surface of the pons, the basilar artery ascends in the midline sulcus. Laterally, as the pontine fibers course posterolaterally to form the middle cerebellar peduncle (brachium pontis), the fibers of cranial nerve V enter (sensory fibers) or emerge (motor fibers) from the pons.

The **medulla oblongata**, the caudal end of the brainstem, extends from the well-demarcated caudal border of the pons to the foramen magnum, where it continues as the spinal cord. It rests on the basilar portion of the occipital bone and is enveloped dorsally by the cerebellum. The external surface of the medulla oblongata has several readily distinguishable features. Ventrally, the **pyramids** containing the dense pyramidal (corticospinal) tracts form two longitudinal ridges on each side of the ventral median fissure. The **olives**, containing the olivary nuclei, are prominent lateral swellings between the dorsolateral and ventrolateral sulci. The medulla consists of a closed portion, which is a continuation of the spinal cord with all the cord's features, as well as an open portion, which forms the floor of the caudal portion of the fourth ventricle. The dorsal surface of the pons forms the floor of the rostral half of the fourth ventricle. On axial MRI through the rostral medulla, the ventrally located pyramids decussate in the anterior median fissure of the medulla and continue into the lateral columns of the spinal cord (lateral corticospinal tracts). Dorsal to the pyramids is the tegmentum of the medulla, which contains gray matter and white matter. The gray matter contains diffuse nuclear areas for sensory and/or motor neurons of cranial nerves VIII–XII, the descending nucleus of cranial nerve V, the reticular nuclear complex, and the prominent motor olivary complex. The most important white matter tracts are the spinothalamic tracts, the medial lemniscus, and the medial longitudinal fasciculus.

THE CEREBELLUM AND CEREBELLAR PEDUNCLES

The **cerebellum** is derived from the metencephalon. It lies dorsal to the pons and medulla and is separated from them by the fourth ventricle. The basic structure of the cerebellum consists of a midline **vermis** and two lateral **hemispheres**. As with the cerebral hemispheres, each lateral hemisphere has a cortex, medullary center, and several nuclear areas, and surrounds a ventricular space. The cortical gray matter is arranged in transverse folds or folia; the medullary center of white matter is composed of afferent and efferent cerebellar fibers. Located within each medullary center, from lateral to medial, are the dentate, emboliform, globose, and fastigial nuclei. The dorsal surface is covered by the **tentorium cerebelli** and its inferior surface overlies the fourth ventricle and the sides of the medulla. Dorsally, the folia of the vermis are not demarcated from that of the left or right hemispheres. On the ventral surface, however, the vermis is clearly separate from the hemispheres. The hemispheres are subdivided into lobes by fissures. Sagittal images are especially good for identifying the many lobules of the vermis, and the superior and inferior medullary velum which form the roof of the fourth ventricle.

Three pairs of **cerebellar peduncles**, which together form the lateral walls of the fourth ventricle, are attached to the ventral aspect of the cerebellum. The middle cerebellar peduncle (brachium pontis) contains afferent fibers, from the contralateral side of the basal pons, that course posteriorly and laterally into the cerebellar hemispheres. The inferior cerebellar peduncle (restiform and juxtarestiform body) consists of afferent and efferent cerebellar fibers. The afferent fibers are derived from the spinal cord (spinal-cerebellar fibers) and brainstem (olivocerebellar, vestibulocerebellar, trigeminocerebellar, and reticulocerebellar fibers); the efferent fibers are derived from the fastigial nucleus. The superior cerebellar peduncle (brachium conjunctivum) consists mainly of efferent fibers derived from the dentate, emboliform, and globose nuclei. These fibers course through the tegmentum of the midbrain, decussate at the midline, and either end in the red nucleus or encapsulate it en route to the ventrolateral nucleus of the thalamus.

MYELINATION OF THE NORMAL BRAIN (Fig. 1.10)

Magnetic resonance imaging is unique in its ability to demonstrate the orderly progression of myelination during the first two years of life, and thus evaluate brain maturity. The significant determinants of the MRI signal intensities of the normal brain are the proton density and relaxation times of the tissues, which, in turn, are dependent on their differential water content. In the mature adult brain, gray matter is 80% to 85% water and white matter is 70% to 75% water. Thus, gray matter is hyperintense to white matter on proton density and T2-weighted images, and hypointense to white matter on T1-weighted images. In the immature unmyelinated brain, however, water concentration is significantly higher in both gray and white matter. Most importantly, the white matter is also more hydrated than the gray matter, the reverse of that in the adult brain. Therefore, the proton densities and relaxation times of white and gray matter are greater than those in the adult, and the adult pattern of signal intensity on T1- and T2-weighted images is inverted. As the brain myelinates and matures, the T1- and T2-relaxation times decrease throughout the brain, doing so most rapidly in the myelinating white matter. As each tract myelinates, the proton density drops and the relaxation times shorten, with the tract gradually taking on the adult appearance relative to the surrounding gray matter. It is this orderly development that permits a relatively accurate assessment of the degree of myelination and, hence, brain maturity.

Myelination begins in utero in the brainstem, generally proceeding centripetally from brainstem to subcortical white matter, and from posterior to anterior. At birth the medulla, dorsal pons, dorsal midbrain, and posterior limb of the internal capsule are myelinated, making them hyperintense to gray matter on T1-weighted images and hypointense on heavily T2-weighted images. By 3 months of age, the remainder of the brainstem has myelinated, as have the middle cerebellar peduncles and the deep cerebellar white matter. By 4 to 6 months of age, the splenium of the corpus callosum has been myelinated. Myelination progresses anteriorly in the corpus callosum, reaching the genu at approximately 6 to 8 months. In the internal capsule, it begins in the posterior limb at birth, the genu at 4 to 6 months of age and, finally, in the anterior limb at approximately 10 months. Myelination of the deep white matter of the frontal lobes and centrum semiovale follows at about 14 to 15 months. By 18 months of age, the adult pattern is complete, except for the subcortical "U" fibers and the periventricular areas adjacent to the trigones of the lateral ventricles. The former are usually completely developed by 5 years of age, whereas the latter myelinate very late and may maintain the immature pattern well into the third decade of life.

While it is not critical to remember myelination milestones in detail, it is worthwhile to acquire a general perspective of the normal at particular ages. This can be accomplished by comparing representative sections through the brain that encompass important myelination landmarks, especially axial sections that include the midpons and middle cerebellar peduncles, the internal capsules, the corpus callosum, and the centrum semiovale and subcortical "U" fibers. These four views are presented in Fig. 1.10 for five infants aged one week, two months, six months, 10 months, and 2 years.

Normal Anatomy of the Brain (Figs. 1.1 to 1.9)

The Brain

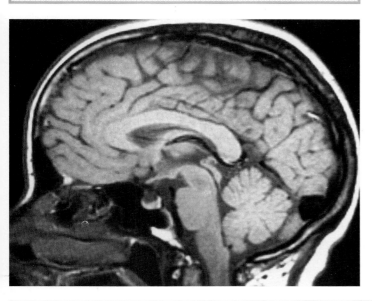

Fig. 1.1 Midline T1-Weighted Sagittal Image The ability to obtain sagittal images is a unique attribute of MRI. The midline sagittal image is ideal for displaying all midline structures to best advantage, including the superior sagittal sinus, the corpus callosum, most of the ventricular system, the brainstem, and the foramen magnum.

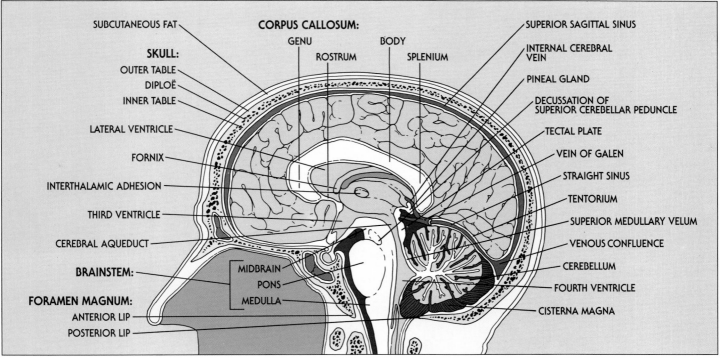

The Brain

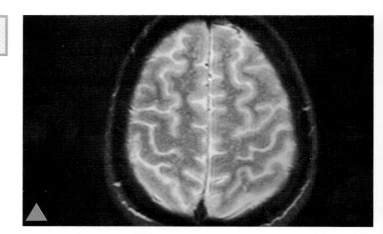

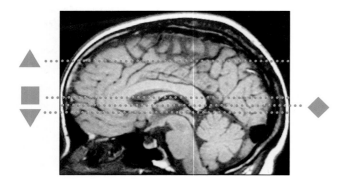

Fig. 1.2 Localizer: Midline T1-Weighted Sagittal Image
The planes of section of four axial images are indicated: through the vertex, the genu and splenium of the corpus callosum, the basal ganglia, and the anterior commissure.

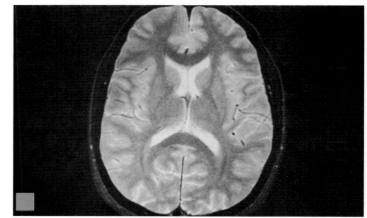

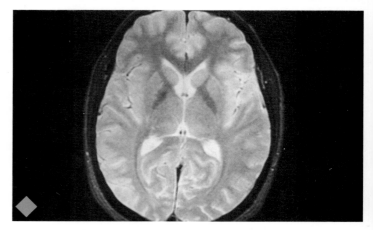

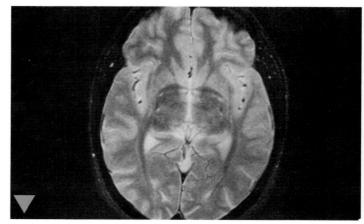

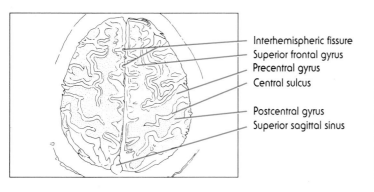

Interhemispheric fissure
Superior frontal gyrus
Precentral gyrus
Central sulcus

Postcentral gyrus
Superior sagittal sinus

Fig. 1.3A T2-Weighted Axial Image at the Level of the Vertex The superior frontal gyrus runs parallel to the interhemispheric fissure until it is interrupted on its posterior margin by the precentral gyrus. The precentral gyrus (sensory cortex) and the postcentral gyrus (motor cortex) can be consistently identified in this manner.

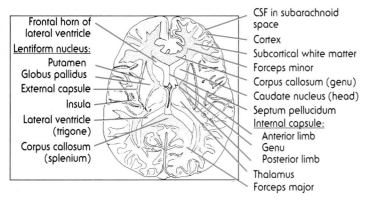

Frontal horn of lateral ventricle
Lentiform nucleus:
  Putamen
  Globus pallidus
External capsule
Insula
Lateral ventricle (trigone)
Corpus callosum (splenium)

CSF in subarachnoid space
Cortex
Subcortical white matter
Forceps minor
Corpus callosum (genu)
Caudate nucleus (head)
Septum pellucidum
Internal capsule:
  Anterior limb
  Genu
  Posterior limb
Thalamus
Forceps major

Fig. 1.3B T2-Weighted Axial Image at the Level of the Genu and Splenium of the Corpus Callosum The large commissural tracts of the corpus callosum and its peripheral extensions, the forceps major and minor, bridge the two hemispheres. The basal ganglia (caudate nucleus and lentiform nucleus) are deep gray matter structures divided by the internal capsule. Peripheral to the basal ganglia are the external and extreme capsules and the insular cortex.

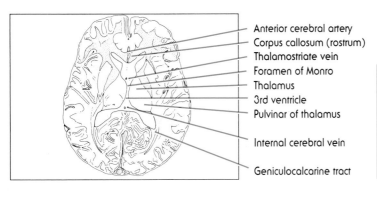

Anterior cerebral artery
Corpus callosum (rostrum)
Thalamostriate vein
Foramen of Monro
Thalamus
3rd ventricle
Pulvinar of thalamus

Internal cerebral vein

Geniculocalcarine tract

Fig. 1.3C T2-Weighted Axial Image at the Level of the Basal Ganglia The foramen of Monro is identified on axial sections as the point where the thalamostriate vein leaves the lateral ventricle. The thalamus is the largest and most posterior of the deep cerebral gray matter nuclei. Note the pulvinar, a segment that overhangs the cerebral peduncle.

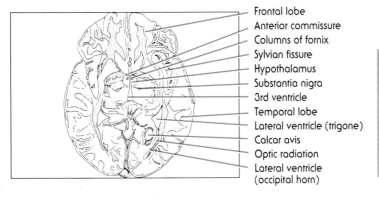

Frontal lobe
Anterior commissure
Columns of fornix
Sylvian fissure
Hypothalamus
Substantia nigra
3rd ventricle
Temporal lobe
Lateral ventricle (trigone)
Calcar avis
Optic radiation
Lateral ventricle (occipital horn)

Fig. 1.3D T2-Weighted Axial Image at the Level of the Anterior Commissure The anterior commissure connects the two temporal lobes. Just posterior to the commissure, the columns of the fornix are located on either side of the third ventricle while the hypothalamus forms the wall of the inferior third ventricle. Posteriorly, the prominent calcar avis indents the medial wall of the occipital horn.

The Brain

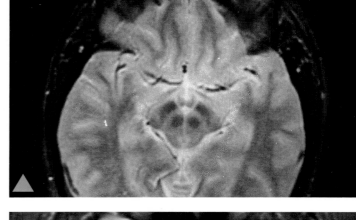

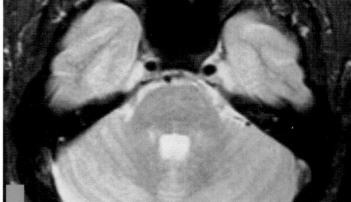

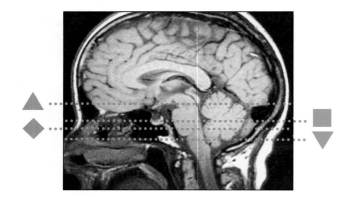

Fig. 1.4 Localizer: Midline T1-Weighted Sagittal Image
The planes of section of four axial images are indicated:
through the midbrain, the midpons, the lower pons and
the medulla.

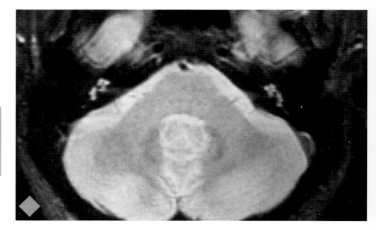

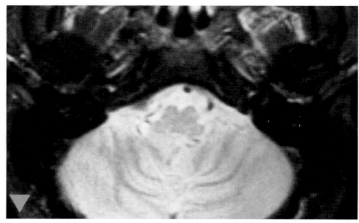

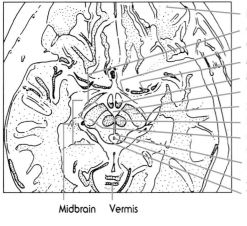

Roof of orbit
Cerebral peduncle
Optic tract
Middle cerebral artery
Mamillary body
Interpeduncular cistern
Substantia nigra
Red nucleus
Corticospinal and
corticopontine tracts
Periaqueductal gray matter
Aqueduct
Tectum

Midbrain   Vermis

Fig. 1.5A T2-Weighted Axial Image at the Level of the Midbrain The internal structure of the midbrain from anterior to posterior consists of: the cerebral peduncle containing the corticospinal tract, the tegmentum containing the substantia nigra and red nucleus, the cerebral aqueduct, and the tectum. The suprasellar and interpeduncular cisterns form the anterior boundary of the midbrain, and the quadrigeminal plate cistern forms the posterior boundary of the midbrain.

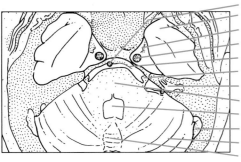

Basilar artery
Temporal lobe
Cavernous sinus
Carotid artery (int.)
Prepontine cistern
Trigeminal nerve
Petrous temporal bone
Pons
4th ventricle
Transverse sinus
Cerebellar hemisphere
Vermis

Fig. 1.5B T2-Weighted Axial Image at the Level of the Midpons The midpons has many projection fibers passing through it, interspersed with small nuclear areas imparting a slightly reticulated appearance. The pons is connected to the cerebellum by the middle cerebellar peduncles and separated from it by the body of the fourth ventricle.

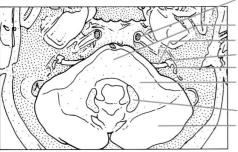

Carotid artery
(horizontal portion)
Pons
Internal auditory canal
Cochlea
Vestibule
Middle cerebellar
peduncle
Dentate nucleus
Cerebellar hemisphere

Fig. 1.5C T2-Weighted Axial Image at the Level of the Lower Pons The basilar artery is anterior to the lower pons and the internal auditory canals are lateral to it. Posterolateral to the recesses of the fourth ventricle lie the comma-shaped dentate nuclei.

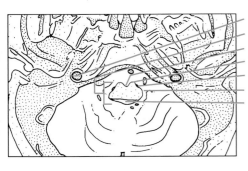

Internal carotid artery
Medulla
Median sulcus
Pyramid
Olive
Foramen of Luschka
Foramen of Magendie

Fig. 1.5D T2-Weighted Axial Image at the Level of the Medulla The medulla is identified by its prominent ventral swellings, the pyramids, which are laterally bounded by the olives. The inferior fourth ventricle empties into the cisterna magna via the midline foramen of Magendie and the paired lateral foramina of Luschka.

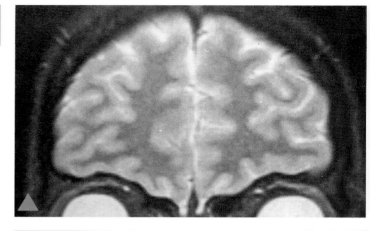

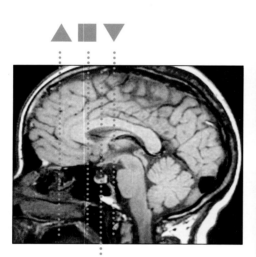

Fig. 1.6 Localizer: Midline T1-Weighted Sagittal Image
The plane of section of four coronal images are indicated: through the olfactory bulbs, the anterior limb of the internal capsule, the thalamus, and the substantia nigra.

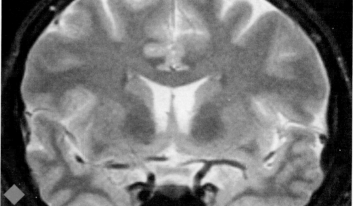

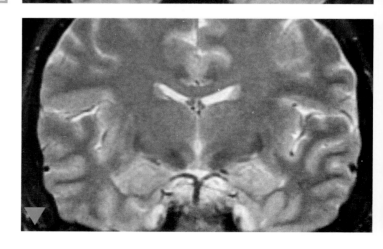

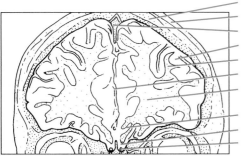

Skull
Subcutaneous fat
Superior sagittal sinus
Cortex
Subcortical white matter
Interhemispheric fissure
Deep white matter
(medullary center)
Gyrus rectus
Olfactory groove
Olfactory bulb

Fig. 1.7A T2-Weighted Coronal Image at the Level of the Olfactory Bulbs   The dark gray medullary center white matter is surrounded by a thin layer of slightly hyperintense gray matter cortex. Inferiorly, on either side of the midline, the olfactory bulbs are within the olfactory grooves of the anterior cranial fossa; superiorly, the superior sagittal sinus is identified as a triangle in cross-section.

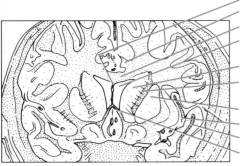

Septum pellucidum
Cingulate gyrus
Corpus callosum (body)
Lateral ventricle
(frontal horn)
Caudate head
Stria (anterior limb of
internal capsule)
Putamen
Sylvian fissure
Temporal lobe
Anterior commissure
(in lamina terminalis)

Fig. 1.7B T2-Weighted Coronal Image at the Level of the Anterior Limb of the Internal Capsule   The internal capsule divides the corpus striatum into the caudate and lentiform nuclei. Several gray matter bridges, or stria, pass between the two structures. The lateral ventricles are separated by the septum pellucidum, and are delimited superiorly by the body of the corpus callosum, which, in turn, is bordered by the cingulate gyrus.

Extreme capsule   Insula   Claustrum

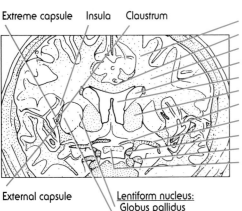

Centrum semiovale
Corpus callosum (body)
Corona radiata
Caudate nucleus
Lateral ventricle
Thalamus
Anterior cerebral artery
Middle cerebral artery
Internal carotid artery
Anterior clinoid process
Optic chiasm

External capsule

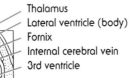

Lentiform nucleus:
Globus pallidus
Putamen

Fig. 1.7C T2-Weighted Coronal Image at the Level of the Thalamus   The large paired thalami are the most posterior of the deep cerebral nuclear structures. The lentiform nucleus is cone-shaped with the globus pallidus being medial and forming the point of the cone. Laterally, the lentiform nucleus is bordered by the external capsule; further laterally, it is bordered by the claustrum, extreme capsule, and insula.

Thalamus
Lateral ventricle (body)
Fornix
Internal cerebral vein
3rd ventricle

Sylvian fissure
Substantia nigra
Posterior cerebral artery
Hippocampus
Basilar artery
Subthalamic area

Fig. 1.7D T2-Weighted Coronal Image at the Level of the Substantia Nigra   The posterior part of the thalamus, the pulvinar, overhangs the substantia nigra in the midbrain. The thalamus forms the floor of the body of the lateral ventricle. The body of the fornix forms the inferomedial wall of the lateral ventricle.

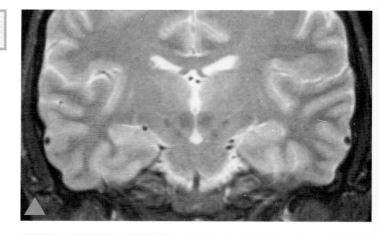

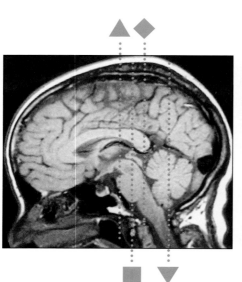

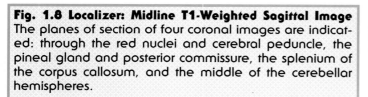

Fig. 1.8 Localizer: Midline T1-Weighted Sagittal Image
The planes of section of four coronal images are indicated: through the red nuclei and cerebral peduncle, the pineal gland and posterior commissure, the splenium of the corpus callosum, and the middle of the cerebellar hemispheres.

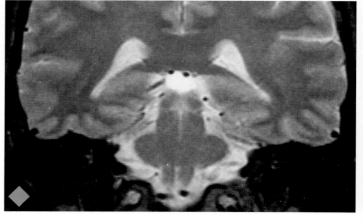

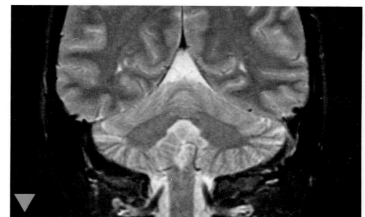

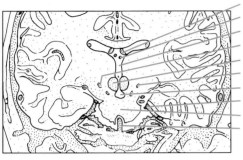

Fornix
Internal cerebral vein
3rd ventricle
Substantia nigra
Red nucleus
Cerebral peduncle
Interpeduncular cistern
Tentorium
Pons
Basilar artery

Fig. 1.9A T2-Weighted Coronal Image at the Level of the Red Nuclei and Cerebral Peduncle   The cerebral peduncles, containing the major descending motor tracts, connect the cerebral hemispheres with the brainstem and form the anterior third of the midbrain. The red nuclei and substantia nigra are distinct nuclear structures in the tegmentum of the midbrain; the red nuclei are medial, and the substantia nigra lateral.

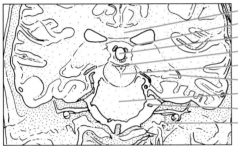

Corpus callosum (body)
Fornix
Pineal gland
Posterior commissure
Midbrain
Hippocampus
Pons
Trigeminal nerve
Internal auditory canal

Fig. 1.9B T2-Weighted Coronal Image at the Level of the Pineal Gland and the Posterior Commissure   The pineal gland is immediately inferior to the paired internal cerebral veins. Beneath it, from superior to inferior, lie the posterior commissure, the midbrain, and the pons.

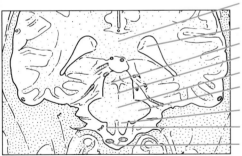

Corpus callosum (splenium)
Lateral ventricle (atrium)
Midbrain
Cerebral aqueduct
Pons
Middle cerebellar peduncle
Pyramid
Medulla
Vertebral arteries

Fig. 1.9C T2-Weighted Coronal Image at the Level of the Splenium of the Corpus Callosum   The thick commissural fibers of the splenium separate the atria of the two lateral ventricles. Inferiorly, the length of the brainstem is laid out, from superior to inferior: the midbrain containing the cerebral aqueduct, the pons, and the medulla containing the pyramids.

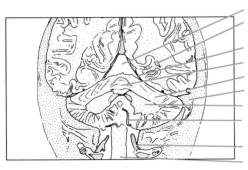

Superior vermian cistern
Lateral ventricle (occipital horn)
Tentorium
Superior vermis
Cerebellar cortex
Transverse sinus
Cerebellar white matter
Posterior inferior cerebellar artery
Vertebral artery
Spinal cord

Fig. 1.9D T2-Weighted Coronal Image at the Level of the Cerebellar Hemispheres   The tentorium separates the cerebral from the cerebellar hemispheres. The surface architecture of the cerebellum, consisting of relatively fine radially oriented folia, is distinctly different from the thick, gyral convolutions of the cerebrum.

Fig. 1.10 Normal Myelination: Birth – 2 Years T2-weighted axial images through the pons and middle cerebellar peduncle, the internal capsule, the corpus callosum, and centrum semiovale of five infants aged 1 week, 2 months, 6 months, 10 months, and 2 years. The same four levels are illustrated for each child, permitting a direct comparison of these key areas at different ages. Myelinated white matter is hypointense to gray matter on this particular sequence; unmyelinated white matter is hyperintense.

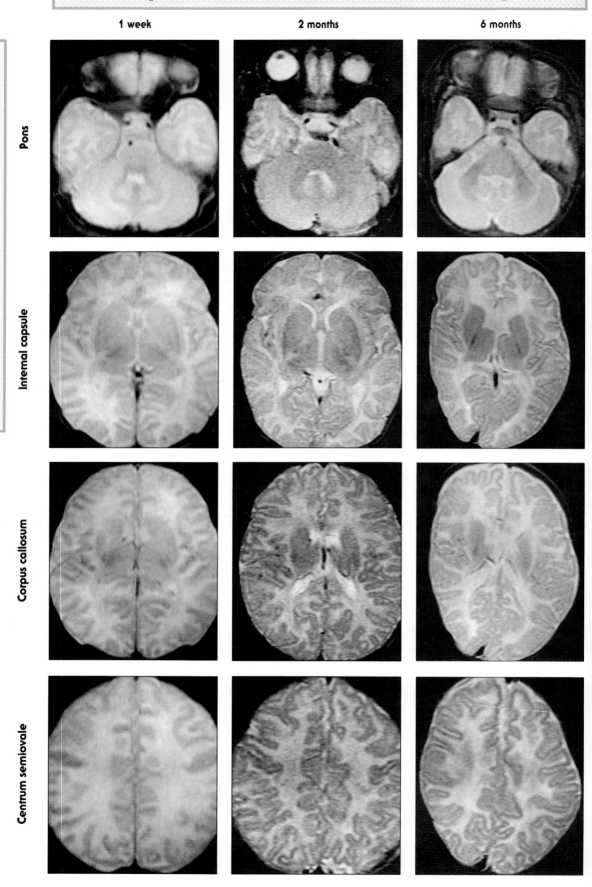

1 week   2 months   6 months

Pons

Internal capsule

Corpus callosum

Centrum semiovale

10 months   **2 years**

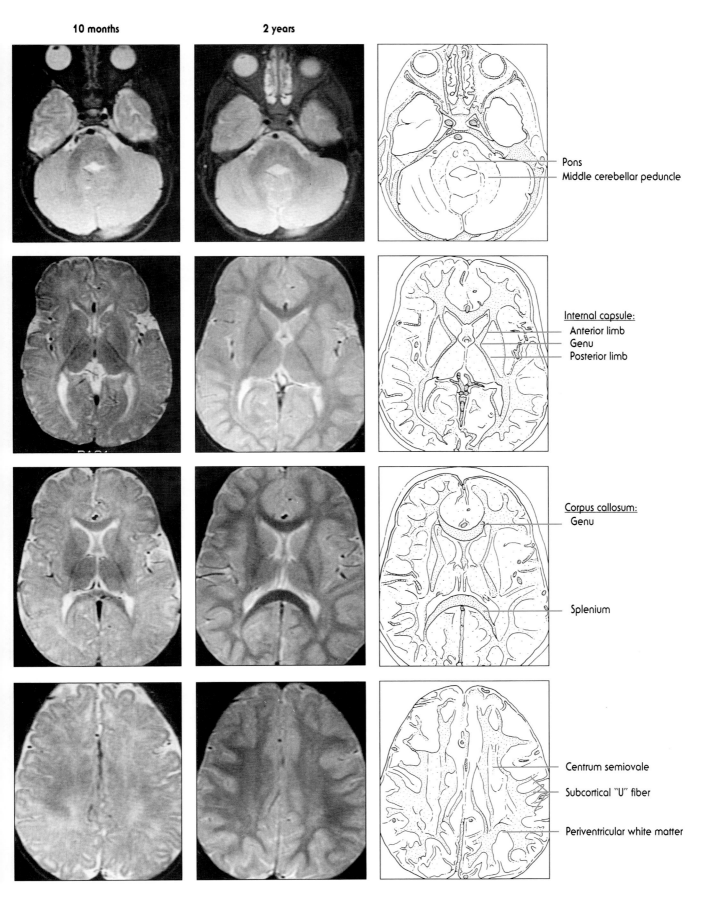

Pons
Middle cerebellar peduncle

Internal capsule:
  Anterior limb
  Genu
  Posterior limb

Corpus callosum:
  Genu

Splenium

Centrum semiovale

Subcortical "U" fiber

Periventricular white matter

TECHNIQUE

The technique for MRI examination of the brain is straightforward, particularly when compared with strategies used for the spine, face, and neck. Figure 1.11 summarizes the recommendations for MR imaging sequences of the brain. A multislice, spin-echo sequence in a circumferential head coil is preferred for virtually all brain examinations; surface coils have little or no role. The choice between axial and coronal images is very much up to individual preference for routine examinations. Certain conditions, however, dictate specific imaging planes. For example, lesions of the vertex, floor of the middle cranial fossa, and the tentorium are best imaged in the coronal plane.

Initial T1-weighted images in the sagittal plane are recommended primarily to exclude midline and foramen magnum pathology. These are followed by an axial, long TR sequence with early and late echoes that yield proton density weighted and T2-weighted images. These long TR images are essential: They are the most sensitive of all sequences in detecting parenchymal abnormalities and thus form the mainstay of MRI diagnosis in the brain. Many significant lesions will be overlooked if only T1-weighted images are used.

The study may stop at this point if it is a "screening" type of examination, or, for example, if the clinical diagnosis is multiple sclerosis or infarction.

Patients being evaluated for tumor, trauma, vascular malformations, or infection should also have a T1-weighted sequence. If a specific area is of concern, such as the posterior fossa, the slices are stacked closely together through the region of interest; otherwise, the T1-weighted sections should encompass the whole brain. Presaturation pulses are useful on T1-weighted images to reduce vascular inflow artifacts.

Supplementary imaging sequences are added with modifications of the plane of section or contrast-weighting when necessary. Gradient echo images are useful for the characterization of suspected aneurysms and vascular malformations. These images highlight patent vascular channels as positive contrast structures because of vascular inflow effects, thereby distinguishing vascular structures from calcific foci, with which they might otherwise be confused. In infants, because of the higher water content of their immature brains, repetition times (TRs) of 2500 to 3000 msec are necessary for adequate T2-weighting.

PATHOLOGY

CONGENITAL ABNORMALITIES

Congenital malformations of the brain include a wide spectrum of complex morphologic abnormalities. These are best understood by grouping them according to the type of developmental defect from which

Fig. 1.11 MRI TECHNIQUE FOR EXAMINATION OF THE BRAIN

Parameter	Sequence			
	No. 1[a] T1-Weighted	No. 2[b] T2-Weighted	No. 3 T1-Weighted	No. 4[c] Gradient-echo
Plane	Sagittal	Axial or coronal	Axial or coronal	Axial or coronal
TR (msec)	400–600	2000–3000	600	100–150
TE (msec)	20	70–100	20	12–20
Flip angle (degrees)	—	—	—	30–50
Slice thickness (mm)	3–5	5	5	5
Matrix	128–256	128–256	256	256
Field of view	24	20–24	20–24	20–24
No. of excitations	1–2	1–2	2	1–2
Gradient moment nulling	No	Yes	No	Yes
Presaturation	Yes	No	Yes	No
Exam time (min)	1–5	8–12	5	0.5–1/slice

[a] Low resolution sufficient for localizer views (e.g., TR 400 msec, MAT 128, NEX 1). For "diagnostic" quality use TR 600 msec, MAT 256, NEX 2.
[b] This long TR sequence usually involves two echoes: a short TE at 20–40 msec for a proton density image and a long TE at 70–100 msec for a T2-weighted image.
[c] Gradient-echo images of the brain usually reserved for vascular lesions (e.g., arteriovenous malformation, aneurysm).

they arise. The most common malformations are due to one of the disorders of neural tube closure, disorders of diverticulation, or disorders of sulcation and migration (Fig. 1.12). Disorders of size, microcephaly, and macrocephaly are straightforward and are thus not discussed here.

The accurate diagnosis of congenital lesions by MRI is due to the ability to acquire both multiplanar images and excellent soft tissue contrast. Generally, T1-weighted images are sufficient for delineation of the anatomic abnormalities, whereas T2-weighted images are best to evaluate the brain parenchyma. The latter technique is useful in clearly separating gray from white matter.

DISORDERS OF NEURAL TUBE CLOSURE

MENINGOENCEPHALOCELE   A meningoencephalocele is a herniation of the meninges and brain tissue through a cranial bony defect. The bony defect may be small in relation to the volume of tissue outside the skull vault. If there is no brain tissue within the herniation, *meningocele* is the preferred and more specific term. Unless MRI or angiography is used, the presence or absence of brain tissue in the hernia can be difficult to determine.

Meningoencephaloceles occur in 0.3%–0.4% of live births. They are either midline, which is the most common, or lateral. The most frequent locations (in order of incidence) of the midline variety are as follows: parietal-occipital, frontal-nasal, and occipital.

Parietal-occipital meningoencephaloceles, which have an internal CSF tract connecting them to the quadrigeminal cistern, are associated with splitting of the tentorium and straight sinus. In rare cases, an elongated third ventricular suprapineal recess may extend into a meningoencephalocele; this is termed a meningoencephalocystode. More rarely, a parietal-occipital meningoencephalocele contains fat; this is termed a lipomeningoencephalocele. Frontal-nasal meningoencephaloceles (Fig. 1.13) are frequently associated with agenesis of the corpus callosum and nearly all occipital ones are associated with the Chiari III malformation. All types may be associated with severe midline anomalies.

Lateral meningoencephaloceles are much less common than the midline type. They are most frequently in the floor of the middle cranial fossa or near the roof of the orbit.

Fig. 1.12 CLASSIFICATION OF CONGENITAL BRAIN MALFORMATIONS

Disorders of Neural Tube Closure
Meningoencephalocele
Chiari malformation
Dandy–Walker syndrome
Agenesis of the corpus callosum

Disorders of Diverticulation
Septo-optic dysplasia
Holoprosencephaly
Lobar
Semilobar
Alobar

Disorders of Sulcation and Migration
Ectopic gray matter
Focal gyral anomalies
Lissencephaly
Schizencephaly

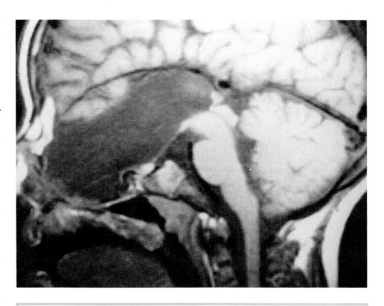

Fig. 1.13 FRONTOETHMOIDAL MENINGOCELE   T1-weighted sagittal image. There is a defect in the floor of the anterior cranial fossa with prolapse of a meningocele downwards through the bony defect into the nasal cavity. A variety of intracerebral midline anomalies are present, including absence of the corpus callosum, septum pellucidum, fornix and lamina terminalis.

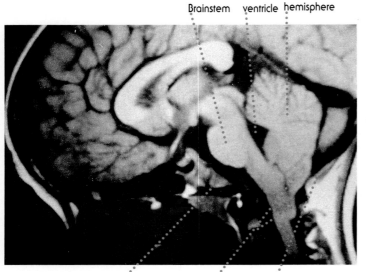

Brainstem — 4th ventricle — Cerebellar hemisphere

Anterior lip of foramen magnum — Low tonsils and vermis — Posterior lip of foramen magnum

Fig. 1.14 CHIARI I MALFORMATION (or TONSILLAR ECTOPIA) T1-weighted sagittal image. The cerebellar tonsils are positioned beneath the plane of the foramen magnum. The brainstem maintains its normal relationship to the foramen magnum. The tonsils, normally ovoid, are triangular in shape.

CHIARI I MALFORMATION   The Chiari I malformation, also referred to as tonsillar ectopia, consists of low positioning of the cerebellar tonsils below the plane of the foramen magnum. There is no spinal dysraphism or associated cranial anomalies. The Chiari I malformation is not associated with hydrocephalus, although hydromyelia is a common finding. Patients often present in adolescence or early adulthood with ataxia, nystagmus, or other gait disturbance. Many remain asymptomatic. A T1-weighted sagittal midline MRI is the best and single most reliable method of establishing a diagnosis. It demonstrates flattened, inferiorly pointed, low tonsillar tissue, and a normal fourth ventricle. Usually there is little or no surrounding subarachnoid space at the level of the foramen magnum. The tip of the tonsils may extend as low as C3 (Fig. 1.14).

CHIARI II MALFORMATION   The Chiari II malformation, or the Arnold–Chiari malformation, is always associated with some form of midline cranial or spinal dysraphism, especially a myelomeningocele. The posterior fossa is always small, and there is tonsillar and/or vermian herniation below the plane of the foramen magnum. The fourth ventricle is small and often elongated, commonly extending below the foramen magnum. The caudal placement of the hindbrain causes folding of the medulla and the cord to form a "cervicomedullary kink." These features are best seen on the T1-weighted sagittal scan. Other features in the posterior fossa include scalloping of the dorsal surfaces of the petrous temporal bones and beaking of the midbrain tectum. The superior cerebellar vermis is often prominent and rises through a widened tentorial hiatus. The shape of the tectum and the apparent vermian hypertrophy are more related to the position and deficiencies of the tentorium rather than a true hypertrophy of the vermis.

In the supratentorial region, the lateral ventricles retain the shape of fetal colpocephaly—large, wide, rounded occipital horns due to the deficiency of the forceps major. The squaring or beaking of the frontal horns is determined by large caudate nuclei that impress upon their infralateral surfaces and deficient forceps minor. This abnormal ventricular shape is by no means limited to the Chiari II malformation and is common in other midline malformations. The shape of the lateral ventricles are well-demonstrated on either axial or coronal scans. Usually there is hydrocephalus due to fourth ventricular outlet obstruction, or obstruction at the tentorial hiatus. There is often callosal hypoplasia or absence and deficiency of the falx cerebri, allowing interdigitation of the hemispheres and polymicrogyria (Fig. 1.15).

CHIARI III MALFORMATION This is a rare but more severe form of hindbrain dysgenesis. The hallmark is a high cervical-occipital encephalocele.

DANDY–WALKER SYNDROME The Dandy–Walker syndrome, also called Dandy–Walker cyst, is characterized by absence of the vermis (complete or partial), hypoplasia of the cerebellum, and cystic dilatation of the fourth ventricle. It is believed that it arises from failure of opening of the foramina of Luschka and Magendie, especially of Magendie (Fig. 1.16).

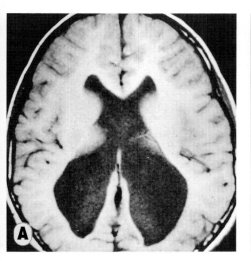 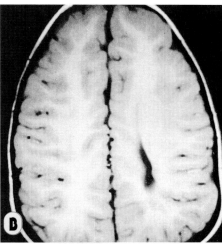 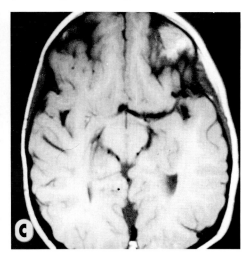

Fig. 1.15 CHIARI II MALFORMATION T1-weighted axial images. **(A)** The lateral ventricles are dilated and have squared frontal horns and dilated occipital horns. The ventricular shape is referred to as colpocephaly. **(B)** The falx is deficient, allowing interdigitation of the gyri of the two hemispheres. **(C)** This image through the midbrain demonstrates classic "beaking" of the tectum. The midbrain is elongated in the anteroposterior direction, and the right and left colliculi are approximated.

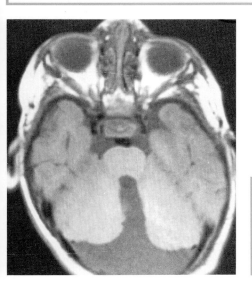

Fig. 1.16 DANDY–WALKER MALFORMATION T1-weighted axial image. The fourth ventricle is in direct communication with the dilated cisterna magna. Normally the vermis separates the two.

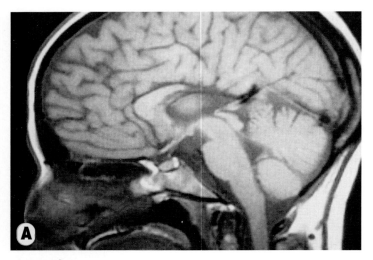

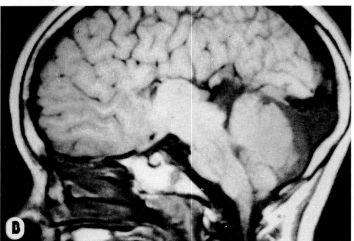

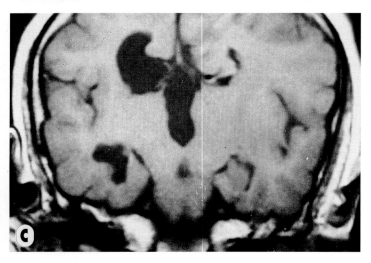

Fig. 1.17 AGENESIS OF CORPUS CALLOSUM (A) T1-weighted sagittal image. In this partial form of corpus callosum agenesis, the anterior half of the corpus callosum is present; the posterior half is absent. **(B)** T1-weighted sagittal image. Complete agenesis. The corpus callosum and cingulate gyrus are absent in their entirety. **(C)** T1-weighted coronal image (same case as B). The third ventricle is displaced upwards and the lateral ventricles are widely separated and dysplastic.

In the Dandy–Walker cyst, the obstruction of the CSF pathway is usually at the outlet of the fourth ventricle, and the lateral ventricles are usually dilated. In the Dandy–Walker variant, there is only partial absence of the vermis involving the inferior part, with no obstruction of the fourth ventricular outlet. The cerebellum is often not hypoplastic, and patients commonly do not have hydrocephalus. The T1-weighted sagittal scan is the best view to demonstrate the aqueduct, the cystic dilatation of the fourth ventricle and absence of the vermis. However, axial images better visualize the hypoplastic cerebellum.

AGENESIS OF THE CORPUS CALLOSUM Agenesis of the corpus callosum is caused by failure of formation, or rarely in utero destruction of the callosal fibers. There can be partial or complete absence of the corpus callosum. Because the corpus callosum develops from anterior to posterior, the congenital partial form is always of the posterior type (Fig. 1.17). Lipomas of the corpus callosum are rare, but when present they are associated (in 50% of cases) with agenesis of the corpus callosum and may have peripheral calcification as well as an azygous anterior cerebral artery.

Prior to the availability of MRI, the coronal CT scan was the most important method of determining the presence or absence of the corpus callosum. Now, the midline T1-weighted sagittal MRI is the single most important scan used to demonstrate the abnormal morphology of the corpus callosum (Fig. 1.17). The absence of callosal fibers is also well demonstrated on coronal views, as are the separation of the lateral ventricles and upward herniation of the third ventricle.

Due to the poorly formed corona radiata and forceps associated with agenesis, the lateral ventricles are oriented parallel to each other (a common finding in most midline anomalies) and their bodies are widely separated. Ectopic gray matter can frequently be seen along the walls of the lateral ventricles.

DISORDERS OF DIVERTICULATION
SEPTO-OPTIC DYSPLASIA This consists of the triad of optic hypoplasia, absence of the septum pellucidum, and hypothalamic dysfunction. It is often regarded as the mildest form of holoprosencephaly. Magnetic resonance imaging is superior to CT in demonstrating the hypoplastic optic nerves, with coronal views providing the single most important projection. The absence of the septum pellucidum results in squared ventricles (especially at the frontal horns) which are similar to those found in the mildest form of holoprosencephaly. The falx cerebri is well-formed in contrast to holoprosencephaly (Fig. 1.18). Hypoplasia of the corpus callosum is common.

HOLOPROSENCEPHALY Holoprosencephaly refers to a congenital abnormality wherein the cerebral hemispheres and lateral ventricles have not separated. It is the result of failure of diverticulation of the hemispheres and is subdivided into three types: lobar, semilobar, and alobar. The lobar type is mildest, semilobar is intermediate, and alobar is the most severe form. These three forms represent different stages in the developmental arrest of hemispheric diverticulation. As in other congenital malformations, MRI is the ideal technique with T1-weighted coronal images being the most useful sequence.

In all three forms of holoprosencephaly, the olfactory bulbs and tracts are absent; the thalami are fused; there is a common lateral ventricle, and there are gyral and sulcal anomalies (Fig. 1.19).

In the lobar type, there is some differentiation of the lateral and third ventricles and some separation superiorly of the thalami, although the ventricles remain a single compartment. The sylvian fissure is formed as are some gyri and sulci.

In both semilobar and alobar types, the thalami are completely fused with a single ventricle consisting of both the lateral and third ventricles. The ventricles on coronal views are shaped like a fat inverted "U." Differentiation between the semilobar and alobar types is often difficult. In the semilobar type, however, the sylvian fissure is formed, whereas in the alobar type it is not. The falx cerebri is absent in both the alobar and semilobar types, and is rudimentary in the lobar type. The most severe forms of holoprosencephaly are associated with a dorsal midline cyst. The differential features are summarized in Figure 1.20.

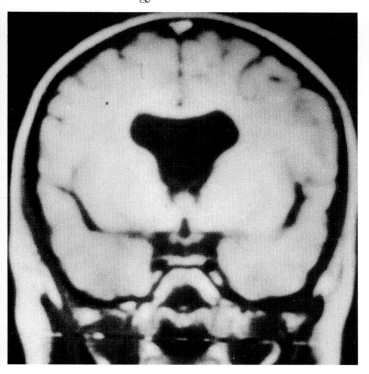

Fig. 1.18 SEPTO-OPTIC DYSPLASIA T1-weighted coronal image. The coronal plane optimally displays this anomaly. The septum pellucidum is absent and the frontal horns are squared. The falx is present, as is the corpus callosum, although it is somewhat hypoplastic.

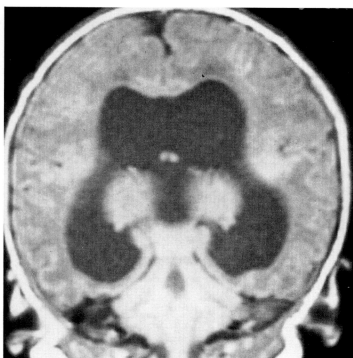

Fig. 1.19 LOBAR TYPE OF HOLOPROSENCEPHALY T1-weighted coronal image. The two lateral ventricles have not separated from one another and are only partially divided from the third ventricle. The sylvian fissures and falx cerebri are present but are rudimentary. (Courtesy of Dr. A.J. Barkovich, University of California, San Francisco)

Fig. 1.20 FEATURES OF HOLOPROSENCEPHALY

Type	Lobar	Semilobar	Alobar
Olfactory bulbs and tracts	Absent	Absent	Absent
Fused thalami	Partial	Total	Total
Separation of lateral and third ventricles	Partial	None	None
Sylvian fissures	Present	Present	Absent
Falx cerebri	Rudimentary	Absent	Absent

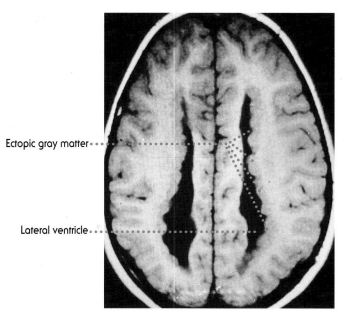

Ectopic gray matter · · ·

Lateral ventricle · · ·

Fig. 1.21 ECTOPIC GRAY MATTER T1-weighted axial image. The T1-weighted axial scan best illustrates the ectopic gray matter tissue in the subependymal region of the lateral ventricles. The wavy margin of the lateral ventricles is caused by the ectopic gray matter. The white matter is also abnormal, consisting of two distinct layers with gray matter in between.

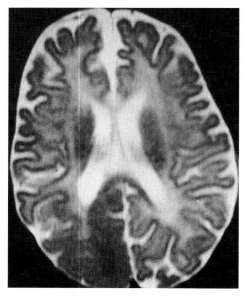

Fig. 1.22 FOCAL GYRATIONAL ANOMALY (FOCAL PACHYGYRIA) T2-weighted axial image. The right occipital lobe, when compared with the rest of the cerebrum, lacks differentiation of normal gray and white matter. There is also lack of sulcation and gyration.

DISORDERS OF SULCATION AND MIGRATION

ECTOPIC GRAY MATTER This is one of the mildest forms of migrational anomalies, often seen with agenesis of the corpus callosum. The ectopic gray matter is visualized as small nodules of tissue protruding into the walls of the lateral ventricles and is best seen on axial T1-weighted images. The signal intensity of these nodules matches that of cortical gray matter on both T1- and T2-weighted images (Fig. 1.21). It is also interesting that often there are two layers of white matter as well as two layers of gray matter. It is therefore likely that there is ectopic white matter as well as ectopic gray matter, reflecting a more generalized disorder of migration than could previously be visualized on CT scans.

FOCAL GYRAL ANOMALIES Gyral anomalies can involve an entire cerebral lobe or a portion of it. In its mildest form, there is a single deep sulcus with associated gray matter that extends deep into the paraventricular white matter. With this form of anomaly, the paraventricular white matter is decreased in size and distorted. On CT especially, this anomaly mimics a mass in the parietal lobe. In the more severe form, the whole lobe is involved and the absence of gyration is associated with poor gray-white matter differentiation (Fig. 1.22). Gyral anomalies are extremely difficult to diagnose accurately on CT scans. The superior soft tissue contrast on MRI greatly facilitates this diagnosis.

LISSENCEPHALY Lissencephaly refers to an abnormally smooth brain surface. There are two forms, agyria and pachygyria. Agyria is complete absence of gyration and infants with this defect have a short life span. On the other hand, pachygyria (broad gyri) can be seen first presenting in patients as late as adulthood. The gyri are large and abnormal. The white matter lacks normal branching, assumes an abnormal shape, and may also have abnormal signal. The cerebrum is smooth, lacks sulcation, and has a smooth gray-white matter interface (Fig. 1.23). The ventricles are mildly dilated and misshaped.

SCHIZENCEPHALY Schizencephaly denotes a cleft in the brain. It is usually bilateral but may be unilateral. The clefts generally separate the frontal, parietal, and temporal lobes, and extend from the subarachnoid space into the lateral ventricles. They are of various sizes and shapes. The most serious mimic severe porencephaly. In schizencephaly, the cleft is lined with gray matter of normal signal intensity (Fig. 1.24). This differentiates schizencephaly from encephaloclastic porencephaly (secondary to vascular insults causing infarction), where the gray matter mantle is absent or abnormal in intensity. Two thirds of the schizencephalies are associated with septo-optic dysplasia.

HEMORRHAGE

Recognition of hemorrhage is critically important in neurodiagnosis. Knowledge of the complex parameters that influence MRI representation of an evolving hematoma is essential. It is important to understand that the relative signal intensity of tissue is principally determined by the T1- and T2-relaxation rates. Comparatively stated, reduction or prolongation of T1- and T2-relaxation times have opposing effects on MRI signal amplitude; that is to say, a shortening of T1 augments MRI signal whereas a shortening of T2 reduces MRI signal.

The presence of certain intra- and extracellular paramagnetic substances that accumulate during the stages of hematoma evolution influences T1 and T2 relaxation and thus the MRI signal, in two important ways: (1) T1 shortening is produced by proton-electron dipole-dipole interactions (PEDD), and (2) T2 shortening is caused by focal field inhomogeneities related to variations in magnetic susceptibility. This second effect is called preferential T2 proton relaxation enhancement (PT2 PRE). Though there is not universal agreement on the nature and effect of these mechanisms, they remain important concepts in understanding the appearance of hematoma. Since a detailed discussion of the mechanisms involved is beyond the scope of this book, the following synopsis is presented.

Paramagnetic molecules that are uniformly distributed and that have direct close access to water protons at the molecular level (e.g., free methemoglobin), cause predominantly T1 shortening through PEDD interactions. A heterogeneous magnetic microenvironment is created by nonuniform distribution of paramagnetic molecules, e.g., sequestration, within red blood cells and macrophages, of blood breakdown products such as deoxyhemoglobin and hemosiderin. Diffusing water protons undergo random local fluctuations in magnetic field strength, causing random fluctuations in precessional frequencies and rapid loss of phase coherence. The net effect is signal loss on T2-weighted images. The MR image of a hematoma thus depends on whether T1-shortening PEDD interactions or T2-shortening PT2 PRE interactions occur, and on which of the two predominates. The interaction that predominates, in turn, depends on the particular heme moiety present (oxyhemoglobin, deoxyhemoglobin, methemoglobin or hemosiderin) and whether it is in free solution or compartmentalized into red blood cells or macrophages.

Immediately following hemorrhage, the collection of blood contains oxyhemoglobin within intact red cells. Oxyhemoglobin has no paramagnetic properties; hence, the signal is due solely to a protein-rich water solution. Increased proton spin density and prolongation of T1- and T2-relaxation values in a fresh

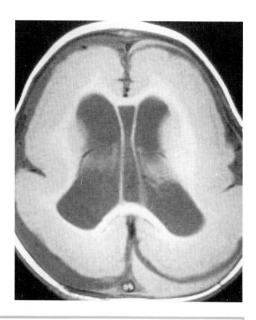

Fig. 1.23 LISSENCEPHALY T1-weighted sagittal image. There is complete lissencephaly. Only the sylvian fissures are present. The lateral ventricles are dysplastic and dilated. The sulci and gyri are absent and there is no subcortical branching of white matter. There is also an old subdural hematoma on the left, an incidental finding.

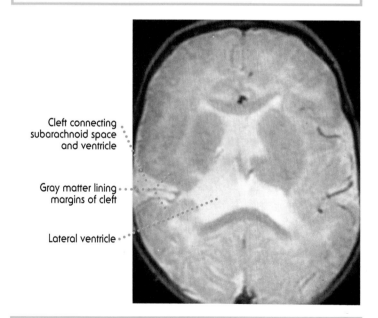

Cleft connecting subarachnoid space and ventricle

Gray matter lining margins of cleft

Lateral ventricle

Fig. 1.24 SCHIZENCEPHALY T2-weighted coronal image. A moderately large cleft on the right extends from the subarachnoid space to the atrium of the lateral ventricle. The cleft is lined by gray matter, which differentiates schizencephaly from hydranencephaly and porencephaly. (Courtesy of Dr. A.J. Barkovich, University of California, San Francisco)

Edema

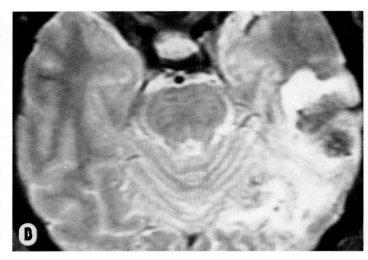

Hematoma
(deoxyhemoglobin)

Fig. 1.25 ACUTE HEMATOMA (18 h OLD, CASE 1)
(A) T1-weighted axial image. This is an intracerebral hemorrhage into an area of venous infarction. The hematoma and the surrounding edema are equally hypointense. At this stage a hematoma is similar to that of any edematous process on T1-weighted images.

Methemoglobin has not yet formed hence there is no hyperintensity. **(B)** T2-weighted axial image. The central portion of the hematoma is markedly hypointense. The surrounding hyperintensity represents edema in the surrounding brain.

Edema

Peripheral clot
(intracellular methemoglobin)

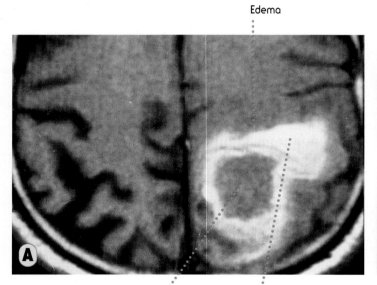

Central clot (deoxy-   Peripheral clot (intracel-
hemoglobin)   lular methemoglobin)

Central clot (deoxy-   Edema
hemoglobin)

Fig. 1.26 ACUTE HEMATOMA (48 h OLD, CASE 2) **(A)** T1-weighted axial image. This is an intratumoral hemorrhage due to melanoma metastasis. The peripheral hyperintensity is due to methemoglobin around the periphery of the clot. **(B)** T2-weighted axial image. The

T2-weighted image remains uniformly hypointense centrally, and is not appreciably different from the younger clot in case 1. Most of the methemoglobin is still intracellular; thus PT2 PRE effects are still apparent and manifest as hypointensity on the T2-weighted image.

hemorrhage are similar to those in any edematous process. Soon thereafter, oxyhemoglobin begins to deoxygenate at a rate dependent on the surrounding oxygen tension. In general, 6–12 hours after the hemorrhage, enough deoxyhemoglobin has accumulated inside erythrocytes to cause sufficient inhomogeneities in magnetic susceptibility to influence the MR signal by shortening the T2-relaxation values of diffusing proton spins. This yields a preferential signal decay (PT2 PRE), which is especially evident on late spin echoes or gradient refocused echoes as a central hypointensity in the clot (Fig. 1.25). With the reduction of deoxyhemoglobin to methemoglobin on or about day two or three, the T1 shortening induced by the unpaired outer electrons in methemoglobin begins to predominate (PEDD). Initially, some compartmentalization of methemoglobin within the red cells can produce T2 shortening; however, as red cells lyse, methemoglobin in free solution yields high signal intensity on both T1- and T2-weighted images. This signal alteration begins at the periphery of the hematoma, moves inward, and persists for several months (Figs. 1.26–1.28).

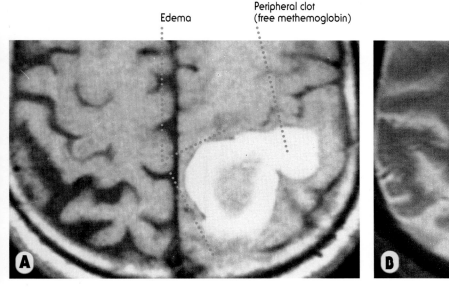
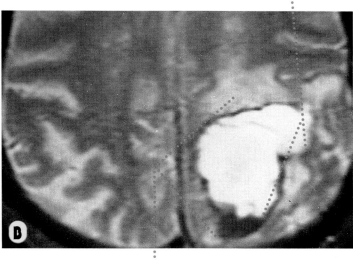

Edema Peripheral clot (free methemoglobin) Hemosiderin-stained brain Edema

Fig. 1.27 SUBACUTE HEMATOMA (2 WEEKS OLD, FOLLOW UP OF CASE 2) (A) T1-weighted axial image. The peripheral hyperintense band is thicker, now almost completely filling the center of the clot. **(B)** T2-weighted axial image. The red cells have lysed and most of the hemoglobin has been reduced to methemoglobin, now in free solution. Consequently, all of the central hypointensity has disappeared. There is also a thin band of hemosiderin-stained brain surrounding the lesion.

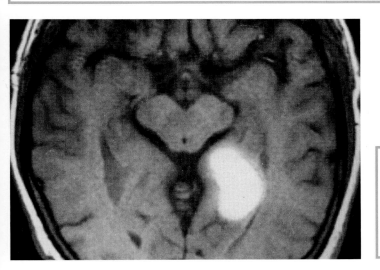

Fig. 1.28 SUBACUTE HEMATOMA (3–4 WEEKS OLD, CASE 3) T1-weighted axial image. The hemorrhage was due to a small, angiographically occult AVM. At this stage the hematoma is uniform, the center completely filled by the advancing peripheral hyperintensity. This appearance and that illustrated in the previous case are characteristic of subacute hematomas.

On or about week three, macrophages appear at the periphery of the clot and begin accumulating hemosiderin, a late breakdown product of hemoglobin. The heterogeneous distribution of hemosiderin causes PT2 PRE on T2-weighted images similar to deoxyhemoglobin, except that it is peripheral rather than central; thus peripheral signal loss is seen late after hemorrhage (Fig. 1.29). Hemosiderin is cleared slowly from the brain and its effects persist for a very long time.

The MR image of the evolving hematoma is clearly different than that seen on CT; however, once understood, the recognition of hemorrhage is greatly improved. This permits formulation of an appropriate differential diagnosis broadly divided into two categories of hemorrhage: traumatic and nontraumatic. The discussion of traumatic hemorrhage is deferred and covered with other traumatic lesions; the causes and features of nontraumatic hemorrhage are presented in Figs. 1.25–1.32.

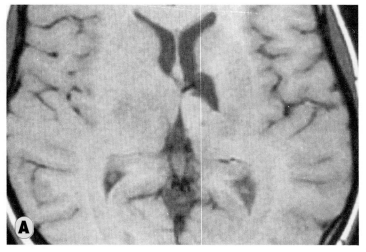

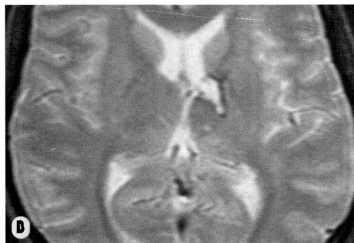

Fig. 1.29 CHRONIC HEMATOMA (6 MONTHS OLD) (A) T1-weighted axial image. All that remains of this hematoma is a small, fluid-filled cleft in the genu of the left internal capsule. **(B)** T2-weighted axial image. The small cleft is surrounded by a hypointense ring. The absence of mass effect and the presence of a hemosiderin ring is typical of an old hematoma.

Fig. 1.30 CAUSES OF NONTRAUMATIC ("SPONTANEOUS") INTRACEREBRAL HEMORRHAGE

Etiology	Features
Hypertension	Most common cause of "spontaneous" hemorrhage. Favored locations: basal ganglia, pons, cerebellum. Basal ganglia hematoma may extend into ventricle.
Infarction	Hematoma develops within infarcted tissue. Venous infarcts especially prone to bleed; may be multiple.
Vascular malformation	AVMs and cavernous hemangiomas associated with bleeding; AVM hemorrhage clinically more significant. AVM may be visible in or adjacent to hematoma as irregular signal void. Cavernous hemangioma characterized by peripheral band of hemosiderin-stained brain.
Neoplasm	Tumoral hemorrhage most frequent with metastatic lesions (especially renal cell carcinoma and melanoma). Mass often visible adjacent to or surrounding hematoma.
Aneurysm	Accompanied by subarachnoid hemorrhage in most cases. The intracerebral hematoma is usually adjacent to aneurysm (thus aiding in aneurysm localization).
Amyloid angiopathy	Disease of elderly; amyloid-like material deposited in small blood vessel walls. Repeated subcortical hemorrhages in varying locations.
Moya-Moya syndrome	Dilated lenticulostriate collaterals prone to rupture. Hematoma usually in basal ganglia. Basal ganglia collaterals may be visible.

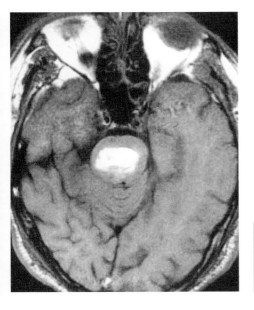

Fig. 1.31 HYPERTENSIVE HEMORRHAGE (APPROXIMATELY 10 DAYS OLD) T1-weighted axial image. The hemorrhage occupies most of the central pons, one of the most common locations for hypertensive bleeds.

Non-hemorrhagic infarct

Subacute intracerebral hemorrhage

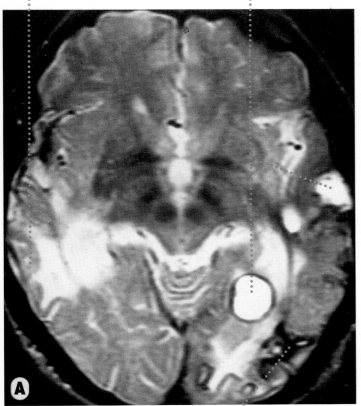

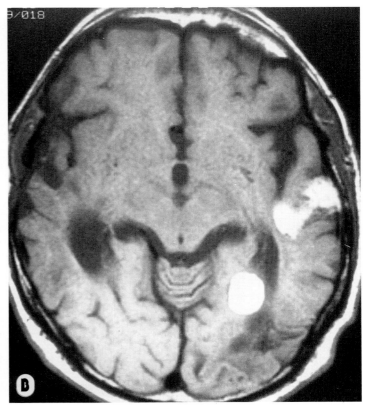

Old intracerebral hemorrhage

Fig. 1.32 AMYLOID ANGIOPATHY **(A)** T2-weighted axial image. This elderly gentleman suffered repeated strokes over a 2-year period. There is evidence in the brain of multiple cortical and subcortical hematomas at different stages of evolution. For example, the irregular hypointense area in the left parieto-occipital cortex, characterized by hypointense signal, indicates remote hemorrhagic infarction. Anterior to this, two other hematomas show the early peripheral hemosiderin formation, indicative of the subacute stage. **(B)** T1-weighted axial image. With this technique, the subacute periventricular hematoma, because of its uniform hyperintensity, is more evident than the old hemorrhage.

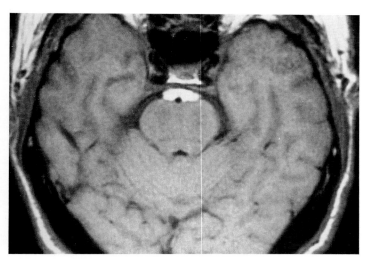

Fig. 1.33 SUBARACHNOID HEMORRHAGE T1-weighted axial image. There is a small localized clot in the prepontine cistern immediately adjacent to the basilar artery.

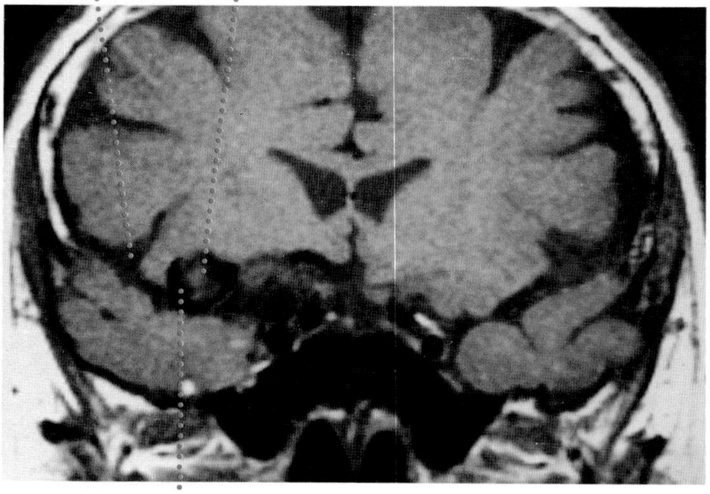

Sylvian fissure   Flow artifact within aneurysm

Aneurysm

Fig. 1.34 RIGHT MIDDLE CEREBRAL ARTERY BERRY ANEURYSM T1-weighted coronal image. There is a 2-cm hypointense lesion in the stem of the right sylvian fissure. The marked hypointensity, usually referred to as a signal void, is caused by blood rapidly flowing through the aneurysm. The central irregular area of gray signal is a flow artifact.

VASCULAR ABNORMALITIES

ANEURYSMS

An aneurysm can be broadly defined as a segment of an artery that has an abnormally increased caliber. The etiology of aneurysms and related pathophysiologic mechanisms can be described as congenital (saccular or berry-type), atherosclerotic, spontaneous/posttraumatic, dissecting, mycotic, or miliary.

SACCULAR ANEURYSMS   Approximately 2% of the adult population harbors saccular aneurysms; 20% of these people have multiple aneurysms. Saccular aneurysms occur almost exclusively in the circle of Willis and are most common at points of branching. The peak incidence of clinical presentation ´of berry aneurysms, with rupture into the subarachnoid space, occurs in the fifth and sixth decades.

Saccular berry-type aneurysms are usually 5 to 10 mm in size before diagnosis. Giant aneurysms, measuring 2 cm or greater in diameter, are less common. Patients with giant aneurysms are less likely to present with subarachnoid hemorrhage; more commonly, symptoms are related to the presence of a space-occupying lesion. Clots in the mural lining of a giant aneurysm may also detach and cause either TIA-like symptoms or even cerebral infarction.

Radiologic evaluation, in particular the algorithm of diagnostic modalities, has not been altered appreciably by MRI for the majority of patients with symptoms caused by the presence, and especially the rupture, of a berry-type aneurysm. Signs and symptoms suggestive of subarachnoid hemorrhage necessitate initial CT of the head. Computed tomography has a very high sensitivity for the diagnosis of subarachnoid hemorrhage due to aneurysm rupture. The increased attenuation of blood in the basal cisterns is usually plainly visible.

Magnetic resonance imaging may occasionally reveal the presence of subarachnoid blood in the acute or subacute phase as a consequence of aneurysm rupture (Fig. 1.33). However, the temporal evolution of blood clot constituents within the subarachnoid space and their MRI signal characteristics are neither predictable nor reliable when compared with the accuracy of CT. In many cases of subarachnoid hemorrhage, MRI is falsely negative. The lumen of a berry aneurysm may be identified by MRI as an area of low signal intensity, known as a "flow void," especially if the lesion measures greater than 5 to 6 mm in diameter (Fig. 1.34). In larger aneurysms, the deposition of concentric layers of laminar thrombus, with differential signal intensities due to the presence of subacute and chronic blood degradation products, may give rise to characteristic crescentic patterns (Fig. 1.35).

ATHEROSCLEROTIC ANEURYSMS In patients with longstanding or severe atherosclerosis, arteries may become elongated and tortuous. The caliber of the vessels enlarge, producing long segments of fusiform swelling. These changes are due to replacement of muscular media with fibrotic tissue and degeneration of the elastic lamina. The segments involved most often are the basilar and the supraclinoid carotid arteries. Neurologic symptoms (e.g., cranial nerve neuropathies) are commonly produced by pressure effects and/or stretching of adjacent neurovascular structures. Rarely, fusiform atherosclerotic aneurysms may serve as a source of embolus due to small thrombi detaching from their walls and migrating distally. Subarachnoid hemorrhage is rare. Detection of dolichoectasia by MRI depends on the demonstration, during routine spin echo sequences, of characteristically enlarged arterial vessels, flow voids, and occasionally thickened mural walls. Thin section images may be of value to demonstrate the effect of these tortuous vessels upon adjacent neurologic structures. The effect is especially pronounced in the posterior fossa, where atherosclerotic fusiform aneurysms may bow medially and posteriorly toward the brainstem, invaginating deeply toward the pontomesencephalic junction (Fig. 1.36). Impingement upon the cisternal segments of the V or VII nerves, due to the irregular branch vessels, may cause syndromes of tic douloureux or hemifacial spasm.

DISSECTING ANEURYSM Dissection most often affects the upper cervical segment of an internal carotid artery. It may be a consequence of trauma, but often occurs spontaneously and with higher frequency in patients with fibromuscular dysplasia or polycystic kidney disease. The vertebral-basilar circulation is also affected, but less prominently.

Carotid dissection must be considered as a possible cause of unexplained cerebral ischemic events or stroke occurring at a premature age, especially in young adults. The dissection typically starts several centimeters distal to the bifurcation of the common carotid artery, extends subintimally over several centimeters toward the skull base, and normally terminates where the internal carotid artery enters the petrous temporal bone. Dissection may occur silently or may produce pain and occasionally a neurologic deficit, related to compression of the pericarotid sympathetic plexus, resulting in a Horner's syndrome. A dissecting channel may secondarily re-enter the true lumen distally, producing a double lumen. More often, the dissection is confined to structures beneath the intima, causing progressive accumulation of hematoma which narrows the true lumen. If the patient has a patent circle of Willis, this may be of no consequence. Occasionally, a devastating hemispheric stroke may occur because of arterial narrowing compounded by hypoperfusion.

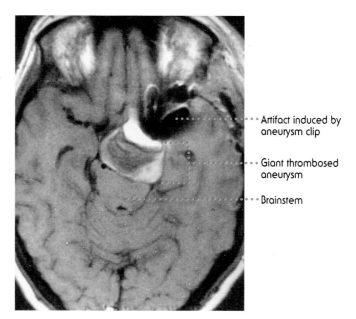

- Artifact induced by aneurysm clip
- Giant thrombosed aneurysm
- Brainstem

Fig. 1.35 THROMBOSED GIANT ANEURYSM OF THE LEFT INTERNAL CAROTID ARTERY T1-weighted axial image. The aneurysm, which occupies the entire suprasellar cistern, displaces the optic chiasm and pituitary infundibulum to the right, the brainstem and basilar artery posteriorly, and the uncus of the left temporal lobe medially. The concentric layers ("onion skinning") within the aneurysm, are a frequent observation in thrombosed aneurysms. The area of reduced signal, anterolateral to the aneurysm, is artifact caused by a surgical clip placed across the aneurysm neck. Such metal clips preclude CT examination due to streak artifact. Aneurysm clips made of titanium are safe for MR imaging. In this case, MRI was extremely useful to demonstrate absence of residual flow within the aneurysm.

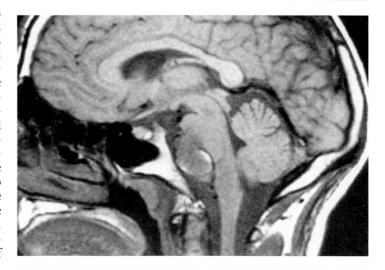

Fig. 1.36 THROMBOSED ATHEROSCLEROTIC BASILAR ARTERY ANEURYSM T1-weighted sagittal image. A large fusiform aneurysm of the basilar artery is filled with thrombus and causes marked compression of the pons and upper medulla.

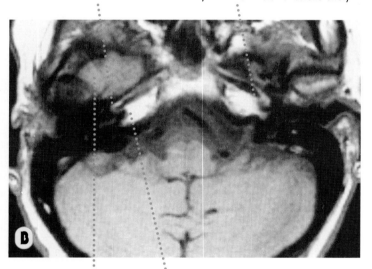

Residual lumen   Subintimal clot   Subintimal clot   Residual lumen

Internal jugular vein   Internal carotid artery   Internal carotid artery

Carotid canal with partially thrombosed carotid artery   Carotid canal with normal "flow void" of carotid artery

Temporal lobe   Petrous apex

Fig. 1.37 SPONTANEOUS BILATERAL CAROTID ARTERY DISSECTION **(A)** T1-weighted axial image through the skull base. Both carotid arteries are abnormal as they enter the skull base. They should be well-defined, circular signal voids. In this case, especially on the right, subintimal clot has caused marked asymmetric concentric narrowing of the vascular lumen. **(B)** T1-weighted axial image through the horizontal carotid canals. Axial sections through the horizontal portions of the carotid canals are valuable for further delineating suspected carotid dissections. On the right, the carotid lumen is almost completely occluded by clot. The left side is normal at this level, indicating that the dissection stopped at the level of the skull base.

Dissection of the internal carotid artery and its secondary effects are often visible in MR images. Careful attention must be directed to the upper cervical and petrous as well as to the cavernous segments of the affected internal carotid artery. Direct visualization of the dissection is usually manifested in the subacute stage by a concentric or eccentric "C-shaped" deposition of hyperintense blood products (subacute methemoglobin or extracellular methemoglobin) deposited beneath the intima (Fig. 1.37). The central flow void is distorted and reduced in cross-sectional diameter. With complete thrombosis, flow void may be absent, replaced by intraluminal thrombus in the entire internal carotid artery up to the ophthalmic artery origin. This imparts obvious asymmetry when comparing the affected cavernous carotid artery with that on the opposite side.

VASCULAR MALFORMATIONS
Vascular malformations are congenital lesions of developmental origin. Four distinct histopathologic types have been described. In decreasing order of occurrence, these are (1) arteriovenous malformation (AVM), (2) cavernous hemangioma, (3) venous angioma, and (4) telangiectasia.

ARTERIOVENOUS MALFORMATION   The AVM is the prototypical vascular malformation of the central nervous system. Embryologically, AVMs are thought to occur as a result of failed involution or incomplete regression of arteriovenous shunts normally present in the primitive fetal cerebral vascular plexus. Although some AVMs are detected incidentally on imaging studies obtained for unrelated reasons, patients usually present in the second or third decades of life with hemorrhage, seizures, headaches, or progressive neurologic deficit.

The following biologic constituents may be encountered in and about an AVM: multiple serpentine vessels, blood pool spaces, hemorrhage, thrombus, calcification, hemosiderin, gliosis, edema, and encephalomalacia. Recognition of a patent AVM on CT or MRI is generally straightforward and dominated by a racemose collection of blood pool spaces that correspond to the abnormal vascular channels in and about the nidus of the AVM. Patent AVMs are usually depicted on MRI with great clarity and specificity. This modality offers the significant advantage of not requiring intravenous infusion of contrast material when screening for an AVM. On routine spin-echo (SE) sequences, most of the vascular channels are depicted as a "flow void," due to turbulent dephasing and high velocity signal loss (Fig. 1.38).

Specially designed flow-sensitive MRI sequences can be utilized to depict patent vascular channels with nearly uniformly bright signal. This is best achieved by single slice, short TR, intermediate flip angle gradient refocused echo (GRE) sequences using flow-compensating gradient modulation (also known as flow compensation) (Fig. 1.38). The use of flow compensation may also be of value to reduce ghost artifacts that may be projected across the phase-encoded direction when using this technique.

Thus, MRI depicts the vessels of an AVM with the relative signal amplitude desired, ranging from virtually complete flow void to uniform brightness, depending upon the MRI pulse sequence prescribed. For instance, hemorrhage in various stages of evolution can simulate flowing blood. Bright signal, due to the presence of methemoglobin, is generally recovered from a subacute blood clot and some stages of thrombus development. This type of signal could simulate the bright signal achieved with flow-sensitive GRE sequences in patent vascular channels.

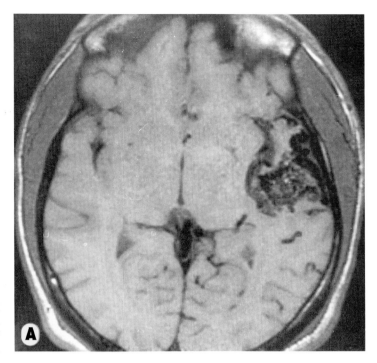

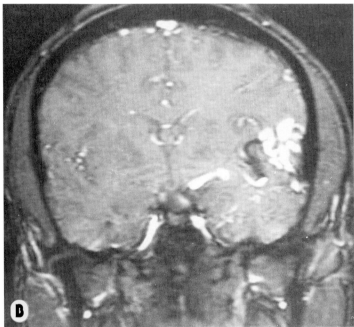

Fig. 1.38 LEFT INTRACEREBRAL ARTERIOVENOUS MALFORMATION **(A)** T1-weighted axial image. The collection of irregular tubular structures with distinct signal voids is typical of an arteriovenous malformation. The size of the nidus can be clearly defined. Enlargement of surrounding vessels is presumptive evidence that these are either the supplying arteries to the malformation or the draining veins. **(B)** Gradient-echo coronal image. The use of sequential single slice gradient-echo images enables the operator to selectively highlight areas of flowing blood. In this case the malformation is highlighted as positive contrast against the surrounding brain.

Specially designed "flow void" sequences with presaturation pulses are optimal for isolating these hemorrhagic sequelae from the patent AVM (Fig. 1.39). The capacity of MRI to distinguish vessels from clot is an asset in preoperative evaluation of AVMs.

CAVERNOUS HEMANGIOMA   A cavernous hemangioma is a developmental and presumably congenital lesion consisting of a variable-sized nidus of thin-walled vascular spaces (sinusoids) without intervening nervous tissue. The surface of the lesion is typically lobulated, imparting a "mulberry-like" appearance. The size varies from several millimeters to several centimeters in diameter. Most are situated in the subcortical regions of the hemispheres, but they can occur superficially along the pial surface of the brain, or within the brainstem or cerebellum.

The sinusoidal spaces of the cavernous hemangioma maintain restricted communication with the afferent vascular system, precluding development of high-flow AV shunts common to AVMs. There are no hypertrophied or enlarged vessels feeding the lesion. Draining veins are usually not evident.

On noncontrast CT scans, approximately 30 percent of cavernous hemangiomas exhibit calcification. These lesions are notable for the lack of mass effect or perifocal edema, except for transient changes associated with internal thrombosis or, more rarely,

Intracerebral hemorrhage

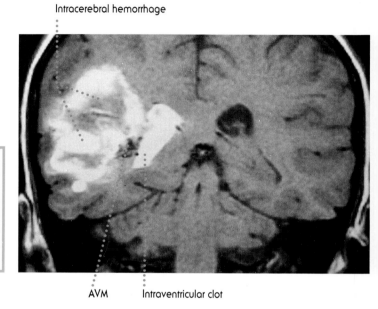

AVM   Intraventricular clot

Fig. 1.39 ARTERIOVENOUS MALFORMATION WITH HEMORRHAGE T1-weighted coronal image. This MR image clearly identifies the nidus of abnormal vessels on the medial aspect of the clot, as well as an intraventricular clot within the right lateral ventricle. On contrast-enhanced CT, both the clot and the AVM were hyperdense and could not be distinguished from one another.

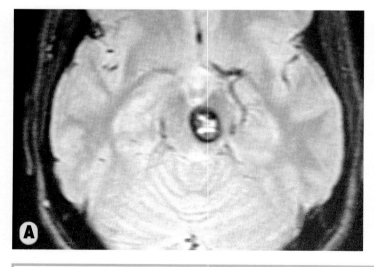

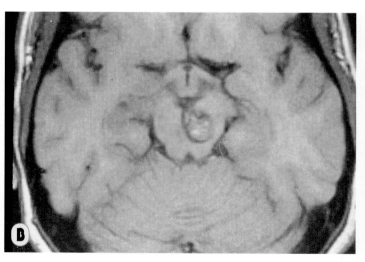

Fig. 1.40 CAVERNOUS HEMANGIOMA   (A) T2-weighted axial image. This patient presented with an intermittent left cranial nerve III palsy. There is a well-defined lesion in the left side of the midbrain characterized by a heterogeneous hyperintense center and a uniform band of surrounding hypointensity. There is no significant mass effect and no surrounding edema. This appearance is virtually pathognomonic of a cavernous hemangioma. (B) T1-weighted axial image. Small areas of hyperintensity are also noted centrally on the T1-weighted image; however, the hypointense surrounding ring is less apparent.

frank hemorrhage. Hemorrhage within cavernous hemangiomas is thought to be self-limiting and, unlike the rupture of an AVM, seldom accounts for a catastrophic event.

On CT, cavernous hemangiomas can mimic the appearance of a glioma (e.g., oligodendroglioma) or meningioma. Both of these lesions classically have calcification, and show significant blood-brain barrier defects upon contrast infusion, yet seldom show significant mass effect or edema. The nonspecific CT depiction of these lesions limits the radiologist's ability to confidently diagnose cavernous hemangioma on the basis of CT alone.

MRI is both more sensitive and specific than CT for the diagnosis of cavernous hemangioma which, on MRI, appears as a "popcorn ball." Central puddles of slowly moving blood and proteinaceous fluid with free methemoglobin account for relative hyperintensity on both T1- and T2-weighted images. Chronic blood products accumulate around the lobulated periphery of the lesion. This somewhat unique pattern of hemosiderin deposition has been attributed to repeated thrombosis and minor hemorrhage, or chronic minute oozing of blood from the incompetent endothelial membranes which would otherwise contain this lesion. Whatever the cause, hemosiderin accumulates within the lysosomes of macrophages in surrounding gliotic brain tissue. The heterogeneous distribution of paramagnetic hemosiderin imparts significant magnetic susceptibility differentials to the perimeter of the lesion. As a result of this magnetic susceptibility effect, water protons diffusing in adjacent hydrated tissue rapidly dephase. This distinctive process is indicated by a uniform, intact ring of signal loss that is often pronounced and which is particularly prominent on heavily T2-weighted (long TR, long TE) SE images at high field strength (Fig. 1.40). Alternately, GRE images can be prescribed for selective sensitivity to these susceptibility effects, at either high field strength or intermediate field strength. The complete intact ring of hemosiderin is an important observation, as are the lack of peripheral edema and mass effect. Nevertheless, other categories of disease, including tumoral hemorrhage, can rarely mimic the MR appearance of a cavernous hemangioma.

VENOUS ANGIOMA   Prior to the advent of CT and MR, venous angiomas were thought to represent rare malformations of the cerebral venous system. However, more recently, this generally benign condition has been recognized with increased frequency, indicating a higher incidence than previously expected. Computed tomography and MRI provide a highly specific means of identifying this type of malformation.

Venous angiomas display an architectural arrangement of multiple enlarged medullary veins that converge and usually drain into a common central vein. This central vein travels toward the ependyma or, more typically, toward the cortex (Fig. 1.41). A paucity of normal surrounding veins has led to speculation that this lesion may represent recruitment and distention of normal medullary veins to compensate for incomplete development of an adult-type cortical

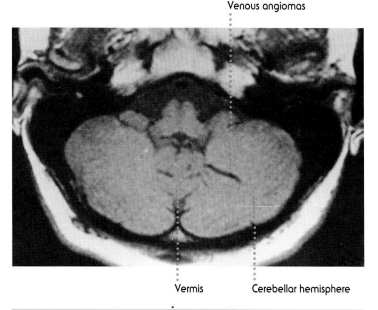

Venous angiomas

Vermis   Cerebellar hemisphere

Fig. 1.41 VENOUS ANGIOMA   T1-weighted axial image. A moderately large vein flows from the central left cerebellar hemisphere to the inferior vermian cistern. There is no mass effect, hemorrhage, or edema. This is the typical appearance of a venous angioma.

venous drainage pattern. There is no arterial participation in this anomaly, no shunting is observed, and the angioma appears in the venous phase, with preservation of a normal circulation time. The three-dimensional architecture of the lesion imparts a pattern that has been described as "umbrella-like," or "caput medusae."

Only rarely have venous angiomas been reported to bleed. Such instances have involved cerebellar venous angiomas in patients presenting with either intracerebral or subarachnoid hemorrhage proximal to a venous angioma. In other patients, the presence of a venous angioma has been alleged to represent the cause of a focal seizure disorder. Nevertheless, on cross-sectional imaging, it appears that the vast majority of vascular lesions that meet diagnostic criteria for a venous angioma represent incidental findings, or a normal variant that is not likely to explain the patient's neurologic signs or symptoms.

CAPILLARY TELANGIECTASIA   This lesion is a pathologic curiosity that is rarely diagnosed on CT or MRI, and which cannot be visualized angiographically. Most recorded cases are identified at autopsy, often as incidental findings. However, the lesion occasionally occurs in association with a slowly progressive neurologic deficit or with a neurologic syndrome that simulates the features of demyelinating disease or chronic degenerative process.

Capillary telangiectasias are small and generally are solitary. They have a predilection for the brainstem, usually the pons. Microscopically, the lesion consists of a tangle of thin-walled, slightly distended capillaries. Capillary telangiectasias presumably account for a small proportion of so called "cryptic" vascular malformations manifested by focal densities or intensities of a vascular nature that are angiographically occult.

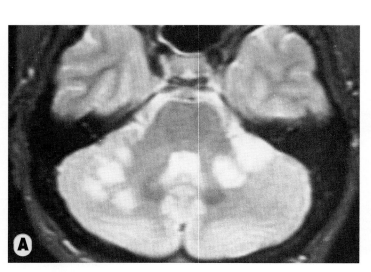

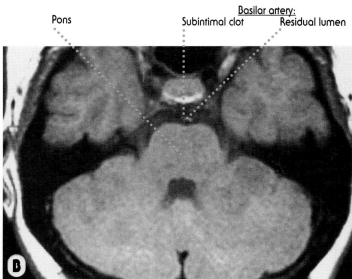

Pons

Basilar artery:
Subintimal clot   Residual lumen

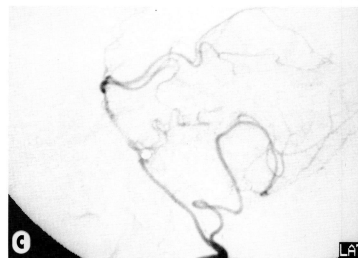

Fig. 1.42 SPONTANEOUS DISSECTION OF THE BASILAR ARTERY **(A)** T2-weighted axial image. This 25-year-old woman presented with onset of acute multiple cranial nerve palsies and ataxia, all preceded by pain in her occiput. Multiple infarcts, due to occlusion of small perforating basilar branches, are visible in both middle cerebellar peduncles. The basilar artery itself appears very small in cross-section. **(B)** T1-weighted axial image. The infarcts are much less evident with this technique, but the wall and lumen of the basilar artery are optimally visualized. Subintimal clot is represented by thickening of the left anterolateral wall of the basilar artery. **(C)** Lateral view of a vertebral angiogram. A long segment of the basilar artery is irregularly narrow, the most frequent appearance of an arterial dissection involving the cerebral vasculature. It is rare to see an actual double lumen or pseudoaneurysm in dissections of cerebral arteries.

ISCHEMIA AND INFARCTION

Its high sensitivity to the brain water changes that accompany early ischemia makes MRI uniquely adapted for the detection of cerebral ischemia. Visualization of the posterior fossa, temporal lobes, and cortex is not limited, as it is with CT, by artifacts from adjacent bone, and, in addition to the evaluation of the cerebral parenchyma, MRI vascular studies are noninvasive (Fig. 1.42). While these attributes would appear to make MRI ideally suited for evaluation of the ischemic brain, there are very important limitations that detract from its utilization for this indication: the MRI environment is such that it is difficult to position and monitor acutely ill patients; motion artifacts arise during the relatively long scan times, and particularly when patients are uncomfortable or uncooperative; and, finally, there are subtleties to reliably detecting acute hemorrhage that are difficult to master. Despite the development of MRI compatible life support equipment, fast scan techniques, and a large body of literature on the MRI appearance of acute hemorrhage, CT continues to be the preferred investigative modality to identify such hemorrhages. Nonetheless, MRI is very useful for the detection and characterization of subacute and chronic ischemic lesions, as well as for the diagnosis of atypical presentations of ischemia.

The feature common to all causes of cerebral ischemia is failure to deliver oxygenated blood in sufficient quantity to maintain normal cerebral metabolism. This metabolic failure triggers a chain of cellular events, beginning with depletion of adenosine triphosphate reserves, impairment of the sodium-potassium pump, and loss of membrane integrity. This leads to a redistribution of extracellular fluid to the intracellular compartment. Cellular swelling ensues (cytotoxic edema). Concomitantly, there is a small increase in total regional water content, accounting for the early visibility of these lesions on MRI. Disruption of the blood-brain barrier follows and results in a more profound transvascular leakage of water and protein into the extracellular space of the affected tissues. This edema further raises tissue pressure, reduces tissue perfusion, and establishes a vicious cycle. Reperfusion of the brain after blood-brain barrier disruption (either through vessel recanalization or clot lysis), and reestablishment of normal perfusion pressures into the diseased vascular bed, further accelerate the process by increasing fluid exudation into the tissue, and by increasing the risk of hemorrhage. The MR image is dominated in these early stages of infarction first by edema, then by mass effect. The affected tissue becomes hyperintense on the T2-weighted image, and adjacent sulci and the ipsilateral ventricle are effaced (Fig. 1.43). The earliest changes are usually visible within 6 hours of vascular obstruction. Mass effect is minimal in the first day, becomes progressively evident over the next several days, and peaks on or about day 5 to 7. By the third week a well-demarcated area of encephalomalacia and focal atrophy become apparent with marked reduction in signal on the T1-weighted image, increase in signal on the proton den-

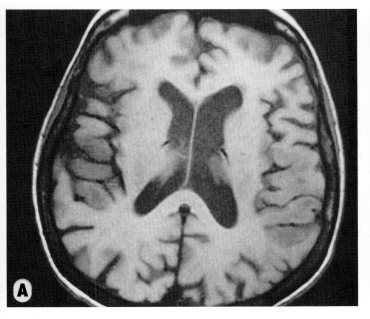
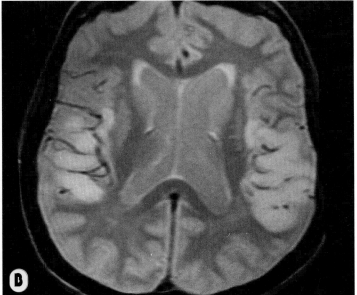

Fig. 1.43 ACUTE MIDDLE CEREBRAL ARTERY INFARCT (BILATERAL) **(A)** T1-weighted axial image. Approximately 24 hours prior to the scan, this patient presented with bilateral strokes clinically localized to the sylvian cortex. The signs of acute infarction demonstrated here are increased hypointensity of the gray matter, thickening of the gray matter mantle, and effacement of the sulci adjacent to the affected gray matter. The underlying white matter is relatively spared. Subsequent angiography demonstrated a widespread vasculitis. **(B)** Proton density axial image. On proton density and T2-weighted images, the infarcted gray matter is hyperintense and more easily visible than on the T1-weighted image. Although more sensitive in the detection of acute infarction, the actual anatomic detail is not as well demonstrated as on the T1-weighted image.

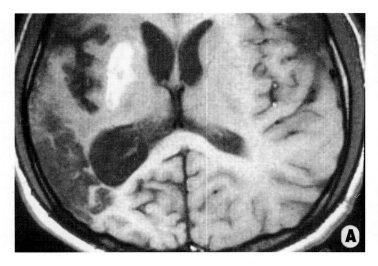

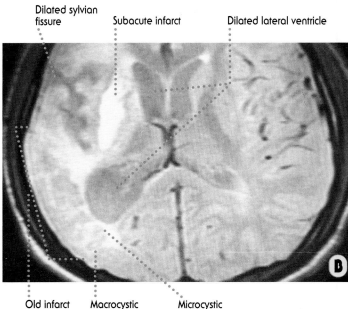

Dilated sylvian fissure   Subacute infarct   Dilated lateral ventricle

Old infarct   Macrocystic encephalomalacia   Microcystic encephalomalacia

Fig. 1.44 OLD RIGHT MIDDLE CEREBRAL ARTERY INFARCT **(A)** T1-weighted axial image. Approximately 1 year prior to this scan, the patient suffered an infarct involving the distal branches of the right middle cerebral artery. More recently there had been a hemorrhagic infarct in the right basal ganglia. The old infarct is characterized by marked hypointensity of the cerebral tissue and dilatation of the overlying sulci. **(B)** Proton density axial image. The peripheral segment of the infarct, the most hypointense area on the T1-weighted image, is almost isointense to brain on the proton density image. Deep to this is an area of distinct hyperintensity. The peripheral area pathologically corresponds to macrocystic encephalomalacia, whereas the deep hyperintense area corresponds to microcystic encephalomalacia. The proton density image is the best for distinguishing between these two components of the lesion. **(C)** T2-weighted axial image. The entire infarct, including the microcystic and macrocystic components, is hyperintense on the T2-weighted image.

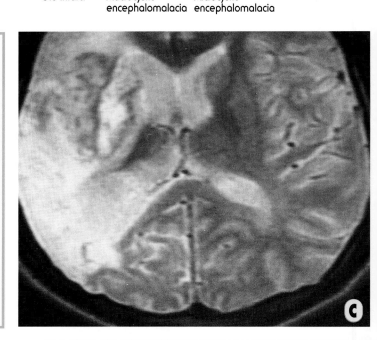

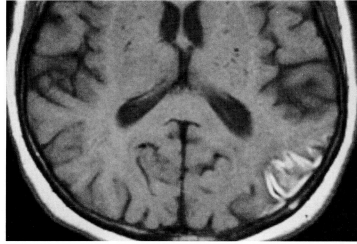

Fig. 1.45 CORTICAL INFARCT WITH PETECHIAL HEMORRHAGE T1-weighted axial image. The hyperintense gyriform ribbon in the left parieto-occipital cortex is diagnostic of a cortical infarct. The high intensity pathologically corresponds to petechial hemorrhage into the infarcted cortex.

sity and T2-weighted image, and sulcal and ventricular enlargement. At 2 to 3 months the necrotic tissue becomes even more demarcated from the surviving parenchyma and may become frankly cystic (Fig. 1.44).

The visualization of hemorrhage in the acutely infarcted brain during day 1 and 2 is difficult due to the variability in appearance of the blood in these early stages. However, between approximately day 3 and day 20, about one third of cortical infarcts show evidence of hemorrhage on MRI, typically as a gyriform ribbon of cortical hyperintensity on the T1-weighted image (Fig. 1.45). The frequency of this finding is generally unappreciated on CT. Pathologically, the MRI correlates very well with the petechial cortical hemorrhage commonly seen in infarction.

Having discussed the common pathogenesis and MRI features of the cerebral infarct, the distinguishing characteristics of different etiologies can be considered (Fig. 1.46).

INFARCTION DUE TO ARTERIAL DISEASE

In the absence of an adequate collateral circulation, occlusion of a major cerebral vessel infarcts a large segment of the brain. Etiologies include atherosclerosis, arterial dissection, subarachnoid hemorrhage-induced vasospasm, or purulent basal meningitis, as well as other rarer causes. The parenchymal lesion that results is notable in that it involves both gray and white matter, has sharp margins, and conforms to a vascular territory or territories (Figs. 1.43–1.45, 1.47). An additional attribute of MRI in this setting is the ability to visualize the major vessels at the base of the brain, within the osseous skull base, and in the neck. Although certainly not a replacement for angiography, this extremely useful attribute of MRI is occasionally instrumental in establishing an unsuspected diagnosis. It has been especially useful in diagnosing arterial dissections (Figs. 1.37 and 1.42).

Cerebral embolism can affect large, medium, or small arteries. The size of the infarction will depend on the vessel occluded and the collateral circulation. As a rule, embolic infarcts are not distinctive from occlusive infarcts except that they are more frequently hemorrhagic and are more often limited to a smaller arterial branch.

Fig. 1.46 ETIOLOGY OF CEREBRAL ISCHEMIA AND INFARCTION

Arterial Disease
Atherosclerosis
Arteriosclerosis
Dissection
Embolism
Arteritis
Vasospasm
Basal meningitis

Venous Disease
Venous occlusion/thrombosis

Systemic Disease
Hypoperfusion
Hypoxia

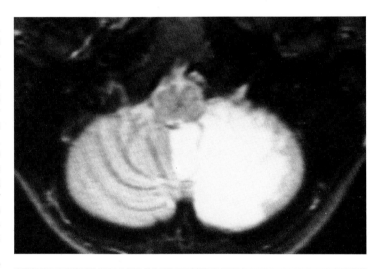

Fig. 1.47 ACUTE LEFT POSTERIOR-INFERIOR CEREBEL-LAR ARTERY INFARCT T2-weighted axial image. The infarct involves the inferior half of the medial aspect of the left cerebellar hemisphere, and the left half of the inferior vermis. The lesion conforms exactly to the territory supplied by the posterior-inferior cerebellar artery. Because of this conformity to a known vascular territory, this image is diagnostic of an infarct. The CT scan through this area was negative, due to the common occurrence of bone artifact through the posterior fossa.

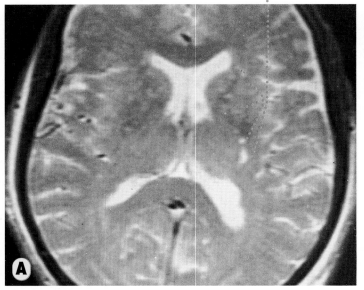

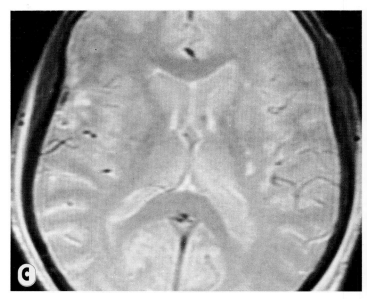

Fig. 1.48 MULTIPLE SMALL BASAL GANGLIA INFARCTS (LACUNES) **(A)** T2-weighted axial image. The small infarcts are visible as foci of increased signal intensity in both basal ganglia, particularly on the left. **(B)** T1-weighted axial image. The lesions are hypointense relative to brain on this image. **(C)** Proton density axial image. The lacunes are hyperintense on the proton density image as well as on the T2-weighted image. This hyperintensity is important in differentiating lesions from normal perivascular spaces, which are isointense on this sequence.

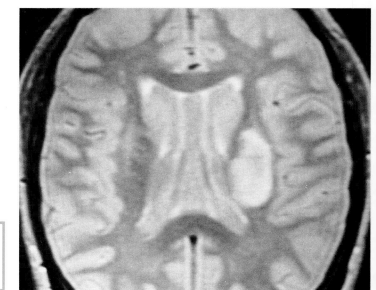

Fig. 1.49 BASAL GANGLIA INFARCT Proton density axial image. There is a well-defined hyperintense lesion in the superior aspect of the left basal ganglia and inferior corona radiata, a common location for cerebral infarcts.

Arteriolosclerosis (atherosclerosis involving the arterioles) occurs in the normal aged population, but the process is accelerated in those with vascular risk factors, particularly hypertension and diabetes mellitus. A common result are lacunar infarcts, which are small, often multiple lesions up to 2 cm in size. There is a predilection for the basal ganglia and internal capsule (Fig. 1.48). Large infarcts may also affect the basal ganglia (Fig. 1.49).

Arteritis is a multifocal process that can involve any vessel, but most commonly affects small and medium sized arteries. Etiologies include the collagen vascular diseases (polyarteritis nodosa, lupus erythematosus, etc.), granulomatous arteritides, and purulent basal meningitis. Constriction or occlusion of the vessels by the inflammatory process results in subsequent infarction of the parenchyma. The important diagnostic points are that a younger age group is affected, the lesions are multifocal, and there may be evidence of a systemic illness (see Fig. 1.43). Angiographic demonstration of multiple arterial irregularities confirms the diagnosis.

INFARCTION DUE TO VENOUS OCCLUSION

Venous occlusion is much rarer than its arterial counterpart. It is principally seen in hypercoaguable states (pregnancy, postpartum, use of birth control pills, polycythemia), inflammatory disease of the paranasal sinusitis, systemic sepsis, and with tumor invasion of the dural venous sinuses. Following venous occlusion and thrombosis, development of cerebral venous hypertension leads to reduced perfusion pressure, regional cerebral edema, and eventually disruption of the blood-brain barrier. There is a high incidence of hemorrhage into these venous infarcts brought on by the maintenance of normal arterial perfusion pressures into a damaged vascular bed, and consequent obliteration of the normal venous drainage. Because of the ability to visualize both the parenchyma and the vessels, MRI is an excellent means of diagnosis. The occluded veins and dural sinuses are clearly visualized tubular structures; the venous infarcts are usually subcortical and often multiple (Fig. 1.50).

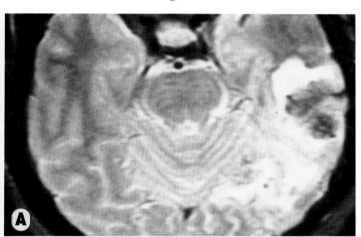

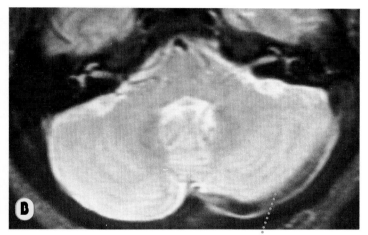

Thrombosed transverse venous sinus

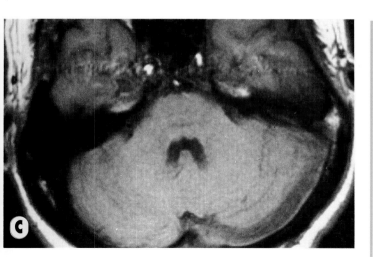

Fig. 1.50 VENOUS SINUS THROMBOSIS WITH INFARCTION **(A)** T2-weighted axial image. This young man presented with aphasia and confusion. Clinically, herpes encephalitis was suspected. The lesion is characterized by a central hypointense area in the left temporal lobe surrounded by a hyperintense area of edema. The central hypointensity is due to the presence of deoxyhemoglobin in an acute clot. **(B)** T2-weighted axial image. The left transverse venous sinus is filled with acute thrombus, which is clearly visible as a markedly hypointense tubular structure. This examination was performed with gradient moment nulling, which causes the normal venous sinuses to be of high signal intensity. Care must be exercised to avoid assigning the hypointensity within this venous sinus to normal flowing blood, rather than to the acute thrombosis which it truly represents. **(C)** T1-weighted axial image. The corresponding T1-weighted image through the venous sinus demonstrates the clot as a moderately hypointense tissue within the venous sinus.

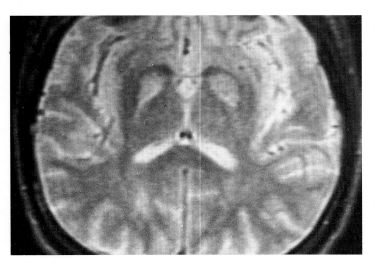

Fig. 1.51 CARBON MONOXIDE POISONING T2-weighted axial image. There are bilaterally symmetric hyperintense lesions in the globus pallidus. This is the most common site of the hypoxic lesions caused by carbon monoxide asphyxiation.

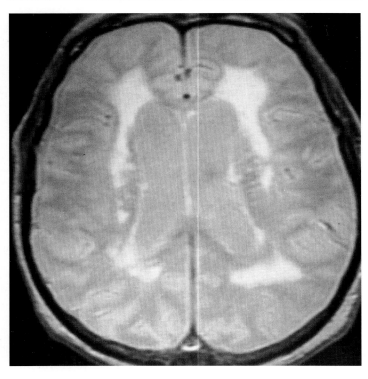

Fig. 1.52 DEEP WHITE MATTER AND PERIVENTRICULAR LESIONS OF THE SENESCENT BRAIN Proton density axial image. Bilateral hyperintense lesions appear adjacent to the lateral ventricles and in the corona radiata. Also referred to as subcortical arteriosclerotic encephalopathy, this is presumed to represent the sequelae of long-term ischemia on the deep white matter.

INFARCTION DUE TO SYSTEMIC DISEASES

Hypoxia and hypoperfusion cause cerebral infarcts that are individually indistinguishable from those caused by arterial lesions. However, the distribution of the infarcts can be distinctive.

Infarction caused by hypoperfusion is frequently seen in the setting of cardiac failure, arrhythmias, or cardiac bypass surgery. The infarcted tissues are usually between the major arterial territories, the so-called "water shed zones," or in terminal vascular areas, such as the basal ganglia, and are often multiple.

Global hypoxia is due to delivery to the brain of poorly oxygenated blood. Respiratory failure is probably the commonest cause of this type of lesion, but it also occurs with drowning, suffocation and asphyxiation. Carbon monoxide poisoning is an interesting example of a relatively specific type of common asphyxiation. Multiple infarcts develop, classically involving the globus pallidus bilaterally (Fig. 1.51).

CHRONIC ISCHEMIC DISEASE

The ubiquitous multifocal deep cerebral lesions demonstrated by MRI in the senescent brain are a problem. Specifically, there are continued questions as to their etiology and clinical significance. Two facts have been established: (1) they become progressively prevalent with increase in age (an estimated one third of the population is affected by age 65), and (2) many of those so affected have no overt clinical deficit. Pathologically these lesions correspond to small foci of gliosis and are probably the result of chronic diffuse ischemia, whether it be due to extracranial stenosis, arteriolosclerosis, repeated hypotensive episodes, or combinations of the three. On MRI they are particularly evident on the proton density and T2-weighted images as small, bilateral, multifocal hyperintense lesions (see Fig. 1.48). Individually they usually do not exceed 5 mm in size, but commonly confluence into larger lesions (Fig. 1.52). The periventricular and deep white matter is most frequently affected. The major problems in differential diagnosis are distinguishing these senescent lesions from atypical presentations of multiple sclerosis and from normal perivascular spaces, both having a similar distribution and appearance of the "lesions."

Perivascular spaces (Virchow–Robin spaces) are normal fluid channels surrounding small perforating arteries. They are more common in those with atherosclerosis but, surprisingly, they are also seen frequently in children. They are usually 2 to 3 mm in diameter, and most often located in the inferior basal ganglia, or adjacent to the parafalcine gray matter. These are fluid-containing spaces as opposed to the gliotic or edematous parenchymal lesions seen in ischemia and demyelination. Therefore, although similar to senescent lesions on T2-weighted (hyperintense) and T1-weighted (hypointense) images, on the proton density image (Fig. 1.53) they are approximately isointense to CSF and to brain. Both lacunes and perivascular spaces are common in the inferior basal ganglia, and a combination of T1-weighted, T2-weighted and proton density MR images is reliable for distinguishing between the two.

Small perivascular spaces

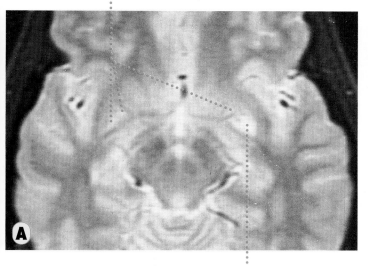

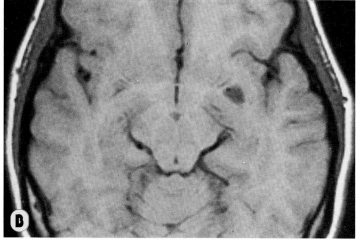

Large perivascular space
with perforating vessel

Basal ganglia   Perforating vessel

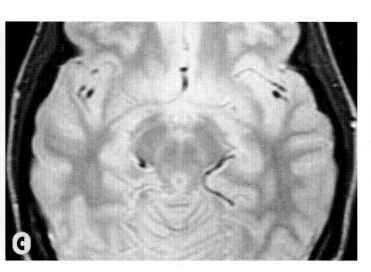

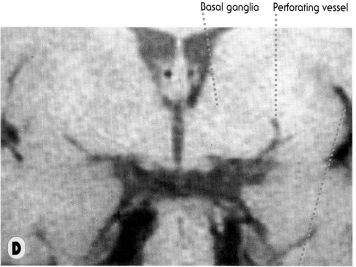

Sylvian fissure

Fig. 1.53 PERIVASCULAR SPACES (VIRCHOW–ROBIN SPACES) **(A)** T2-weighted axial image. As with the lacunes illustrated previously, the fluid-containing perivascular spaces are hyperintense relative to brain on T2-weighted images. **(B)** T1-weighted axial image. On the T1-weighted image, the perivascular spaces are typically hypointense relative to brain. Interestingly, a small vessel is visible within one of these perivascular spaces. **(C)** Proton density axial image. This technique best distin-guishes the small infarct from the perivascular space. The perivascular space is not visible because it has the same signal intensity as CSF. On this particular sequence, CSF is isointense to brain and therefore not distinct from the brain. **(D)** T1-weighted coronal image. An example of one of the perforating lenticulostriate arteries is particularly well seen on the left. It is around these small vessels that Virchow–Robin spaces are found.

The lesions of multiple sclerosis, particularly if late onset or atypical multiple sclerosis is suspected, are absolutely indistinguishable in most instances. If the patient is under 40 years of age, multiple sclerosis is by far the most likely diagnosis; the opposite is true for those over 60 years of age. It is in the 40- to 60-year-old age group that the diagnosis is particularly difficult. Multiple sclerosis plaques tend to be larger, some usually exceeding 5 mm in diameter, and more often involve the brainstem and cerebellar hemispheres. In many instances paraclinical tests, such as evoked potentials and CSF banding, must be closely correlated with the clinical history, physical findings and MR images.

NEOPLASMS

The annual incidence of intracranial tumors is between 5 and 15 per 100,000. These tumors can be divided into two large groups: primary intracranial tumors and metastases.

Fig. 1.54 INTRAAXIAL NEOPLASMS

	% of Primary Intracranial Tumors[a]	Location[b]	No. of Lesions[c]	Edema	Mass Effect
Glial Tumors					
Astrocytomas					
Low-grade	20				
Children		I	Si	0	+
Adults		Su	Si	+	+
High-grade	35	Su	Si[a,e]	++	++
Oligodendroglioma	5	Su	Si	+	+
Tumors of Primitive Bipotential Cells					
Medulloblastoma	5	I	Si[e]	0	+
Ganglioglioma	<1	Su	Si	0	+
Blood Vessel Tumors					
Hemangioblastoma	1	I	Si[f]	0	+
Reticuloendothelial Tumors					
Lymphoma	1	Su	Si[a]	+	+
Tumors of Maldevelopment					
Lipoma	1	Su or I	Si	0	0, +
Metastases	NA	Su or I	Si or M	++	++

0, uncommon; +, common; ++, very common; NA, not applicable.

[a]Multifocal tumors occur.
[b]Su, supratentorial; I, infratentorial.
[c]Si, single; M, multiple.
[d]F, fine; C, coarse.
[e]Propensity to spread via CSF may result in multiple lesions.
[f]Multiple tumors common in von Hippel–Lindau disease.
[g]Mural nodule enhances.

In adults, the largest group of primary intracranial tumors consists of gliomas, followed by meningiomas, acoustic neuromas and pituitary adenomas (acoustic neuromas and pituitary adenomas are discussed in the next chapter). The reported incidence of intracranial metastases varies widely. Metastases account for over 50% of intracranial tumors in some autopsy series, to less than 20% in surveys of general hospitals. Among children, primary brain tumors are second only to leukemia in cancer incidence. Metastases in children are rare.

The pathologic classification of intracranial tumors is conventionally based on tumor histology and cell of origin. This type of classification scheme is only of limited use in radiology. It is easier to reach a radiologic diagnosis based on tumor location, the number of lesions present and patient age, than it is to attempt to define the histologic type based on the MRI characteristics (Figs. 1.54 and 1.55). The general features on MRI of tumors and the tissues associated with tumors are considered separately from specific tumors.

Fig. 1.54 INTRAAXIAL NEOPLASMS (cont'd)

Cyst	Necrosis	Calcium^d	Hemorrhage	Vessels	Enhancement
++	0	0, F	0	0	+^{g}
0	0	0, F	0	0	0
0	++	0	+	+	++
0	0	0, F, C	+	0	0
0	0	0	0	0	++
+	0	0, F, C	0	0	+
++	0	0	0	++	+^{g}
0	0	0	0	0	0, +
0	0	0	0	0	0
0	+	0	+	+	++

0, uncommon; +, common; ++, very common; NA, not applicable.

^{a}Multifocal tumors occur.
^{b}Su, supratentorial; I, infratentorial.
^{c}Si, single; M, multiple.
^{d}F, fine; C, coarse.
^{e}Propensity to spread via CSF may result in multiple lesions.
^{f}Multiple tumors common in von Hippel–Lindau disease.
^{g}Mural nodule enhances.

GENERAL FEATURES OF INTRACRANIAL NEOPLASMS

SIGNAL INTENSITY   MRI signal intensity is in itself a poor guide by which to differentiate between intracranial tumors or, for that matter, between tumors and other pathologies. The vast majority of tumors contain more water than the normal brain and, thus, are generally characterized by increased proton density as well as increased T1 and T2 relaxation times. These increases result in their typical alteration of MRI signal intensity: hypointensity on T1-weighted images and hyperintensity on proton density and T2-weighted images. The magnitude of signal alteration correlates somewhat with the rapidity of tumor growth and malignancy, but this correlation is poor and is not an accurate diagnostic tool in the individual case.

The following generalizations about signal intensity are, however, valid. Most tumors are hypointense on T1-weighted images and hyperintense on T2-weighted images; most are more obvious on the T2-weighted images. The major exceptions are tumors that contain fat (lipomas, dermoids, and teratomas),

Fig. 1.55 EXTRAAXIAL NEOPLASMS[a]

	% of Primary Intracranial Tumors	Location[b]	No. of Lesions[c]	Edema	Mass Effect
Surface Tumors					
Meningioma	20	Su	Si	0, +, ++	+
Intraventricular Tumors[e]					
Ependymoma	5			0	+
Children		I	Si[f]		
Adults		Su	Si		
Choroid Plexus	<1	Su (Children)	Si	0	++
Papilloma		I (Adults)	Si		
Choroid Plexus	<1	S	Si	+	+
Carcinoma					
Colloid Cyst[g]	<1	Su	Si	0	0
Meningioma	<1	Su	Si	0	+
Astrocytoma	<1	Su	Si	+	+
Pineal Region Tumors[e]					
Germ Cell Tumors	<1	Su	Si[f]	0	+
Germinoma					
Teratomas					
Pineal Cell Tumors	<1	Su	Si		+
Pinealocytoma				0	
Pinealoblastoma				+	
Astrocytomas	<1	Su	Si	0	+
Tumors of Maldevelopment					
Dermoid/Epidermoid	<1	Su or I	Si	0	0, +
Leptomeningeal Metastases[e]	NA	Su or I	Si or M	0, +	0, +

0, uncommon; +, common; ++, very common; NA, not applicable.

[a]Excluding cranial nerve and parasellar tumors.
[b]Su, supratentorial; I, infratentorial.
[c]Si, single; M, multiple.
[d]F, fine; C, coarse.
[e]Often cause hydrocephalus.
[f]Propensity to spread via CSF may result in multiple lesions.
[g]Occurs exclusively in anterior third ventricle.
[h]Complex, irregular cysts.

tumors that have hemorrhaged, and melanoma metastases. The signal intensities of these unusual tumors stem from fundamental MRI principles: fat is bright on T1-weighted images and dark on T2-weighted images; the signal intensity of hemorrhage depends on the age of the bleed; and melanin is dark on T2-weighted images and bright on T1-weighted images.

CEREBRAL EDEMA   Cerebral edema is the excess accumulation of water in the brain and is a common accompaniment of brain diseases. Three distinct patterns of cerebral edema are recognized on imaging studies of the brain: vasogenic, cytotoxic, and periventricular.

Vasogenic edema is initiated by a loss of integrity of the blood-brain barrier. Vascular hydrostatic pressure then causes plasma filtrate to enter the extracellular space and diffuse along the relatively loosely organized white matter tracts. Radiologically, it is characterized by finger-like extensions into the subcortical "U" fibers and down along the main white

Fig. 1.55 EXTRAAXIAL NEOPLASMS^a (cont'd)

Cyst	Necrosis	Calcium^d	Hemorrhage	Vessels	Enhancement
0	0	0, F, C	0	+	++
0, +	0	0, F, C	0	0	+
0	0	0, F, C	0	0	++
0	+	0, F, C	0	0	++
+	0	0, F, C	0	0	+
0	0	0, F, C	0	0	++
0	0	0	0	0	+
0	0	0, F, C	0	0	++
0	0 / +	0, F, C	0	0	+
0	0	0	0	0	+
+^{h}	0	0, F, C	0	0	0
0	0	0	0	0	++

0, uncommon; +, common; ++, very common; NA, not applicable.

^{a}Excluding cranial nerve and parasellar tumors.
^{b}Su, supratentorial; I, infratentorial.
^{c}Si, single; M, multiple.
^{d}F, fine; C, coarse.
^{e}Often cause hydrocephalus.
^{f}Propensity to spread via CSF may result in multiple lesions.
^{g}Occurs exclusively in anterior third ventricle.
^{h}Complex, irregular cysts.

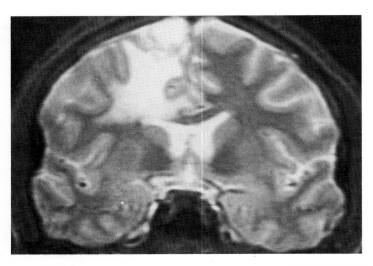

Fig. 1.56 VASOGENIC EDEMA T2-weighted coronal image. A 2-cm metastatic tumor in the vertex of the right cerebral hemisphere is immediately adjacent to the superior sagittal sinus. Deep to the metastasis there is a large area of edema in the white matter of the right cerebral hemisphere.

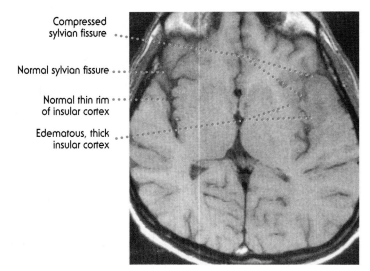

Compressed sylvian fissure

Normal sylvian fissure

Normal thin rim of insular cortex

Edematous, thick insular cortex

Fig. 1.57 CYTOTOXIC EDEMA T1-weighted axial image. There is an infarct involving the left temporal lobe and left insula. The lesion is characterized by thickening of the cortex and hypointensity of the cortex, both due to edema. Cytotoxic edema features selective involvement of the cortex with sparing of the underlying white matter. This is particularly well contrasted to the previous case of vasogenic edema, where the exact opposite is seen.

matter pathways (Fig. 1.56). It generally is less marked in the cortex and basal ganglia and usually does not involve the corpus callosum or the commissures, probably because these structures are relatively compact and resist the spread of edema. Virtually any lesion that occurs in, abuts on, or compresses white matter can incite vasogenic edema, but it is particularly common with neoplasms, and focal inflammation.

Cytotoxic edema results from impaired cellular metabolism. The sodium-potassium pump fails and water accumulates in the cells. It involves both white and gray matter. It is most often seen with early cerebral infarction (Fig. 1.57).

Periventricular edema is the accumulation of water that occurs around the ventricles when the normal egress of CSF from the ventricles to the basal cisterns is obstructed. It is most evident around the frontal and occipital horns of the lateral ventricles (Fig. 1.58). Regardless of the type of edema, the effect on relaxation times is the same—increased proton density and prolonged T1 and T2 relaxation, resulting in marked hyperintensity on proton density and T2-weighted images, and hypointensity on T1-weighted images.

The majority of intraaxial tumors (especially glioblastoma multiforme and metastases) and some extraaxial tumors (large meningiomas in particular) have associated vasogenic edema. The prolonged relaxation times caused by the edematous fluid often result in an MRI signal intensity similar to that of the tumor itself; the two may not be clearly separable in some cases. In most cases, however, the degree of intensity alteration is not exactly the same, usually being greater in the edematous areas. This distinguishes the tumor nidus, relatively hypointense on T2-weighted images, from the edema (Fig. 1.59). The demarcation is less evident on T1-weighted images. Intravenous contrast enhancement (gadolinium-DTPA) is of considerable benefit in these circumstances, permitting a more confident separation between the enhancing tumor and the nonenhancing edema.

MASS EFFECT The hallmark of a neoplasm is that it occupies space, or has mass effect. Mass effect is indicated by enlargement of the affected structure, by displacement of adjacent structures, and by compartmental shifts (for example, uncal herniation). Mass effect is due mostly to the volume of the tumor itself, but it is increased by concomitant edema (Fig. 1.60). Tumors that grow rapidly and incite the most edema have the greatest mass effect.

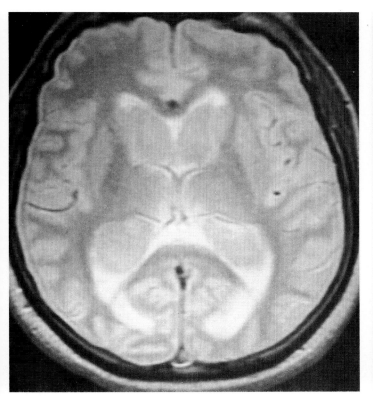

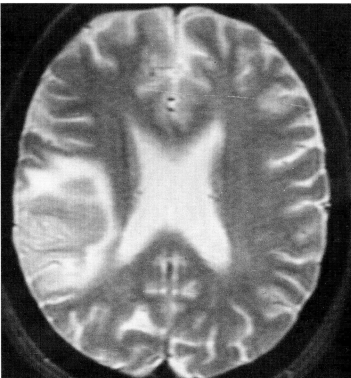

Fig. 1.58 PERIVENTRICULAR EDEMA Proton density axial image. This young man had obstructive hydrocephalus due to a posterior fossa tumor. The tumor obstructed the ventricular system, causing marked dilatation of the lateral ventricles and fluid egress from the ventricles into the parenchyma of the brain. This is particularly well seen on the proton density image as an area of hyperintensity, most marked at the tips of the frontal and occipital horns. The bilaterality, and the relatively smooth outline of the edematous area, are most characteristic of the edema seen with obstructive hydrocephalus.

Fig. 1.59 GLIOMA WITH SURROUNDING EDEMA T2-weighted axial image. There is a 4-cm glioma in the posterior aspect of the right sylvian fissure. It is just slightly hyperintense to the normal white matter of the brain, but is surrounded by an area which is markedly hyperintense. This hyperintense area is the vasogenic edema previously described (see Fig. 1.56). In instances such as this, the edema and the gross margin of the tumor are clearly separable. However, it should be understood that microscopically the tumor usually extends beyond this margin.

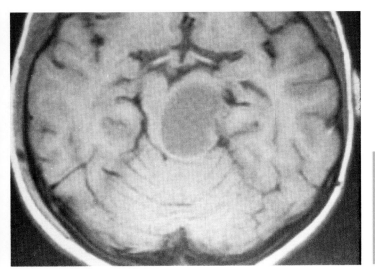

Fig. 1.60 MASS EFFECT T1-weighted axial image. There is a large, well-defined glioma in the left cerebral peduncle. The tumor causes marked expansion of the peduncle, compression of the contralateral peduncle, and displacement posteriorly of the quadrigeminal plate. It also encroaches anteriorly on the suprasellar cistern.

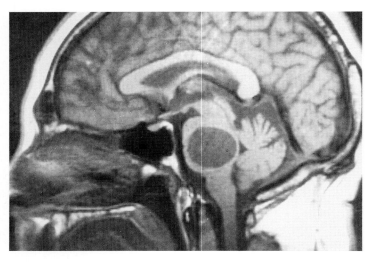

Fig. 1.61 CYSTIC PONTINE ASTROCYTOMA T1-weighted sagittal image. Cysts are characterized by a well-defined, uniform margin and a homogeneous internal architecture. In most cases on T1-weighted images, cysts, even those caused by tumors, are similar to CSF in intensity.

CYSTS AND NECROSIS Liquid or near-liquid centers identify these two entities. As might be expected, the high regional water content results in MRI signal intensity approaching that of CSF—very dark on T1-weighted images and very bright on T2-weighted images. Because the effect on MRI signal intensity is so similar, regions of necrosis and cysts, even those caused by tumors, may be indistinguishable from one another if only signal intensity is considered. Internal architecture and boundary morphology is important. Cysts are internally homogeneous and have smooth, thin walls (Fig. 1.61). Regions of necrosis are heterogeneous and have irregular, thick margins (Fig. 1.62).

Tumors that typically have large cystic components are the juvenile cerebellar astrocytoma and the hemangioblastoma. Both tumors are found principally in the cerebellar hemispheres, the astrocytoma in young children and the hemangioblastoma in young adults, particularly those with von Hippel-Lindau disease (Fig. 1.63). Dermoid and epidermoid tumors are often referred to as dermoid and epidermoid cysts. They fulfill the pathologic definition of cysts in that they have acellular centers contained within

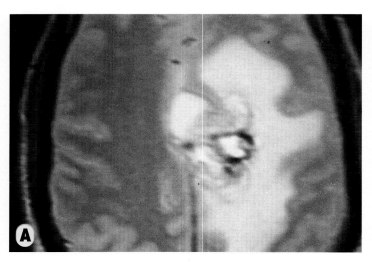

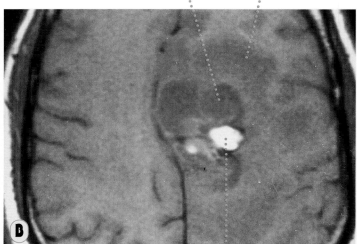

Tumor necrosis   Peritumoral edema

Intratumoral hemorrhage

Fig. 1.62 GLIOBLASTOMA WITH HEMORRHAGE AND NECROSIS **(A)** T2-weighted axial image. An irregular tumor in the medial aspect of the left cerebral hemisphere is surrounded by a large area of edema. Centrally within this glioblastoma there is a hemorrhagic area encircled by an irregular hemosiderin ring. In contrast to the peripheral hemosiderin ring seen with cavernous hemangiomas, the hemosiderin ring in this case is of irregular thickness and does not completely surround

the lesion. Furthermore, it is surrounded by an area of abnormal signal intensity. This type of hemorrhage is indicative of a malignant tumor. **(B)** T1-weighted axial image. Peripheral to the intratumoral hemorrhage there is a multilobulated hypointense region pathologically corresponding to areas of necrosis. The necrotic portion of the tumor has an irregular outline, is internally heterogeneous and, although hypointense, is not as dark as fluid in simple cysts.

epithelially lined walls, but their appearance on MRI is more complex than that of other cysts. The dermoid tumor may contain fat, calcium, hair, or keratin and the MRI is correspondingly complex. The epidermoid contains desquamated squamous epithelium and keratin. Its signal intensity is just slightly brighter than CSF on T1-weighted images and slightly darker than CSF on T2-weighted images, with subtle internal septae and an irregular outline.

Tumor necrosis occurs in rapidly expanding neoplasms and, therefore, is usually limited to the more highly malignant tumors. It is most commonly seen in glioblastomas and metastases, but may occur in several other malignant tumors (Fig. 1.62).

CALCIFICATION   False negatives of faintly calcified lesions are common with MRI. The difficulty in visualizing calcification is, in fact, a well-recognized deficiency. Calcium does not contribute to signal intensity but does replace tissue that otherwise might. Its effect on intensity is therefore basically a null effect—if it is finely dispersed its presence, and the lesion itself, will be overlooked (Fig. 1.64). Dense calcification is noticeable as an area devoid of signal

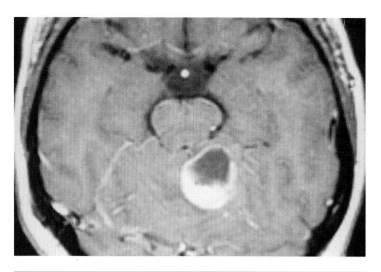

Fig. 1.63 HEMANGIOBLASTOMA (CONTRAST-ENHANCED STUDY)   T1-weighted axial image following gadolinium-DTPA infusion. The hemangioblastoma is identified as a partially cystic, partially solid mass in the superior vermis on the left side. The solid component demonstrates marked contrast enhancement. Hemangioblastomas are one of the few benign intraaxial tumors that demonstrate such profuse enhancement.

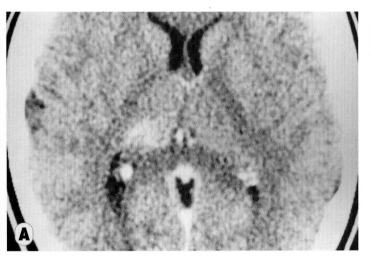

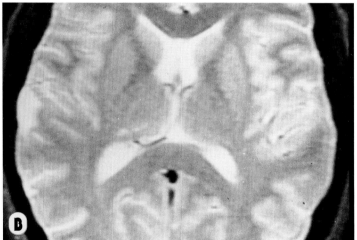

Fig. 1.64 FINE CALCIFICATION IN A LOW-GRADE ASTROCYTOMA   (A) CT scan. There is a slightly calcified lesion in the posterior half of the right thalamus. This lesion showed sequential enlargement over a number of years and presumably represents a low-grade astrocytoma. **(B)** T2-weighted axial image. The thalamic lesion is not evident on the MRI scan. False negatives are common on MRI with such faintly calcified lesions.

(black) (Fig. 1.65). Lesions with intermediate densities of calcification may or may not be detected.

Calcification occurs in those tumors that are relatively slow growing. Among intraaxial tumors, oligodendrogliomas and gangliogliomas, although both relatively uncommon, have a high incidence of MRI visible calcification. Of the extraaxial tumors, craniopharyngiomas, meningiomas, and dermoids frequently calcify. Many other tumors have CT evidence of calcium; only a fraction of these will be apparent on MRI.

HEMORRHAGE   Hemorrhage in intraaxial neoplasms is much more frequent than in extraaxial neoplasms. Approximately 10% of intraaxial tumors will have evidence of new or remote bleeding. The incidence is highest among metastatic lesions, in particular melanoma, renal cell carcinoma, thyroid carcinoma and choriocarcinoma. Glioblastoma and oligodendroglioma are the primary tumors most likely to bleed.

The appearance of hemorrhage depends principally on the age of the bleed and the proportion of the

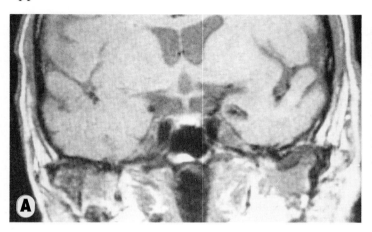
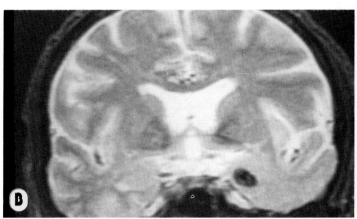

Fig. 1.65 DENSELY CALCIFIED LEFT TEMPORAL LOBE ASTROCYTOMA   (A) T1-weighted coronal image. There is a markedly hypointense ovoid nodule in the uncus of the left temporal lobe. **(B)** T2-weighted coronal image.

The lesion is uniformly hypointense, having a signal intensity similar to that of bone. This case illustrates the combination of signal intensities to be expected from a densely calcified lesion.

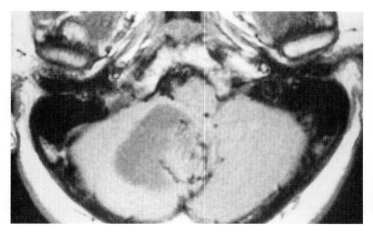
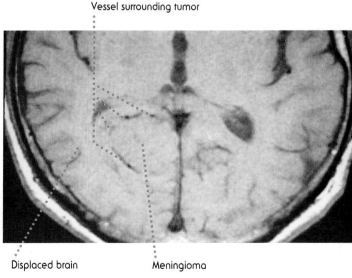

Vessel surrounding tumor

Displaced brain   Meningioma

Fig. 1.66 HEMANGIOBLASTOMA   This is a common appearance of a hemangioblastoma. There is a large cystic component in the right cerebellar hemisphere and a large, solid nodule containing many small vessels.

Fig. 1.67 TUMOR VESSELS   T1-weighted axial image. There is a 4-cm parafalcine meningioma directly posterior to the atrium of the right lateral ventricle. The tumor itself is difficult to see due to its isointensity relative to surrounding brain. However, it is clearly outlined by several small vessels draped over its surface. Such vessels are commonly seen with meningiomas.

tumor involved. In most cases the hematoma occupies only a portion of the neoplasm. Tumor can usually be identified beyond the margin of the clot (see Fig. 1.62). This is an important diagnostic sign and distinguishes hemorrhagic tumors from other parenchymal hemorrhages due to hypertension, trauma, and vascular malformations.

TUMOR VESSELS   Blood vessels have inherently high visibility on MRI due to the natural contrast provided by the flow void of the vascular channels. The detection of abnormal vessels in and adjacent to tumors is a useful differential diagnostic sign. The only other intracranial lesion in which they are seen with any frequency is the AVM. These are different from neoplasms in that the vessels completely define the lesion—no other component is visible; with tumors, a solid component is also present. Large vessels leading to or from a tumor are typical of a

hemangioblastoma (Fig. 1.66) and are frequent with glioblastomas and meningiomas. In glioblastomas they are irregular and eccentrically placed in or adjacent to the tumor, and in meningiomas they are usually draped over the surface of the tumor (Fig. 1.67).

ENHANCEMENT   Gadolinium-DTPA is an intravenously injected paramagnetic contrast agent that behaves analogously to iodinated agents used in computed tomography. It assesses the integrity of the blood-brain barrier. Enhancement is most profound when there is no blood-brain barrier or when its permeability is increased. Among intraaxial tumors, enhancement is usually a sign of relatively aggressive biologic behavior. For example, enhancment is more profound with high grade astrocytomas and medulloblastomas than with low grade astrocytomas or oligodendrogliomas (Figs. 1.68 and 1.69). Notable exceptions to this general rule are the juvenile cystic

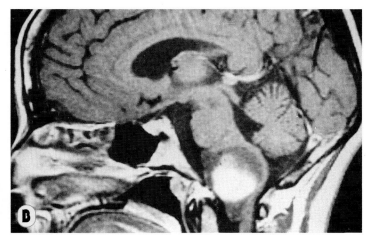

Fig. 1.68 BRAINSTEM GLIOBLASTOMA   (A) T1-weighted sagittal image. In the anterior half of the medulla, there is a large tumor mass fungating into the basal cisterns anteriorly and into the anterior subarachnoid space of the spinal canal. **(B)** T1-weighted sagittal image, con-

trast enhanced. Following gadolinium-DTPA there is irregular central enhancement of a portion of the tumor. This degree of enhancement in an intraaxial lesion usually indicates an aggressive histology. Low-grade intraaxial tumors enhance minimally, if at all.

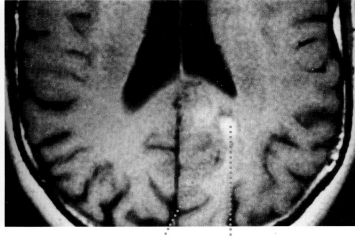

Astrocytoma   Contrast enhancement

Fig. 1.69 LOW-GRADE ASTROCYTOMA CONTRAST-ENHANCED STUDY   T1-weighted axial image following gadolinium-DTPA infusion. There is a relatively well-defined mass in the posterior aspect of the occipital lobe and a faint area of enhancement involves a portion of the tumor.

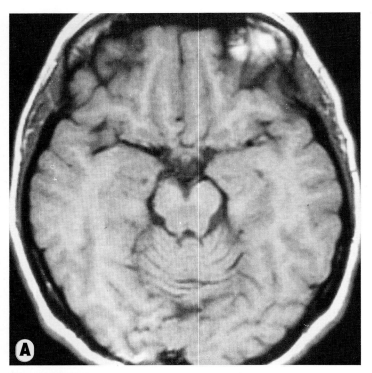

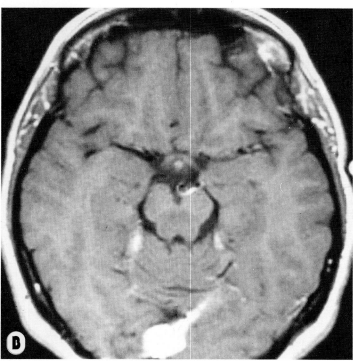

Fig. 1.70 TENTORIAL MENINGIOMA **(A)** T1-weighted axial image. The tumor, positioned directly anterior to the torcula, was entirely overlooked on a noncontrast study. **(B)** T1-weighted axial image, contrast-enhanced. Following gadolinium-DTPA the meningioma is easily identified by profuse contrast enhancement.

astrocytoma and the hemangioblastoma. Although they are benign tumors, both display intense enhancement (see Fig. 1.63), at least of their mural nodules.

The extraaxial tissues within the cranium (leptomeninges, ependyma, choroid plexus, pineal gland) do not have a blood-brain barrier and, therefore, normally enhance. It follows that extraaxial lesions also enhance regardless of benignancy or malignancy (Fig. 1.70). A few extraaxial tumors, such as dermoids, epidermoids, and lipomas, do not enhance simply because they are avascular.

FEATURES OF SPECIFIC NEOPLASMS

INTRAAXIAL TUMORS
GLIAL TUMORS   Gliomas include astrocytomas, glioblastomas, and oligodendrogliomas. In the broadest sense they also include ependymomas, but these are usually located within the ventricle and are included in the category of intraventricular neoplasms. As a group, glial tumors account for well over half of all primary intracranial tumors.

The juvenile cystic astrocytoma, with a median presentation age of 5 years, is the commonest brain tumor of childhood. The MRI features are quite specific: a well-defined mass located in the cerebellar hemisphere, with a large cyst and a small mural nodule that enhances intensely with intravenous contrast. Childhood cystic astrocytomas are relatively benign tumors which, as a rule, are cured with surgical excision. The other glioma seen in childhood is the brainstem glioma, which is more malignant and occurs in older children, usually during the early teens. There is generally enlargement of the brainstem, often with a poor margin between the tumor and the normal brainstem (Fig. 1.71). The tumor may fungate into the cistern, creating an exophytic component. The exophytic portion can be surgically removed, but total removal of the tumor is impossible. Radiotherapy is the primary treatment modality. Sagittal MRI is particularly useful prior to radiotherapy, as it clearly delineates the cephalocaudad extension of the tumor.

Adult gliomas span the entire spectrum of histology from the low-grade, extremely slow-growing astrocytoma and oligodendroglioma through to the extremely malignant, high-grade tumor, the glioblastoma multiforme. The feature common to both low- and high-grade tumors is that neither is particularly well-demarcated from normal parenchyma. The edges of the tumor interdigitate and merge with the surrounding brain. The low-grade tumors have less edema, less mass effect, more frequently have calcification (particularly oligodendrogliomas), and do not enhance (Fig. 1.72; also see 1.59, 1.64, 1.65, and 1.69). Glioblastomas have much more edema and mass effect, frequently with necrotic areas, foci of hemorrhage, and enlarged surrounding vessels (Fig. 1.73, also see 1.62 and 1.68).

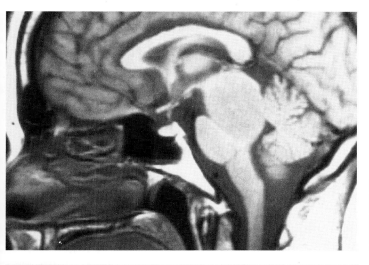

Fig. 1.71 BRAINSTEM GLIOMA T1-weighted sagittal image. The large, well-defined mass, occupying the entire midbrain and tegmentum of the pons, is pathognomonic of a brainstem glioma.

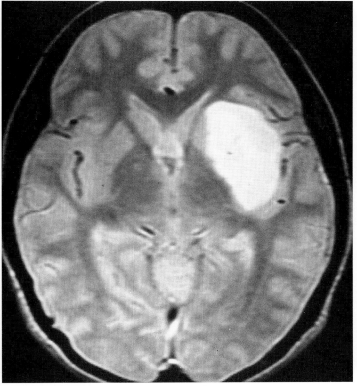

Fig. 1.72 LOW-GRADE ASTROCYTOMA T2-weighted axial image. There is no surrounding edema, no necrosis, and no unusual tumor vessels. This appearance is most consistent with that of a low-grade astrocytoma; however, in some cases even high-grade tumors, such as glioblastomas, can have a similar "benign" appearance.

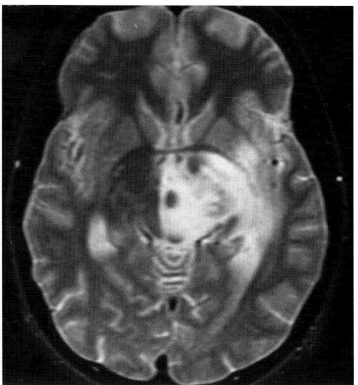

Fig. 1.73 GLIOBLASTOMA T2-weighted axial image. An irregular, ill-defined area of hyperintensity in the left half of the midbrain extends upward through the thalamus, into the temporal lobe and optic radiation. The poorly defined margin makes it difficult to separate tumor from surrounding edema. This type of appearance is most consistent with a high-grade tumor.

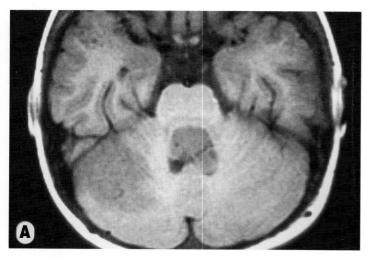

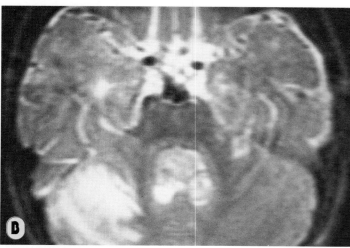

Fig. 1.74 MEDULLOBLASTOMA (CHILD) (A) T1-weighted axial image. There is a tumor filling the fourth ventricle, as well as a second lesion in the right cerebellar hemisphere. In the child, the differential diagnosis is between medulloblastoma and ependymoma; the presence of the second lesion favors the former. **(B)** T2-weighted axial image. Both tumors are once again identified. The second lesion indicates spread of the malignancy through CSF pathways. The child had a third lesion in a parafalcine location within the cerebral hemisphere (not shown). The multiple lesions favor medulloblastoma as the diagnosis, subsequently proven at surgery.

TUMORS OF PRIMITIVE BIPOTENTIAL CELLS

Medulloblastomas are highly malignant tumors of children and young adults and are found predominantly in the posterior fossa. Recently they have been reclassified as primitive neuroectodermal tumors (PNET). They arise in residual germinative cells which are the embryonic precursors of the external granular layer. In children they are usually found midline, in the superior vermis, but can occur anywhere in the cerebellar hemispheres (Fig. 1.74). A minority (about 25%) appear in young adults; these occur laterally in the cerebellar hemispheres (Fig. 1.75). Medulloblastomas show a tremendous propensity to disseminate through the cerebrospinal fluid, and up to 50% have already spread beyond the primary site by the time of clinical presentation. Surprisingly, for a highly malignant tumor, it may be difficult to see on MRI. Its intensity closely resembles that of normal vermis on both T1- and T2-weighted images but has a mass effect. The tumor expands the vermis, frequently extending to the fourth ventricle, kinking the aqueduct, and causing obstructive hydrocephalus. Its spread through the subarachnoid space is difficult to recognize on unenhanced MRI, since the only evidence may be small surface nodules or loss of normal surface morphology. Gadolinium-DTPA is essential for accurate diagnosis and staging as the tumor enhances prominently.

Gangliogliomas are most frequently found in children and are slow-growing, well-circumscribed tumors with both glial and neuronal elements. There is a predilection for involvement of the temporal lobes (Fig. 1.76). Calcification is frequently noted on CT, a finding often entirely overlooked on MRI. A minority of these tumors have cystic components. In a young person, the combination of a cystic component and calcification in a temporal lobe suggests the possibility of ganglioglioma.

TUMORS OF BLOOD VESSELS The most important tumor in this group is the hemangioblastoma. The hemangioblastoma, usually found in young adults, is a benign tumor composed of thin-walled blood vessels. Ten to twenty percent are multiple and occur as part of von Hippel–Lindau disease. Most are found in the cerebellar hemispheres; rarely is the brainstem or even the cerebrum involved. Two different types of morphology are seen on MRI. Most are cystic lesions with a small mural nodule (Fig. 1.77). The others are enhancing nodules without a cyst (Fig. 1.78). Large vessels are seen in or adjacent to both types of lesions. Visualization of the triad of cyst, mural nodule and large vessels is specific for the diagnosis of hemangioblastoma. Very small lesions may go undetected on noncontrast MRI. As might be expected from the marked vascularity of these lesions, there is intense enhancement with paramagnetic contrast agents (see Fig. 1.75). Gadolinium-DTPA is particularly indicated to avoid overlooking these smaller lesions in cases of known von Hippel–Lindau disease.

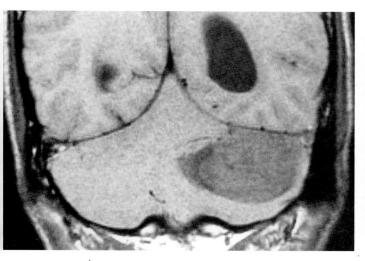

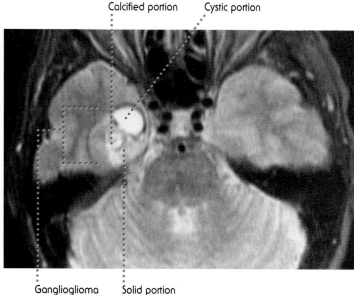

Calcified portion   Cystic portion

Ganglioglioma   Solid portion

Fig. 1.75 MEDULLOBLASTOMA (ADULT) T1-weighted coronal image. There is a large tumor in the left cerebellar hemisphere extending superiorly to the tentorial surface. There is also tumor invasion of the left transverse sinus, indicated by the absence of the expected signal void.

Fig. 1.76 GANGLIOGLIOMA T2-weighted axial image. Several components of the tumor are evident: the cystic component is anterior, a small calcified portion is posterolateral to the cyst and, posterior to both, is a slightly hyperintense solid tumor component.

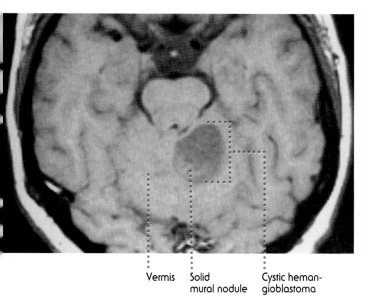

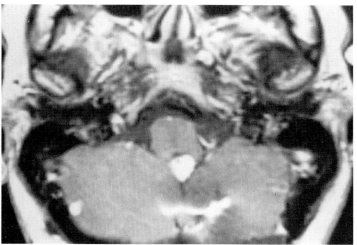

Vermis   Solid   Cystic heman-
          mural nodule   gioblastoma

Fig. 1.77 HEMANGIOBLASTOMA T1-weighted axial image. There is a predominantly cystic tumor, with a solid nodule along its posteromedial wall, in the superior portion of the left vermis.

Fig. 1.78 HEMANGIOBLASTOMA T1-weighted axial image, contrast-enhanced. Multiple enhancing nodules are seen in the cerebellum. Surgery confirmed the presence of multiple hemangioblastomas, diagnostic of the von Hippel–Lindau syndrome. Previous surgery accounts for the posterior pseudomeningiocele.

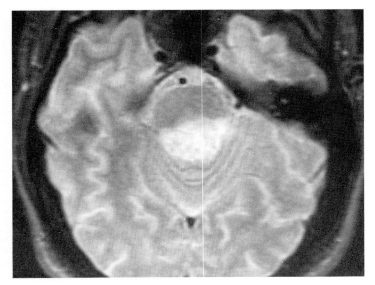

Fig. 1.79 LOCALIZED LYMPHOMA T2-weighted axial image. A well-defined 2- to 3-cm mass of increased signal in the tegmentum of the pons compresses the fourth ventricle. The differential diagnosis for this appearance is quite broad and would include glioma and lymphoma. At autopsy this lesion was found to be a lymphoma.

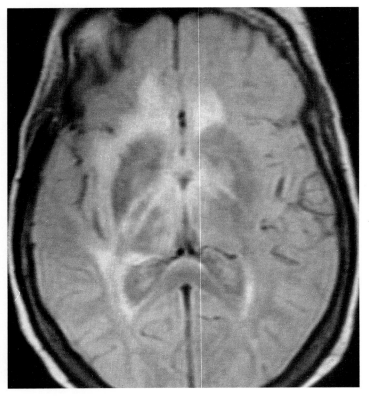

Fig. 1.80 INFILTRATING LYMPHOMA Proton density axial image. There is a diffusely infiltrating lesion involving the base of the brain. The lesion extends around both ventricles, and infiltrates both the internal and external capsules. Biopsy demonstrated this to be a lymphoma.

LYMPHOMA Lymphoma may originate in the central nervous system or, as is more common, involve the central nervous system as part of a systemic illness. Non-Hodgkin's lymphoma is much more common than Hodgkin's disease in the central nervous system; primary occurrence of Hodgkin's disease in the brain is particularly rare.

Lymphoma in the brain takes one of two forms—a localized mass (Fig. 1.79) or, more frequently, a diffusely infiltrating lesion (Fig. 1.80). It is one of the few tumors where multiple parenchymal lesions are frequent (the others being metastases and multicentric glioblastoma). Lymphoma has no distinguishing features on MRI apart from its tendency to involve the corpus callosum and to cross the midline (see Fig. 1.80). Hemorrhage is extremely rare. The disease is much more common in immunocompromised individuals, in particular in those with the acquired immune deficiency syndrome.

TUMORS OF MALDEVELOPMENT Intracranial lipomas are rare. Half or more are in the corpus callosum and are associated with callosal anomalies. The others are found in the quadrigeminal plate, suprasellar cistern, and cerebellar vermis. Lipomas are benign and, with the exception of callosal lipomas, are invariably small. They are characterized by uniformly bright signal on T1-weighted images (Fig. 1.81). Dermoids and epidermoids are discussed with extraaxial tumors.

METASTASES In autopsy series, metastases are the commonest intracranial neoplasms in adults, but they are much less prevalent in general hospitals. Bronchial and breast carcinomas are the commonest sources. Multiplicity is the sine qua non of metastatic disease (Fig. 1.82). However, even a single intracerebral metastasis is more common in adults than all but a few primary brain tumors. Consequently, metastatic tumor is always high in the differential diagnosis of any intracerebral mass. Unfortunately, the solitary metastasis is indistinguishable from primary brain tumors. Other than multiplicity, there are few distinguishing features. One is rapid growth on sequential scans; the other is a relatively large amount of edema with even small metastatic foci (Fig. 1.83).

EXTRAAXIAL NEOPLASMS
Regional classification facilitates the differential diagnosis of extraaxial tumors. On that basis, they are herein divided into the following categories: surface tumors of the meninges, intraventricular tumors, pineal tumors, parasellar tumors, and skull base

tumors. The last two groups are discussed with the skull base in the next chapter. Tumors of maldevelopment and metastases are included in this regional classification, but it is clear that they occur in a variety of locations. The classification of the ventricles and pineal gland as extraaxial, while not entirely correct, is useful for radiologic differential diagnosis. Some intraaxial neoplasms are included because of their tendency to grow exophytically and thereby mimic extraaxial tumors.

SURFACE TUMORS OF THE MENINGES   Meningiomas account for about 20% of intracranial tumors in adults with a peak incidence in the fifth decade; they are the commonest extraaxial tumor and the commonest benign tumor within the cranial vault. Their malignant counterpart, the meningosarcoma, is extremely rare and is mentioned only in passing. The majority of meningiomas are supratentorial, with a particularly high incidence over the convexity, alongside the falx, or adjacent to the sphenoid ridge. They are slow-growing, well-circumscribed tumors that can assume a variety of shapes: flat (meningioma-en-plaque), broad-based, or pedunculated. Those over the convexity and alongside the falx are usually broad-based; basal meningiomas have a tendency to assume an en plaque configuration.

About three quarters of meningiomas have MRI relaxation characteristics similar to cerebral cortex

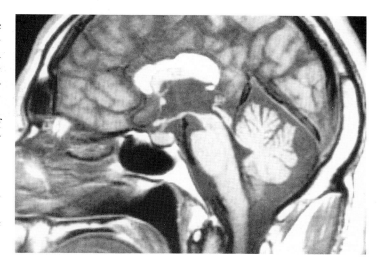

Fig. 1.81 CORPUS CALLOSUM LIPOMA   T1-weighted sagittal image. A well-defined hyperintense lipoma occupies most of the corpus callosum, the most common intracranial site of these lesions. This appearance is pathognomonic of a lipoma.

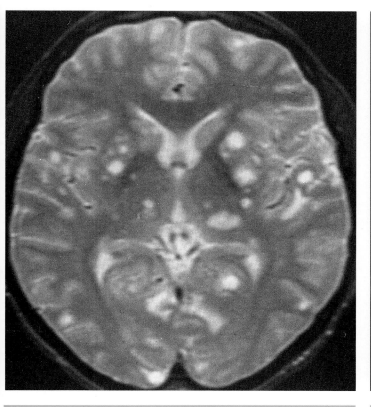

Fig. 1.82 MULTIPLE BREAST METASTASES   T2-weighted axial image. Numerous nodules are present throughout both cerebral hemispheres of this patient with a known primary breast carcinoma. In this clinical setting, this appearance is pathognomonic of cerebral metastases.

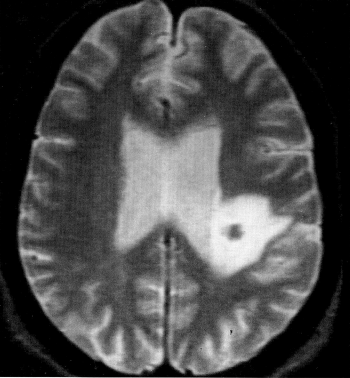

Fig. 1.83 SOLITARY METASTASIS   T2-weighted axial image. A 7-mm nodule, adjacent to the body of the left lateral ventricle, is surrounded by a large area of edema.

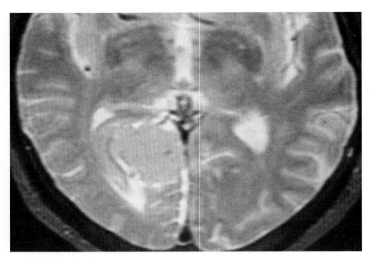

Fig. 1.84 MENINGIOMA   T2-weighted axial image. There is a well-defined tumor mass posterior to the atrium of the right lateral ventricle and abutting the falx cerebri. The signal intensity is only slightly hyperintense to the cortex. The extraaxial location and the near isointensity with brain indicate the diagnosis of meningioma.

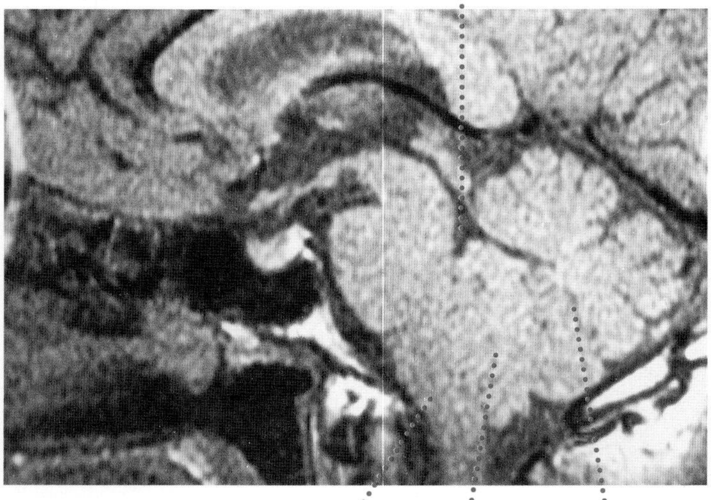

Proximal 4th ventricle

Brainstem   Ependymoma   Cerebellum

Fig. 1.85 FOURTH VENTRICLE EPENDYMOMA   T1-weighted sagittal image. A tumor mass fills the inferior three quarters of the fourth ventricle and extends inferiorly through the foramen of Magendie into the cisterna magna.

and are isointense to cortex on all MRI pulse sequences (Fig. 1.84). The remainder are moderately hyperintense on T2-weighted images. Brain edema is surprisingly common with meningiomas given that the tumor does not invade the brain. Cysts, necrosis, and hemorrhage are all rare. Calcification is common, occurring in about one quarter of tumors, but difficult to appreciate on MRI. Vessels are often distinctly visualized draped over the tumor periphery or radiating through the tumor center. Marked, uniform contrast enhancement is a characteristic feature (see Fig. 1.67).

INTRAVENTRICULAR TUMORS   Ependymomas, although accounting for less than 5 percent of the total of intracranial tumors, are the commonest intraventricular tumors in children and adults. As with parenchymal glial tumors, they are primarily above the tentorium in adults but usually below the tentorium, in the fourth ventricle in children. Ependymomas are relatively benign, slow-growing, circumscribed tumors. Because of their intraventricular location, hydrocephalus is common. Ependymomas are somewhat similar to cortex in MRI signal intensity. Cysts and necrosis are frequent; calcification, although present in about one quarter of cases, is rarely visible on MRI. The intraventricular location is the most valuable differential diagnostic sign (Fig. 1.85). Ependymomas in the fourth ventricle often protrude laterally with tongue-like extensions into the cerebellopontine angle cistern or inferiorly into the subarachnoid space, entering the cisterna magna through the foramen of Magendie.

Tumors of the choroid plexus are rare. Children are more frequently affected than adults. The benign variety, the papilloma, is usually in the lateral ventricle (children) or the fourth ventricle (adults); it does not invade the brain. The tumor is typically multilobulated (Fig. 1.86); cysts are frequent as is calcification. Hydrocephalus is a characteristic but not invariable feature, and may be secondary to increased CSF secretion by, or hemorrhage from, the tumor. Choroid plexus carcinoma is even rarer. The MR image of the carcinoma is generally indistinguishable from the benign papilloma. However, invasion of the brain, or the presence of cerebral edema around the tumor, should suggest the possibility of malignancy (Fig. 1.87).

Meningiomas can rarely arise primarily in the ventricle. Mesenchymal cellular rests in the choroid plexus of the lateral ventricle are the usual cells of origin. The MRI appearance is exactly analogous to the more common surface variety (Fig. 1.88). Colloid cysts, containing gelatinous material, are benign epithelial cysts of developmental origin located exclusively in the anterior third ventricle. Hydrocephalus is common due to obstruction of the foramen of Monro. The most consistent MRI features of colloid cysts are their location, spherical shape, and well-defined margins (Fig. 1.89). The signal intensity in these lesions is variable, ranging from hyperintensity to hypointensity on either T1- or T2-weighted images.

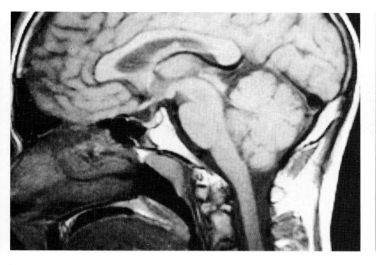

Fig. 1.86 CHOROID PLEXUS PAPILLOMA (ADULT) T1-weighted sagittal image. There is a slightly lobulated, well-defined tumor mass filling the fourth ventricle. There is no evidence of invasion of the surrounding brain. The differential diagnosis is between a choroid plexus papilloma and ependymoma. At surgery a papilloma was found and completely excised.

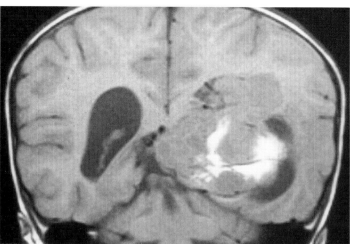

Fig. 1.87 CHOROID PLEXUS CARCINOMA (CHILD) T1-weighted coronal image. There is a huge multilobulated tumor with areas of hemorrhage in the atrium of the left lateral ventricle. The tumor invades the periventricular areas of the brain, indicating its malignant nature.

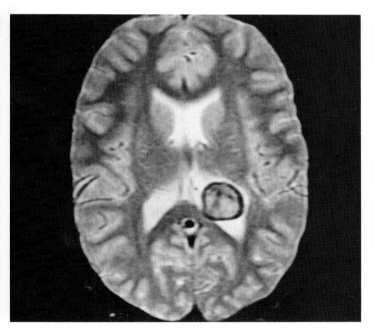

Fig. 1.88 INTRAVENTRICULAR FIBROBLASTIC MENINGIOMA T2-weighted axial image. A very well-defined, spherical tumor occupies the trigone of the left lateral ventricle. It is hypointense peripherally, an appearance indicative of a benign intraventricular tumor. The differential diagnosis is between a papilloma and a meningioma. At surgery this was found to be a fibroblastic meningioma. A useful feature in distinguishing it from a papilloma is that papillomas are usually lobulated in outline.

Lateral ventricle Colloid cyst Fornix Corpus callosum

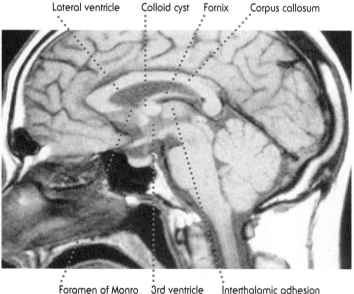

Foramen of Monro   3rd ventricle   Interthalamic adhesion

Fig. 1.89 COLLOID CYST OF THE THIRD VENTRICLE T1-weighted sagittal image. There is a 1-cm, spherical, well-defined lesion in the anterior third ventricle. The nodule is approximately isointense to brain.

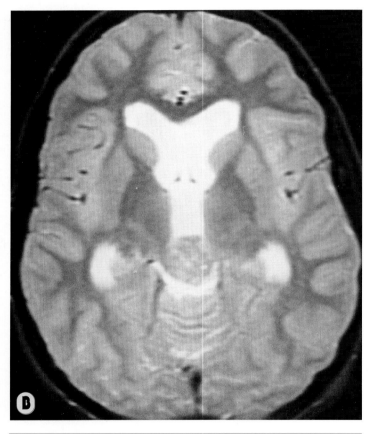

Dilated lateral and 3rd ventricles   Germinoma   Compressed aqueduct   Tectum

Fig. 1.90 PINEAL GERMINOMA **(A)** T1-weighted sagittal image. A well-defined ovoid tumor in the pineal gland compresses the cerebral aqueduct, causing obstructive hydrocephalus. **(B)** T2-weighted axial image. The tumor is identified in the pineal gland as slightly hyperintense to white matter with some heterogeneous internal signal. The ventricles are dilated due to obstruction of the cerebral aqueduct.

PINEAL REGION TUMORS   The cells of the pineal parenchyma, pinealocytes, are modified nerve cells which give rise to two histologic types of neoplasms. The pinealocytoma is a relatively low-grade tumor. In common with other pineal region tumors, it has a tendency to disseminate via the CSF. The pinealoblastoma is a malignant tumor which probably arises from primitive precursors of pinealocytes. Both tumors are uncommon and do not have any distinguishing features on MRI.

The most common tumor to occur in the pineal gland is of germ cell, not pineal cell origin. Tumors of germ cell origin are subclassified as germinomas or as teratomatous (embryonal cell carcinoma, choriocarcinoma and teratoma). Germinomas have a strong predilection to occur in young males, usually in their teenage years (Fig. 1.90). They can also occur primarily in, or spread to, the suprasellar region. Cerebrospinal fluid dissemination is an early feature of the tumor. Calcification is frequent but very difficult to appreciate on MRI, as with so many other intracranial tumors. Plain radiographs or CT are recommended. The much rarer teratomatous tumors are distinctive only if fat is present.

TUMORS OF MALDEVELOPMENT   Several important examples of maldevelopmental tumors are encountered in neurodiagnosis. Although not frequent, they are of sufficient incidence and distinctive appearance to merit illustration. Of particular importance are craniopharyngioma, arachnoid cyst, dermoid, epidermoid, and lipoma. The essential feature of all these tumors is that they are benign, extraaxial (excluding most lipomas), and may occur in a variety of locations despite the predisposition of each to certain areas. Because these tumors are usually found adjacent to the skull base or sella turcica (excluding lipomas), they are included in the subsequent chapter. Lipomas have already been discussed with other intraaxial tumors.

METASTASES   Metastases from tumors, both within and external to the central nervous system, can involve the leptomeninges, the ependyma, the choroid plexus and the pineal gland. However, extraaxial involvement is less common than parenchymal metastatic disease. The central nervous system primaries most often involving the leptomeninges and ependyma are the medulloblastoma (PNET), ependymoma, glioblastoma multiforme, lymphoma and germinoma; bronchial and breast carcinomas are the commonest nonneurologic tumors to do so.

Extraaxial tumor deposition takes one of two forms, distinct nodules or diffuse infiltration. If deposits are small, there is usually no direct evidence of leptomeningeal carcinomatosis but hydrocephalus, a manifestation of tumor cells obstructing the arachnoid villi, is often present. With progression, the meningeal coverings become thick and occasionally nodular; if the ependyma is involved, it is hyperintense and irregular (Fig. 1.91). This is particularly noticeable on the proton density images. Diagnosis is greatly facilitated by intravenous contrast, which demonstrates diffuse meningeal and/or ependymal enhancement.

INFECTION

PARENCHYMAL INFECTION

Infection of the brain may be caused by most bacteria, fungi, parasites, or viruses. While the majority of clinically important infections are caused by relatively few of these microorganisms, these infections require consideration and are reviewed below.

Despite somewhat different pathologic processes, the resultant imaging characteristics of bacterial and fungal infections are very similar. They are, therefore, considered as a single group, with noted exceptions, using bacterial infection as the prototype.

Bacterial infection frequently gains access to the brain by direct spread from the paranasal or mastoid sinus, or by hematogenous seeding from distant infected foci. Less common modes of entry into the brain are by penetrating trauma, particularly with retained foreign bodies, and surgery. Infection develops in the brain adjacent to the direct access site; in hematogenous seeding, there is a geographic predilection toward these areas of highest regional blood flow, especially the region of the brain supplied by the middle cerebral artery and its branches.

Initially, a localized inflammatory reaction occurs surrounded by edema, the so-called "cerebritis" stage (Fig. 1.92). Subsequently, central tissue necrosis develops. Within 1 to 2 weeks, new blood vessels form around the lesion and fibroblasts begin to lay down reticulin and collagen, the precursors of an

Dilated lateral and 3rd ventricle

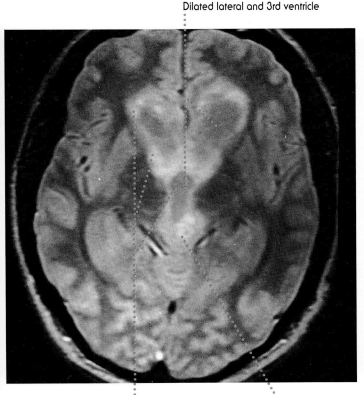

Subependymal tumor spread   Pineal tumor

Fig. 1.91 MALIGNANT ASTROCYTOMA OF THE PINEAL GLAND WITH SUBEPENDYMAL SPREAD Proton density axial image. As in the previous case there is a well-defined tumor in the pineal gland. However, the third ventricle and frontal horns of the lateral ventricle are surrounded by irregular areas of high signal intensity. This indicates the spread of subependymal tumor. This appearance should be contrasted with the smooth hyperintensity seen in simple obstructive hydrocephalus.

Fig. 1.92 CEREBRITIS T2-weighted axial image. There is a huge lesion occupying the anterior half of the right cerebral hemisphere. It is characterized by a central area of reduced signal completely surrounded by extensive vasogenic edema which permeates the white matter of the right cerebral hemisphere. Separation of the central component and the edema is extremely poorly defined, a characteristic of cerebritis prior to abscess formation.

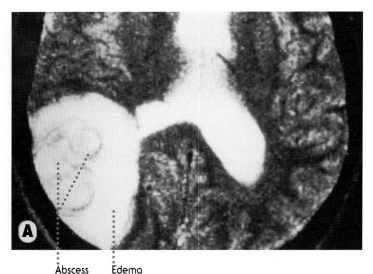

Abscess   Edema

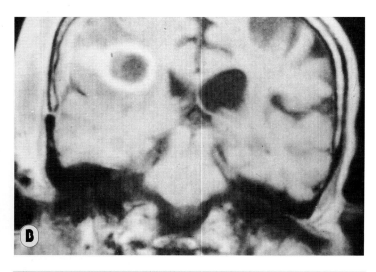

Fig. 1.93 GRAM NEGATIVE ABSCESS **(A)** T2-weighted axial image. In the posterior aspect of the right temporal lobe, there is a well-defined cortically based lesion surrounded by vasogenic edema. **(B)** T1-weighted coronal image, contrast enhanced. Following infusion of gadolinium-DTPA, the abscess wall is enhanced and the low intensity necrotic center is highlighted as an area of reduced signal. (Courtesy of Dr. W. Dillon, University of California, San Francisco)

abscess wall. By 2 to 3 weeks the process has usually evolved into a mature abscess consisting of a necrotic center, a fibrous wall, and surrounding edema. On MRI the fluid center is hypointense on the T1-weighted images and hyperintense on T2-weighted; the wall is a low signal rim; and the edematous surrounding brain is hyperintense on T2-weighted images. The rim enhances with contrast (Fig. 1.93).

Aspergillus, Candida and *Cryptococcus* are the three important fungal infections to consider because of their relatively high clinical incidence. For the most part they are indistinguishable from each other and from bacterial infections, except that they may occasionally develop a well-defined capsule. *Cryptococcus* is unique in its predilection to involve ependymal and meningeal surfaces, often accompanied by hydrocephalus.

There are two notable cerebral parasitic infestations, toxoplasmosis and cysticercosis. *Toxoplasma gondii* is now the commonest parasitic infection of the brain. In adults its incidence is virtually confined to the immunocompromised host. It can cause diffuse encephalitis or localized abscesses. The morphology of the individual toxoplasma abscess is indistinguishable from bacterial abscesses but toxoplasmosis has some characteristic features in its tendency to multiplicity, and a predilection for the basal ganglia (Fig. 1.94).

Cysticercosis is caused by the pork tapeworm. The central nervous system is the most common site of extraintestinal involvement, with the parasite lodging in one or more sites, including the choroid plexus, the basal cisterns, and the brain substance. The classic parenchymal lesions are cysts with well-defined walls, and a scolex attached to one wall (Fig. 1.95). The cyst fluid is identical to CSF intensity and the cyst's wall is very thin, making it difficult to visualize. As a result, cysts in the cisterns and ventricles are usually evident only indirectly, either as hydrocephalus or by local displacement of normal brain structures. Multiplicity in all forms of the disease is common (Fig. 1.96).

Herpes simplex is the most important cause of viral encephalitis. The radiology is characteristic and early treatment is effective. The CT scan is usually normal during the initial stage of herpes simplex encephalitis. MRI appears to be the most sensitive imaging means by which to establish an early diagnosis and determine the anatomic location of the lesion. The latter is particularly important if biopsy confirmation is contemplated. The MRI appearance of early herpes simplex encephalitis is that of a predominantly cortical temporal lobe lesion with selective gray matter

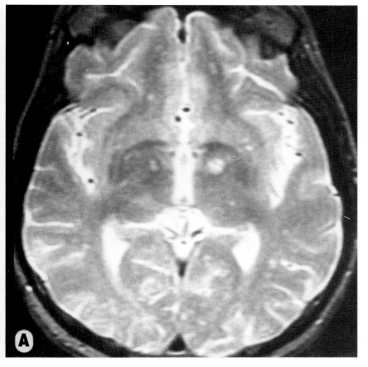

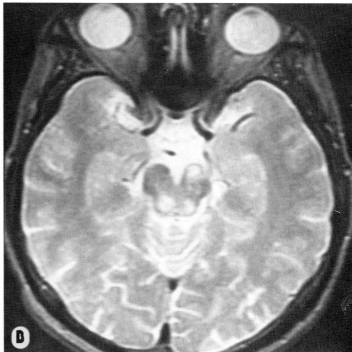

Fig. 1.94 TOXOPLASMOSIS T2-weighted axial images. These images through the basal ganglia **(A)** and midbrain **(B)** demonstrate multiple bilateral high intensity lesions. The patient had acquired immune deficiency syndrome.

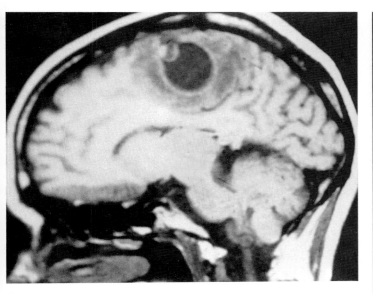

Fig. 1.95 NEUROCYSTICERCOSIS T1-weighted sagittal image. There is a large cyst in the cerebral hemisphere. The scolex of the pork tapeworm forms a bilobed nodule on the cyst's anterosuperior wall. Visualization of a scolex within a cyst is pathognomonic of cysticercosis.

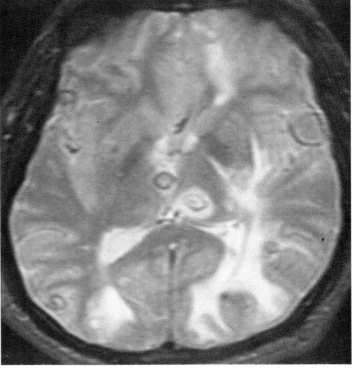

Fig. 1.96 NEUROCYSTICERCOSIS T2-weighted axial image. Both cerebral hemispheres are occupied by multiple well-defined lesions, some surrounded by edema, many circumscribed by black rings. While not pathognomonic of cysticercosis, this appearance is highly suggestive.

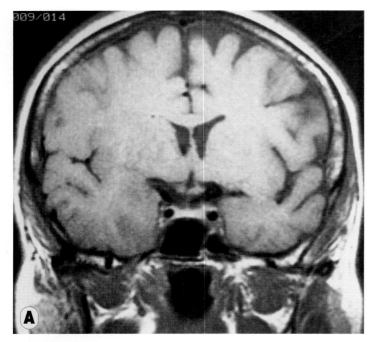

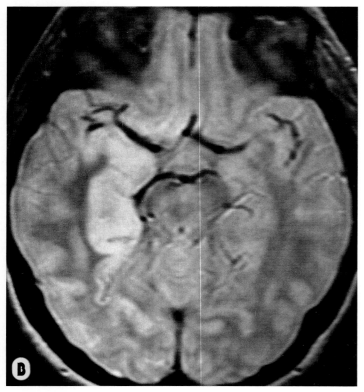

Fig. 1.97 HERPES SIMPLEX ENCEPHALITIS **(A)** T1-weighted coronal image. The cortex of the right temporal lobe is edematous and swollen on its inferior and medial aspects. **(B)** T2-weighted axial image. There is striking high intensity in the medial temporal lobe cortex, on the right, with sparing of the temporal lobe white matter.

involvement and sparing of underlying white matter. Magnetic resonance imaging shows the gray matter mantle to be thickened and edematous (Fig. 1.97); CT is usually normal at this stage. Later there is spread to the subcortical white matter, and occasionally progression to bilateral lesions and to hemorrhage.

Unusual manifestations of viral brain infections include atrophy and demyelination. The slow viruses (e.g., Jakob–Creutzfeldt syndrome) typify the former. Magnetic resonance imaging shows minimal focal abnormalities, but ventricular and sulcal enlargement are profound. Progressive multifocal leukoencephalopathy (PML) is an example of the latter and is covered in the section on demyelinating disease.

MENINGITIS AND VENTRICULITIS
Any microorganism can cause inflammation of the meninges and/or ependyma. Diagnosis can be based on a clinical history of headache, fever, and neck stiffness, augmented with lumbar puncture and CSF analysis. Computed tomography or MRI may be performed prior to lumbar puncture to exclude other pathology, or during the course of the disease to assess for complications. The imaging findings are usually limited to thickening and enhancement of the meninges and, occasionally, to hydrocephalus.

EPIDURAL ABSCESS AND SUBDURAL EMPYEMA
Epidural abscesses form between the dura and the periosteum of the inner table of the skull. Because these two tissue layers are tightly adherent, the extent of the abscess is usually limited. Subdural empyemas, on the other hand, occur in the potential space deep to the dura and are usually much more extensive. Both conditions are rare. The most common predisposing causes are paranasal sinusitis, trauma, and surgery.

The findings in the two are quite different. Extradural abscesses are usually obvious. They are adjacent to an infected sinus or mastoid process and are biconvex in shape. Subdural empyemas are spread out over the surface of the brain, often interhemispheric, and are more difficult to see. In both epidural and subdural infections, the purulent material is brighter than CSF on the T1-weighted images. They may be darker or brighter than CSF on the T2-weighted image, depending on the degree of T2-weighting.

TRAUMA

Head injury may result in focal or diffuse injury to the brain. Focal lesions include extraaxial hematomas, frank intraparenchymal hematomas, and parenchymal contusions. Diffuse injuries are the result of widespread shearing of the brain substance and are grouped together under "diffuse axonal injuries." Secondary complications also occur following head trauma and are caused primarily by compartmental shifts induced by space occupying hematomas or brain edema. For example, transtentorial herniation of the uncus can result in compression of the posterior cerebral artery and lead to infarction of the occipital lobe, or diffuse cerebral edema may reduce cerebral perfusion pressure and cause generalized hypoxic damage.

Magnetic resonance imaging has limited utility in the management of acute head injuries for many reasons. Most importantly, the acute head injury is difficult to manage in the MR environment, the strong magnetic field precluding the introduction of many life-support paraphernalia into the imaging room and the restricted space of the magnet bore limiting accessibility to the patient. Furthermore, the modality is relatively slow and the images less sensitive than CT in the detection of hemorrhage.

Conversely, CT plays a central role in these patients, providing an expeditious and accurate means of diagnosing most of the sequelae of head injury, in particular intra- and extraaxial hematomas. Computerized tomography can also detect cortical contusion and diffuse axonal injuries, but is less sensitive in detecting extent and severity of the latter lesions. Magnetic resonance imaging, however, is more sensitive in the diagnosis of cortical contusion and axonal injury, but, because these lesions do not significantly affect acute patient management, MRI is best deferred past the acute stage. Following the acute phase, MRI is useful in staging the extent and the severity of the injuries, thereby aiding in formulating the prognosis for the patient.

The MRI signal characteristics of hemorrhage at different stages of evolution have already been discussed; however, it is important to review the morphology of traumatic lesions. **Epidural hematomas** are typically in the temporal or frontal regions and underlie a skull fracture that has lacerated a meningeal artery. The hydrostatic force of the extravasating blood strips the tightly adherent dura from the skull, resulting in a localized collection, typically biconvex in shape.

Subdural hematomas are not confined by a tightly adherent dura and spread freely in the potential space between the dura and arachnoid. On cross-sectional images they have a concave inner margin, which conforms to the shape of the brain surface, and may over time become convex (Fig. 1.98).

Traumatic **subarachnoid hemorrhage** is difficult to detect by MRI. It is extremely common but usually minimal in degree and plays a small role in the management of the patient.

Intraparenchymal hematomas are discrete collections of frank blood in the brain and are distinguished from contusions, which are characterized by petechial bleeding dispersed finely into the neural tissue. In head trauma, several types of these injuries may coexist.

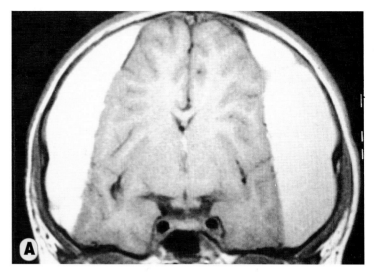

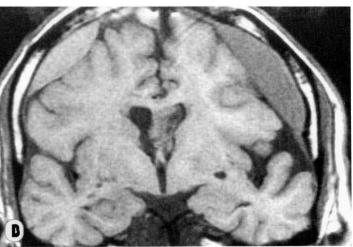

Fig. 1.98 BILATERAL SUBACUTE AND CHRONIC SUBDURAL HEMATOMAS (A) T1-weighted coronal image. These subacute hematomas are uniformly hyperintense bilaterally. Their outlines are characterized by a convex external margin and a concave internal margin. The intensity and shape are typical of subacute (1–4 weeks) subdural hematomas. (B) T1-weighted coronal image. There are moderately large bilateral subdural hematomas. In contrast to case (A), the intensity of the hematomas is approximately equal (right) or hypointense (left) to brain, features of chronic organized hematomas. The hematomas resulted from shunting of obstructive hydrocephalus caused by an intraventricular tumor (visible in this section).

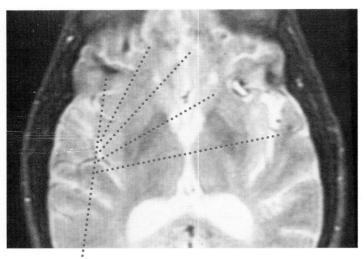

Diffuse gray-white shear injury

Fig. 1.99 DIFFUSE AXONAL INJURY T2-weighted axial image. Multiple small bifrontal lesions at the gray-white junction are predominantly characterized by hypointense rings, some with a hyperintense center. These represent shear injury at the gray-white junction. (Courtesy of Dr. W. Dillon, University of California, San Francisco)

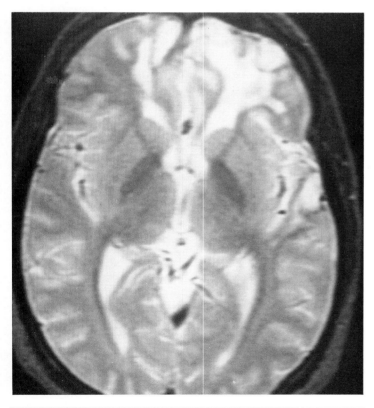

Fig. 1.100 BIFRONTAL CONTUSIONS T2-weighted axial image. Both frontal lobes have wedge-shaped lesions involving both white and gray matter. The patient had been in an automobile accident approximately four months prior to this scan. This appearance, particularly the bifrontal nature, is typical of a contusion.

Diffuse axonal injury is characterized by diffuse, multiple, small white matter and subcortical lesions, usually ovoid in shape and radially oriented (Fig. 1.99). Small central areas of hemorrhage are occasionally seen within individual lesions. The lobar subcortical white matter, the corpus callosum and the brainstem are most often affected. The gray matter is spared.

Contusions are primarily lesions of the gray matter and, like diffuse axonal injuries, tend to be multiple. If the surface of the brain is disrupted they are more properly termed lacerations. Contusions are most frequent in the frontal and temporal lobes, and most commonly involve the crown of a gyrus (Fig. 1.100).

T1- and T2-weighted sequences should be performed in the evaluation of every traumatized patient. The T2-weighted images are the most sensitive technique for detection of traumatic lesions in general, and the T1-weighted process aids in determination of the presence or absence of hemorrhage. It is also advisable to obtain images in at least two planes, to avoid partial averaging effects at the various surfaces of the brain. The coronal image is particularly useful in determining compartmental shifts, such as subfalcine herniation of the cingulate gyrus or transtentorial herniation of the uncus.

WHITE MATTER DISEASE

Diseases of the white matter are classified as **de**myelinating (myeloclastic) or **dys**myelinating. Demyelinating diseases are characterized by destruction of normal myelin; dysmyelinating disorders by abnormally formed myelin or myelin that cannot be maintained in its normal state due to some enzymatic or metabolic defect.

DEMYELINATING DISEASE
Demyelinating diseases are characterized pathologically by destruction of myelin sheaths accompanied by an inflammatory response in the surrounding neural tissue. Three major types can be identified on the basis of clinical findings and pathology: (1) multiple sclerosis, (2) acute disseminated encephalomyelitis, and (3) acute necrotizing hemorrhagic encephalomyelitis. Demyelination also occurs following toxic, infectious, or ischemic insults.

MULTIPLE SCLEROSIS Multiple sclerosis (MS) is by far the commonest demyelinating disease encountered in clinical practice. Although the etiology is unknown, there is a definite geographic, racial, and age distribution of the disease. It is commonest in young adult Caucasians in temperate climates, and is rare in non-Caucasian races and in the tropics.

Multiple sclerosis can affect any part of the central nervous system. The histopathology of affected areas in the acute stages of the disease is characterized by selective destruction of myelin sheaths (sparing the underlying axons) and perivenous inflammation. Later in the course of the disease gliosis predominates. Clinically, the initial presentations most frequently consist of visual loss, diplopia, and paresis or paresthesia, but virtually any neurologic deficit, alone or in combination, is possible. The course of the disease is characterized by unpredictable relapses and remissions. Indeed, definitive diagnosis requires documenting two temporally and anatomically distinct lesions. Magnetic resonance imaging is an excellent diagnostic aid, particularly early in the course of the disease and in atypical clinical presentations when evidence of two or more lesions is lacking. Demonstration of the typical plaques, in conjunction with the appropriate clinical or laboratory findings, supports the diagnosis. The MRI findings alone, however, should never be considered diagnostic.

Magnetic resonance imaging is a very sensitive indicator of the presence of MS, showing typical lesions in over 90 percent of definite cases. This compares with less than 50 percent for CT and 60 to 80 percent for evoked potentials and CSF oligoclonal banding. The most sensitive MRI technique is a long TR spin-echo sequence with early and late echoes (e.g., TR = 2500 msec, TE = 40 and 80 msec), yielding proton density and T2-weighted images, respectively.

The former displays the high intensity periventricular plaques with the highest degree of contrast relative to adjacent CSF in the ventricles; the latter is best for deep white matter plaques and remains the most sensitive means of detecting MS lesions.

The plaques vary in size from less than 1 mm to several centimeters. They may be distinct isolated lesions or they may be confluent. Typically they are multiple and bilateral with periventricular distribution. Half occur adjacent to the lateral ventricles, particularly near the trigones; the remainder occur in the centrum semiovale, the internal capsules, the corpus callosum, brainstem, and cerebellar hemispheres (Fig. 1.101). In general, the presence, number, and location of the MRI-visible plaques correlates poorly with the clinical localization of the lesions and the severity of the disease. This is particularly true of the periventricular lesions.

Dating lesions is difficult. Both new and old lesions appear similar on spin-echo MRI. On contrast-enhanced MRI, new lesions are more likely to enhance than old lesions (Fig. 1.102). Successive examinations may reveal decrease in lesion size dur-

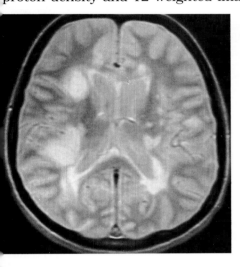
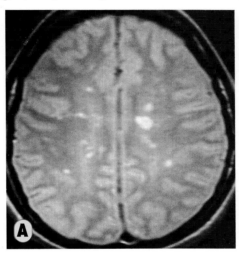
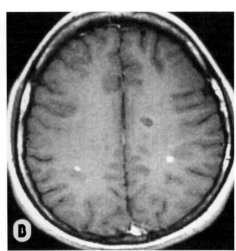

Fig. 1.101 MULTIPLE SCLEROSIS Proton density axial image. There are multiple bilateral plaques in the deep white matter and in the periventricular areas. They vary in size from 2 mm to 3 cm, some confluent with one another.

Fig. 1.102 MULTIPLE SCLEROSIS (A) T2-weighted axial image. These multiple bilateral lesions of various sizes typify multiple sclerosis. **(B)** T1-weighted axial image, contrast-enhanced. Only two of the lesions demonstrated on the T2-weighted image enhance with gadolinium-DTPA. These are presumed to be the most recent lesions with an active disruption of the blood-brain barrier. The largest lesion, quite hypointense on the T1-weighted image, is thought to represent an area of cystic gliosis and indicate an old lesion. It is important to note that the noncontrast enhanced T2-weighted image demonstrates the most lesions.

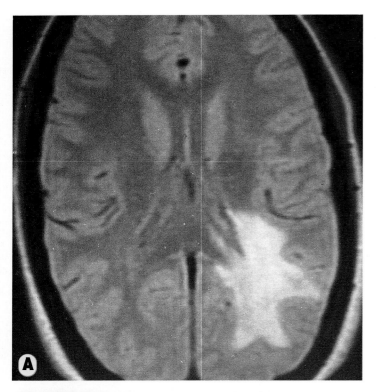

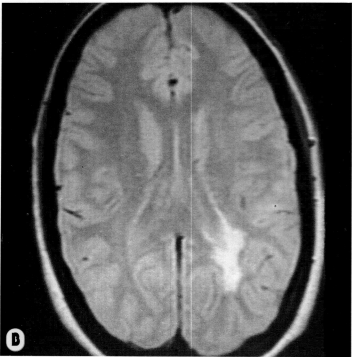

Fig. 1.103 SOLITARY MULTIPLE SCLEROSIS PLAQUE
(A) Proton density axial image. This patient presented with a partial visual field defect. The MRI demonstrates a large lesion around the atrium of the left lateral ventricle. The differential diagnosis was between tumor and demyelination. No treatment was given and no biopsy was performed. **(B)** Proton density axial image (3-month follow-up). The lesion is markedly smaller. The spontaneous involution is typical of multiple sclerosis and rules out a diagnosis of neoplasm.

ing clinical remission, and appearance of new lesions with subsequent exacerbations (Fig. 1.103). In severe or longstanding disease, cerebral atrophy becomes apparent.

The major difficulty in differential diagnosis is distinguishing demyelination from other small white matter lesions, particularly perivascular spaces and small infarcts. Perivascular spaces have a fairly distinctive distribution and appearance. Small white matter infarcts are more problematic, as both the distribution and appearance of the individual lesions overlap considerably with MS. Multiple sclerosis plaques are on average larger, but considerable overlap exists and differential diagnosis may be impossible, especially in the elderly.

ACUTE DISSEMINATED ENCEPHALOMYELITIS
Acute disseminated encephalomyelitis (ADE) is a clinicopathologic term that refers to a monophasic illness pathologically characterized by demyelination with perivascular inflammation. The lesions are multifocal and bilateral, and tend to be asymmetric. The disease usually follows an acute viral illness, especially measles, or vaccination. It is probably a hypersensitivity response. The patient may be only minimally and transiently affected, or the illness may be severe, resulting in permanent neurologic impairment or death. Magnetic resonance imaging demonstrates multifocal or confluent white matter lesions identical to those of MS. The main differentiating feature is that the illness does not remit and relapse.

ACUTE NECROTIZING HEMORRHAGIC ENCEPHALOMYELITIS   This is a catastrophic illness that usually occurs a few days after an upper respiratory tract infection. There is massive necrosis of brain tissue with multiple small hemorrhages. Onset is sudden and progression to death is rapid. The MRI resembles that of extensive MS or ADE; some of the plaques may have visible areas of necrosis or hemorrhage.

OTHER DEMYELINATING DISORDERS   Therapeutic doses of cranial irradiation produce a variety of abnormalities in the brain; however, the effects of irradiation are observed on MRI only after the cumulative dose to the brain exceeds 4000 rads. Furthermore, there is usually a 6- to 9-month delay between treatment and observed effect. The effect of radiation on the brain parenchyma is indirect. The primary change is in the media of small and medium-sized arteries, which undergo hyaline proliferation and thereby partially occlude the vascular lumen. The parenchyma then undergoes anoxic demyelination. The individual radiation-induced lesions are hyperintense on T2-weighted images and are indistinguishable from other demyelinating lesions. The distribution of involvement takes one of three forms: periventricular, multifocal, or geographic (Fig. 1.104). The geographic form, with sharp borders paralleling that of the radiation ports, is the most distinctive type of radiation-induced demyelination (Fig. 1.105).

Intrathecal methotrexate therapy, especially when administered in conjunction with cranial radiation, can cause widespread demyelination or a disseminated necrotizing leukoencephalopathy. Clinically there is a progressive, profound neurologic deficit. Magnetic resonance imaging shows diffuse white matter hyperintensity on T2-weighted images, particularly around the ventricles, with sparing of the gray matter (Fig. 1.106). This appearance is not specific for methotrexate/radiation leukoencephalopathy, and is often seen in other demyelinating disorders as well as in several leukodystrophies.

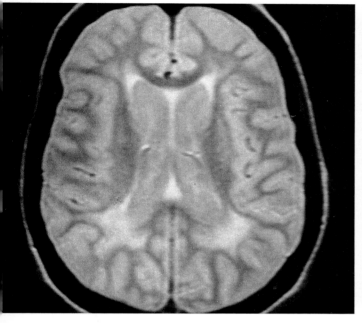

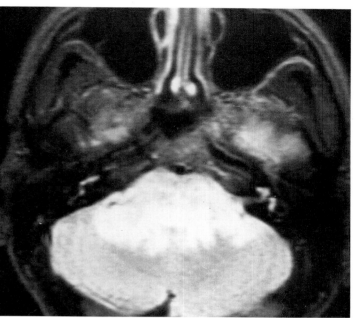

Fig. 1.104 RADIATION-INDUCED DEMYELINATION Proton density axial image. This patient had received whole head radiation for treatment of an intracerebral tumor (not shown). There are bilaterally symmetric high intensity lesions adjacent to the atria and frontal horns of both ventricles.

Fig. 1.105 RADIATION-INDUCED DEMYELINATION T2-weighted axial image. A large high intensity lesion occupies the entire pons and anterior halves of the middle cerebellar peduncles bilaterally. The striking feature is the relatively straight posterior border of this lesion. This patient had received localized radiation to the thalamus and upper brainstem for a thalamic glioma.

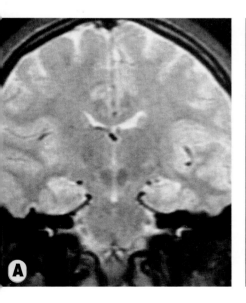

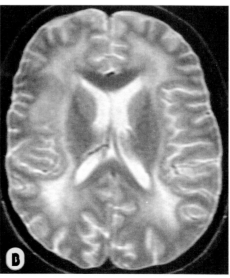

Fig. 1.106 COMBINED RADIATION/METHOTREXATE LEUKOENCEPHALOPATHY (A) T2-weighted coronal image. This patient had acute lymphocytic leukemia. This baseline MRI was performed prior to the initiation of chemotherapy to exclude the possibility of intracerebral disease. The scan is normal. **(B)** T2-weighted axial image. This 6-month follow-up demonstrates marked bilateral demyelination throughout the white matter.

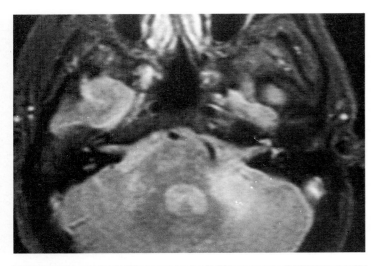

Fig. 1.107 PROGRESSIVE MULTIFOCAL LEUKOEN-CEPHALOPATHY T2-weighted axial image. This HIV-positive patient has a high-intensity lesion in the left middle cerebellar peduncle, as well as several smaller lesions in the opposite peduncle and the pons. The differential diagnosis is among lymphoma, PML and opportunistic infection. There are no consistent distinguishing features between these lesions, although multiplicity favors toxoplasmosis.

Modifications in intrathecal methotrexate therapy were introduced in response to this complication, and the incidence of methotrexate leukoencephalopathy has decreased significantly since the late 1970s.

Progressive multifocal leukoencephalopathy (PML) is another unusual demyelinating illness. It is caused by papovavirus infection. It occurs in immunocompromised individuals, in particular, in patients with disseminated malignancies or acquired immune deficiency syndrome, and following organ transplantation. Brain biopsy demonstrates multiple areas of demyelination, with minimal perivascular infiltration (in contrast to MS) and distinctive intranuclear inclusions in the oligodendroglia. The oligodendroglia are damaged by the virus and rendered incapable of maintaining the myelin sheath. The lesions progress steadily, with death in several months. On MRI, single or multiple intraparenchymal lesions are evident on T2-weighted images as regions of hyperintensity (Fig. 1.107). Most lesions are supratentorial, although infratentorial lesions are becoming more frequently identified.

Central pontine myelinolysis (CPM) and Marchiafava–Bignami syndrome (MBS) are two rare focal forms of demyelination that are seen predominantly in alcoholics, although neither may actually be due to the direct effects of alcohol. Central pontine myelinolysis is defined by the presence of a central pontine lesion (Fig. 1.108), but the basal ganglia and

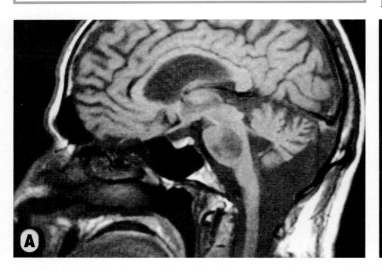

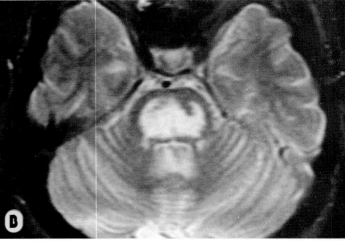

Fig. 1.108 CENTRAL PONTINE MYELINOLYSIS **(A)** T1-weighted sagittal image. There is a well-defined low-intensity lesion in the central pons. This patient became symptomatic during correction of hyponatremia. **(B)** T2-weighted axial image. Most of the pons is affected. Smaller lesions were present in the thalami bilaterally (not shown).

thalamus may also be affected. Patients are profoundly ill and their prognosis is dismal. Most are hyponatremic at presentation; the pontine lesion usually becomes apparent as the electrolyte disturbance is corrected.

Marchiafava–Bignami is characterized by a region of demyelination in the body of the corpus callosum. Italian red wine drinkers are the group principally affected. The intrinsic characteristics of the individual CPM and MBS lesions are identical to those of MS. The most useful differential diagnostic features are the clinical history and the site of the abnormality.

DYSMYELINATING DISEASES (LEUKODYSTROPHIES)

The leukodystrophies are predominantly diseases of infancy and childhood, but, in some cases, the onset of the illness is as late as early adulthood. Differential diagnosis between the various leukodystrophies is primarily by clinical and laboratory means. There is little to distinguish between them on MRI. In most leukodystrophies, and some demyelinating disorders, MRI demonstrates diffuse bilateral white matter abnormalities as regions of hyperintensity on T2-weighted images (Fig. 1.109). A few leukodystrophies are known to have distinctive features. For example, in Alexander's and Canavan's diseases, there is brain enlargement in addition to the white matter lesions. In adrenoleukodystrophy, the lesions are striking in their preferential distribution to the visual and auditory pathways. The other leukodystrophies have few, if any, distinctive features.

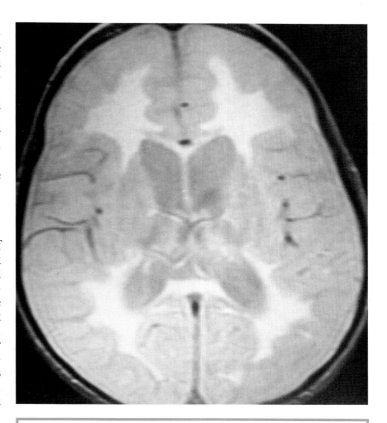

Fig. 1.109 METACHROMATIC LEUKODYSTROPHY Proton density axial image. The scan demonstrates bilateral symmetric involvement of the deep white matter.

NEUROECTODERMAL SYNDROMES (PHAKOMATOSES)

The phakomatoses are a group of genetically determined diseases in which distinctive central nervous system lesions are associated with lesions of the skin or eye, and with tumors elsewhere in the body. The commonest syndromes are tuberous sclerosis, Sturge–Weber disease, neurofibromatosis, and von Hippel–Lindau disease. Any of these may occur sporadically with no antecedent family history, but tuberous sclerosis, neurofibromatosis, and von Hippel–Lindau disease also have well-established Mendelian dominant patterns of inheritance.

TUBEROUS SCLEROSIS (BOURNEVILLE'S DISEASE)

The majority of cases of tuberous sclerosis are sporadic; in others it is inherited as an autosomal dominant. Incomplete expressions of the syndrome are common, in particular by periventricular hamartomas. Whether these represent "formes frustes" of tuberous sclerosis is questionable. The classic clinical syndrome consists of epilepsy, mental retardation, and subungual fibromas. The central nervous system lesions consist of hamartomas (tubers) in the cortex, subependymal region, and in the deep white matter. There is a definite predisposition for giant cell astrocytomas to arise from these nodules, particularly in the subependymal areas.

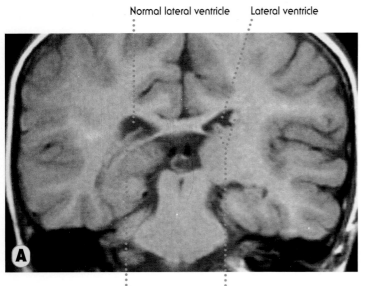

Normal lateral ventricle   Lateral ventricle

Choroid plexus   Subependymal tubers

Subependymal tubers   Cortical tubers

Fig. 1.110 TUBEROUS SCLEROSIS **(A)** T1-weighted coronal image. Two small nodules, subependymal tubers, protrude into the left lateral ventricle and are approximately equal in signal intensity to the white matter. **(B)** Proton density axial image. Multiple periventricular tubers are evident, as well as several cortical and subcortical abnormalities. Subcortical lesions are characterized by distortion of the gyral architecture and high intensity "U's" deep to these gyri. This appearance is relatively specific for cortical hamartomas.

The lesions of tuberous sclerosis are readily evident on MRI. The subependymal lesions, best seen on T1-weighted images, are small nodular projections into the ventricles. They have the same intensity as gray matter on both T1- and T2-weighted images (Fig. 1.110). Interval enlargement of any of these are suggestive of degeneration into a giant cell astrocytoma. The cortical tubers are most evident on T2-weighted images as moderately hyperintense lesions in the cortex and subcortical white matter representing convolutional foci of sclerosis (see Fig. 1.110). These subcortical lesions show little tendency to undergo neoplastic transformation. The deep glial nodules are uncommon. Of note is that on CT the subependymal nodules are frequently calcified. The calcification is generally not visible on MRI.

NEUROFIBROMATOSIS (VON RECKLINGHAUSEN'S DISEASE)

There are two relatively distinct variants of this disease: peripheral neurofibromatosis (type I) and central neurofibromatosis (type II). In type I neurofibromatosis (von Recklinghausen's disease), patients have optic nerve gliomas, cerebral gliomas and hamartomas, extracranial neurofibromas, and cutaneous pigmentation (café-au-lait spots). Type II neurofibromatosis (central neurofibromatosis) consists of cranial nerve schwannomas and meningiomas, and spinal neurofibromas: there are few, if any, cutaneous manifestations. The presence of bilateral acoustic neurinomas is specific for the diagnosis of central neurofibromatosis.

Central nervous system tumors are frequently multiple in both variants. The meningiomas and parenchymal gliomas found in neurofibromatosis are not distinctive in any way from those occurring sporadically in the "normal" population. Schwannomas may affect any cranial nerve, but most commonly nerves V and VIII are involved. These cranial nerve tumors are best analyzed on T1-weighted images, which provide the highest contrast between the enlarged nerve and surrounding CSF. The optimal plane of section depends on the specific nerve involved. Coronal or axial sections are optimal for acoustic tumors; a combination of coronal and oblique sagittal images (along the long axis of the optic nerve) are preferred for optic gliomas.

Atypical glial rests and malformative lesions (hamartomas) are not evident on CT. Thus, prior to the advent of MRI, they were generally appreciated only at pathology. With MRI, these lesions are discovered in one quarter to one third of patients with von Recklinghausen's disease. They are unusual in appearance, seen only on T2-weighted images. They are visible as hyperintense areas without mass effect and may be in any area of the brain, but are particularly frequent in the basal ganglia or brainstem, optic radiations or cerebellum, and in the posterior fossa (Fig. 1.111). Most are asymptomatic. Unfortunately, these hamartomas cannot readily be discerned from gliomas. Interval follow-up examination is valuable, since hamartomas do not enlarge and gliomas typically do, although slowly in some cases.

ENCEPHALOTRIGEMINAL ANGIOMATOSIS (STURGE–WEBER SYNDROME)

Sturge–Weber syndrome consists of a meningeal venous malformation, cerebral cortical calcification, and an angioma of the face. The meningeal vascular malformation cannot be detected on CT or MRI because of the small size of the vessels involved and the lack of significant arteriovenous shunting. Characteristic calcification in the underlying cortex is best appreciated on CT and, indeed, is often visible on plain radiographs of the skull. The cortical calcification is difficult to visualize on MRI, but close inspection will reveal a gyriform ribbon of reduced signal intensity within the cortex (Fig. 1.112). There is a reported association of angiomas of the choroid plexus on the involved side. These cause enlargement and high signal intensity in the involved choroid plexus.

VON HIPPEL–LINDAU DISEASE

The central nervous system manifestations of von Hippel–Lindau disease are frequently multiple hemangioblastomas of the cerebellum and spinal cord, and angiomas of the retina. Nonneurologic manifestations of the disease include cysts in multiple abdominal organs (liver, pancreas, kidney), renal cell carcinoma, and pheochromocytoma.

The cerebellar tumors are relatively distinctive in appearance, consisting of a small nodule projecting into a relatively large cyst. With contrast administration the nodule and the cyst wall enhance intensely (see Figs. 1.69, 1.77, 1.78). Large vessels are often visualized in or adjacent to the tumor. In some cases, the cystic component is absent. The eye should always be closely inspected if a hemangioblastoma is detected in the cerebellum. A retinal angioma in someone with a hemangioblastoma establishes the diagnosis of von Hippel-Lindau disease, as does the occurrence of multiple hemangioblastomas.

HYDROCEPHALUS

Hydrocephalus is defined as a net accumulation of CSF in the ventricles due to an excess of CSF production relative to CSF absorption. Hydrocephalus must be distinguished from atrophy, wherein there is enlargement of intracranial CSF spaces secondary to a loss of brain substance. In hydrocephalus, the ventricles are enlarged but the sulci remain normal or become flattened. In atrophic ventriculomegaly, all of the CSF spaces are enlarged. In practice this distinction is not always clear, particularly in the elderly who may develop slowly progressive hydrocephalus on a background of atrophic ventricular and sulcal enlargement.

Almost all cases of hydrocephalus are due to a pathological obstruction of the CSF circulatory pathway. In this sense all hydrocephalus is "obstructive," with one notable exception, that being the choroid plexus papilloma. For diagnostic purposes, it is useful to classify hydrocephalus into two major types: communicating and noncommunicating.

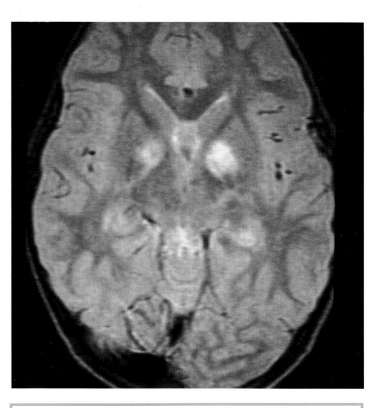

Fig. 1.111 NEUROFIBROMATOSIS, HAMARTOMAS T2-weighted axial image. There are bilateral lesions of high signal intensity in the globus pallidus. The lesion on the left is larger. They are thought to represent hamartomas or atypical glial cell rests and generally are not evident on CT.

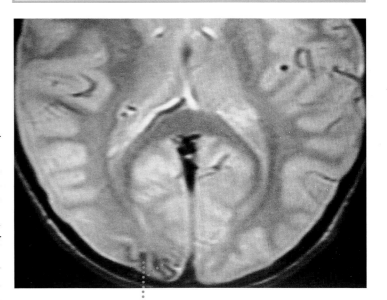

Calcification in cortex

Fig. 1.112 STURGE–WEBER DISEASE T2-weighted axial image. There is a gyriform ribbon of low signal intensity in the right occipital cortex with slight enlargement of the overlying sulci. The low signal intensity represents calcification in the brain underlying a small venous angioma.

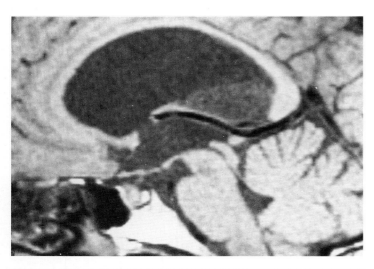

Fig. 1.113 AQUEDUCT STENOSIS T1-weighted sagittal image. There is marked narrowing of the distal cerebral aqueduct and dilatation of the lateral ventricle, third ventricle and proximal aqueduct. MRI localizes the lesion responsible for the hydrocephalus by demonstrating the transition point from dilated to nondilated CSF pathway. Of importance is that no tumor can be identified at the point of obstruction.

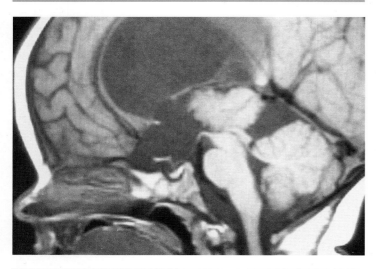

Fig. 1.114 PINEAL GERMINOMA WITH OBSTRUCTIVE HYDROCEPHALUS T1-weighted sagittal image. A large pineal region tumor is compressing the tectum of the midbrain and the aqueduct. The lateral and third ventricles are dilated; the fourth ventricle and the cerebral aqueduct remain normal size. In this case MRI demonstrates both the site and cause of obstruction.

Noncommunicating hydrocephalus is caused by lesions that obstruct the CSF pathway within the ventricular system, thereby interrupting the normal egress of CSF from the ventricles to the subarachnoid space. This is also referred to as intraventricular obstructive hydrocephalus (IVOH). In communicating hydrocephalus, the obstruction is outside the ventricles (i.e., within the subarachnoid space), hence its alternate designation as extraventricular obstructive hydrocephalus (EVOH). In communicating hydrocephalus, CSF may leave the ventricles freely but either cannot reach the sites of absorption at the arachnoid villi, or cannot be normally absorbed at the arachnoid villi.

In general, in communicating hydrocephalus all ventricles dilate, although the fourth ventricle may not dilate to the same extent as the lateral and third ventricles because of the relatively confined space of the posterior fossa. In noncommunicating hydrocephalus, the ventricular system dilates only proximal to the obstruction. Obstructive lesions at the inferior fourth ventricle cause dilatation of the entire ventricular system and, thus, it may be impossible to distinguish communicating hydrocephalus from that caused by a lesion at the outlet of the fourth ventricle. Choroid plexus papillomas may also cause a pattern of ventricular enlargement identical to that seen in communicating hydrocephalus. Choroid plexus papillomas actively secrete fluid into the ventricular system and are the one cause of hydrocephalus that is due to overproduction rather than obstruction of CSF circulation. This is uncommon.

In general, a T1-weighted midline sagittal image is ideal for determining the specific site of obstruction, usually evident as the transitional point between a proximally dilated and a distally normal ventricular system (Figs. 1.113 and 1.114). To elucidate the nature of the obstructing lesion, the sagittal image is supplemented by axial or coronal sections (either T1- or T2-weighted) through the obstruction to provide images as greatly detailed as possible (Fig. 1.114). Subarachnoid hemorrhage and meningitis are the most frequent overall causes of hydrocephalus, and they can cause obstruction of the system at any and multiple sites by debris or postinflammatory adhesions. Here MRI will clearly demonstrate the hydrocephalic pattern of ventricular dilatation, but, notably, no obstructing mass will be seen. Congenital lesions causing hydrocephalus include webs across the cerebral aqueduct (benign aqueductal stenosis) and the Chiari malformation (adhesions at the outlet foramina of the fourth ventricle or occlusion of CSF space at the tentorial hiatus). In children and in adults, tumors in and adjacent to the ventricles are important causes of hydrocephalus. The specific histologic type of tumor causing the hydrocephalus varies by site. For example, colloid cysts occur in the anterior third ventricle, hypothalamic gliomas and craniopharyngiomas in the mid- and posterior third ventricles, pineal neoplasms and tectal gliomas about the aqueduct, and ependymomas and medulloblastomas in the fourth ventricle. The tumor need not be intraventricular; parenchymal neoplasms frequently compress the ventricular system or kink the aqueduct sufficiently to block CSF circulation (Fig. 1.115).

In hydrocephalus, the parenchymal abnormalities seen on MRI depend not only on the location and cause of the obstruction, but also on the rapidity with which the process takes place. If the process is acute, there is no opportunity for compensatory mechanisms to act. Typically, there is a striking accumulation of CSF around the ventricles, particularly immediately adjacent to the frontal and occipital horns. These zones of fluid accumulation, or periventricular edema, are hyperintense on proton density and T2-weighted images. They are most clearly seen on the proton density image, wherein the white periventricular edema is contrasted against the relatively low intensity ventricular CSF. This zone of hyperintensity is less marked along the remaining ventricular margin (see Fig. 1.115). This periventricular edema is quite labile, so that it resolves quickly following ventricular decompression by shunting, usually within 24 hours. In chronic forms of hydrocephalus, compensatory mechanisms have had time to act so that, even though the ventricles may be more dilated than in acute hydrocephalus, the periventricular changes are less marked. Usually they are limited to a relatively thin band of hyperintensity along the entire ventricular margin with no particular preponderance in any one zone (Fig. 1.116).

There are two specific forms of chronic hydrocephalus which warrant special discussion. These are "normal pressure hydrocephalus" and "arrested hydrocephalus."

Normal pressure hydrocephalus (NPH) is a form of chronic hydrocephalus in which CSF pressure is within the physiologic range, but a slight pressure gradient persists between the ventricles and the brain. It is due to an incomplete block of the CSF pathway, usually within the subarachnoid space. The ventricles are enlarged and the brain is damaged by sustained stretching of periventricular tissue. The ventricles may enlarge further with time.

The classical clinical triad in NPH consists of dementia, incontinence and ataxia. Both CT and MRI may show ventriculomegaly disproportionate to any sulcal enlargement that may coexist. If the ventriculomegaly can be documented to progress with time, the sequence of scans showing progressive ventricular enlargement are diagnostic of NPH. However, successive exams often do not demonstrate progressive interval enlargement, and, on a single examination, it is difficult to distinguish NPH from atrophic ventriculomegaly. Parenchymal changes around the ventricles are of little diagnostic help, as they are commonly present in asymptomatic, elderly individuals. Patients with extensive white matter lesions do poorly; this is presumably due to concurrent cere-

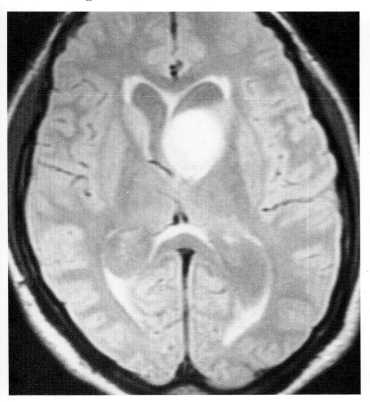

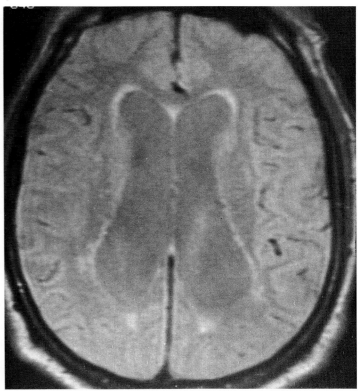

Fig. 1.115 ASTROCYTOMA WITH OBSTRUCTIVE HYDRO-CEPHALUS *Proton density axial image. A large astrocytoma, in the lateral wall of the left lateral ventricle, encroaches upon the ventricular lumen and obstructs the foramen of Monro. Localized areas of periventricular edema cap the frontal and occipital horns.*

Fig. 1.116 CHRONIC HYDROCEPHALUS *Proton density axial image. This patient has congenital benign aqueductal stenosis. There is marked dilation of the ventricles, but only a thin rim of high signal outlines the entire ventricular system, typical of the parenchymal changes in chronic forms of hydrocephalus.*

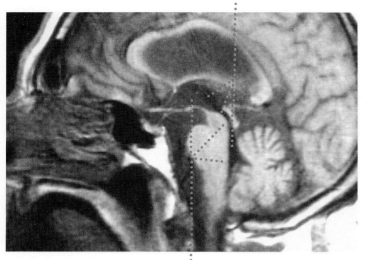

Accentuated flow void

Dilated 3rd ventricle, aqueduct
and 4th ventricle

Fig. 1.117 NORMAL PRESSURE HYDROCEPHALUS T1-weighted sagittal image. This patient presented with dementia, ataxia, and incontinence. The entire ventricular system is dilated without evidence of any obstructing lesion. There is a striking flow void in the posterior third ventricle, aqueduct and fourth ventricle, thought to be a sign of normal pressure hydrocephalus.

brovascular ischemia rather than to periventricular changes which are unreliable predictors of therapeutic outcome to shunting. There has been some speculation that analysis of CSF flow patterns will be of diagnostic value in NPH. It has been postulated that in the noncompliant brain of the NPH patient, the flow of CSF through the aqueduct goes through greater amplitude excursions than is normal, and this manifests itself as an accentuation of the flow void that is normally seen in the aqueduct. This finding, however, remains to be proven (Fig. 1.117). Notwithstanding, the diagnosis of NPH requires very close correlation between clinical findings and imaging results, with the best diagnostic test for NPH remaining a clinical improvement following ventricular shunting.

Arrested hydrocephalus is a type of chronic hydrocephalus where the CSF pressure has been restored to normal after a period of sustained elevation, and no gradient remains between the ventricles and the brain tissue. It is most commonly seen with obstructive lesions outside the ventricles, particularly in children. Examination may show that the dilated ventricles have returned to normal size, remain enlarged, or, most importantly, that there has been no further interval enlargement. The MRI appearance is similar to other forms of chronic hydrocephalus. It is the temporal sequence of sequential ventricular enlargement, followed by arrest, which is important diagnostically.

BIBLIOGRAPHY

BOOKS

Ferner H, ed. *Eduard Pernkopf atlas of topographical and applied human anatomy*, vol 1. Baltimore: Urban and Schwarzenberg, 1980.

Nieuwenhuys R, Voogd J, van Huijzen C. *The human central nervous system, a synopsis and atlas*. Berlin: Springer-Verlag, 1981.

Okazaki H. *Fundamentals of neuropathology*. New York: Igaku-Shoin, 1983.

Russell DS, Rubinstein LJ. *Pathology of tumors of the central nervous system*, 5th ed. Baltimore: Williams and Wilkins, 1989.

JOURNAL ARTICLES AND BOOK CHAPTERS

Atlas SW, Grossman RI, Goldberg HI, et al. MR diagnosis of acute disseminated encephalomyelitis. *JCAT* 1986;10:798.

Atlas SW, Grossman RI, Gomori JM, et al. Hemorrhagic intracranial malignant neoplasms: spin-echo MR imaging. *Radiology* 1987;164:71.

Atlas SW. Intracranial vascular malformations and aneurysms. Current imaging applications. *Radiol Clin North Am* 1988;26(4):821–837.

Barkovich AJ, Chuang SH, Norman D. MR of neuronal migration anomalies. *AJNR* 1987;8:1009.

Barkovich AJ, Kjos BO, Jackson DE Jr, et al. Normal maturation of the neonatal and infant brain: MR imaging at 1.5 T. *Radiology* 1986;166:173.

Barkovich AJ, Norman D. MR imaging of schizencephaly. *AJNR* 1988;9:297.

Berry I, Brant-Zawadzki M, Osaki L, et al. Gd-DTPA in clinical MR of the brain. II. Extra-axial lesions and normal structures. *AJNR* 1986;7:789–793.

Bradley WG. Flow phenomenon in MR imaging. *AJR* 1988;150:983.

Braffman BH, Zimmerman RA, Trojanowski JQ, et al. Brain MR: pathologic correlation with gross and histopathology. 1. Lacunar infarction and Virchow-Robin spaces. *AJNR* 1988;9:621.

Braffman BH, Zimmerman RA, Trojanowski JQ, et al. Brain MR: pathologic correlation with gross and histopathology. 2. Hyperintense white matter foci in the elderly. *AJNR* 1988;9:629.

Brant-Zawadzki M, Berry I, Osaki L, et al. Gd-DTPA in clinical MR of the brain. I. Intra-axial lesions. *AJNR* 1986;7:781–788.

Breger RK, Papke RA, Pojunas KW. Benign extra-axial tumors: contrast enhancement with Gd-DTPA. *Radiology* 1987;163:427.

Bydder G, Kingsley D, Brown J, et al. MR imaging of meningiomas including studies with and without gadolinium-DTPA. *J Comput Assist Tomogr* 1985;9(4):690–697.

Byrd SE, Bohan TP, Osborn RE, et al. CT and MR evaluation of lissencephaly. *AJNR* 1988;9:923.

Curnes JT, Laster DW, Ball MR, et al. Magnetic resonance imaging of radiation injury to the brain. *AJNR* 1986;7:389.

Davis PC, Friedman NC, Fry SM, et al. Leptomeningeal metastasis: MR imaging. *Radiology* 1987;163:449.

Drayer BP. Imaging of the aging brain: part I—normal findings. *Radiology* 1988;166:785.

Drayer BP. Brain infarction. In: Stark DD, Bradley WG, eds. *Diagnostic categorical course in MR imaging*. Oak Brook: Radiological Society of North America, 1988;39–52.

Dubowitz LMS, Pennock J, Johnson MA, et al. High-resolution magnetic resonance imaging of the brain in children. *Clin Radiol* 1986;37:113.

Gomori JM, Grossman RI, Goldberg H, et al. Intracranial hematomas: imaging by high-field MR. *Radiology* 1985;1157:89–93.

Gomori JM, Grossman RI, Goldberg HI, et al. Occult cerebral vascular malformations. High field MR imaging. *Radiology* 1986;158:707–713.

Gomori JM, Grossman RI. Head and neck hemorrhage. In: Kressel HY, ed. *Magnetic resonance annual*. New York: Raven Press, 1987;71–112.

Guilleux M-H, Steiner RE, Young IR. MR imaging in progressive multifocal leukoencephalopathy. *AJNR* 1986;7:1033.

Hecht-Leavitt C, Gomori JM, Grossman RI, et al. High-field MRI of hemorrhagic cortical infarction. *AJNR* 1986;7:581.

Hesselink JR, Dowd CF, Healy MR, et al. MR imaging of brain contusions: a comparative study with CT. *AJNR* 1988;9:269.

Horowitz AL, Kaplan R, Sarpel G. Carbon monoxide toxicity: MR imaging in the brain. *Radiology* 1987;162:787.

Hurst RW, Newman SA, Cail WS. Multifocal intracranial MR abnormalities in neurofibromatosis. *AJNR* 1988;9:293.

Jack CR Jr, Mokri B, Laws ER Jr, et al. MR findings in normal-pressure hydrocephalus: significance and comparison with other forms of dementia. *JCAT* 1987;11:923.

Kilgore DP, Strother CM, Starshak RJ, et al. Pineal germinoma: MR imaging. *Radiology* 1986;158:435.

Kjos B, Brant-Zawadzki M, Kucharczyk W, et al. Cystic intracranial lesions: magnetic resonance imaging. *Radiology* 1985;155:363–369.

Kucharczyk W, Lemme-Plaghos L, Uske A, et al. Intracranial vascular malformations: MR and CT imaging. *Radiology* 1985;156:383–389.

Kucharczyk W, Brant-Zawadzki M. Magnetic resonance imaging of cerebral ischemia and infarction. In: Kressel HY, ed. *Magnetic resonance annual*. New York: Raven Press, 1987;49–70.

Marshall VG, Bradley WG Jr, Marshall CE, et al. Deep white matter infarction: correlation of MR imaging and histopathologic findings. *Radiology* 1988;167:517.

McMurdo SK Jr, Moore SG, Brant-Zawadzki M, et al. MR imaging of intracranial tuberous sclerosis. *AJNR* 1987;8:77.

Post MJD, Tate LG, Quencer RM, et al. CT, MR, and pathology in HIV encephalitis and meningitis. *AJNR* 1988;9:469.

Price AC, Runge VM, Nelson KL. CNS—neoplastic disease. In: Runge VM, ed. *Enhanced magnetic resonance imaging*. St. Louis: CV Mosby, 1989;139–177.

Price AC, Runge VM, Nelson KL. CNS—nonneoplastic disease. In: Runge VM, ed. *Enhanced magnetic resonance imaging.* St. Louis: CV Mosby, 1989;178–192.

Uhlenbrock D, Seidel D, Gehlen W, et al. MR imaging in multiple sclerosis: comparison with clinical, CSF, and visual evoked potential findings. *AJNR* 1988;9:59.

von Schulthess GV, Higgin CB. Blood flow imaging with MR: spin-phase phenomena. *Radiology* 1985;157:687–695.

chapter two

the
skull base

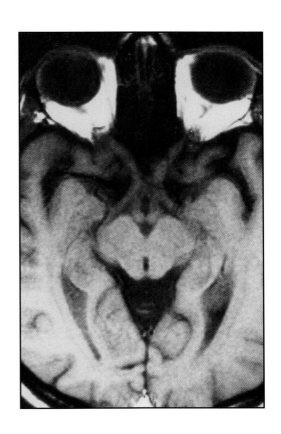

WALTER KUCHARCZYK   KEVIN LEE   E.G. BERTRAM

Normal Anatomy of the Skull Base (Fig. 2.1)

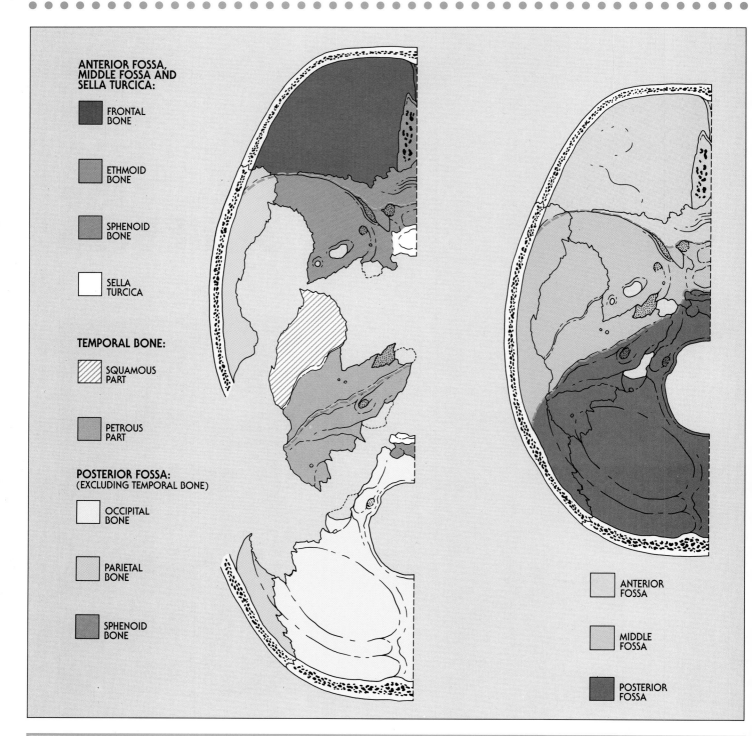

ANTERIOR FOSSA, MIDDLE FOSSA AND SELLA TURCICA:

- FRONTAL BONE
- ETHMOID BONE
- SPHENOID BONE
- SELLA TURCICA

TEMPORAL BONE:

- SQUAMOUS PART
- PETROUS PART

POSTERIOR FOSSA:
(EXCLUDING TEMPORAL BONE)

- OCCIPITAL BONE
- PARIETAL BONE
- SPHENOID BONE

- ANTERIOR FOSSA
- MIDDLE FOSSA
- POSTERIOR FOSSA

Fig. 2.1 Schematic View of the Intracranial Surface of the Skull Base The anterior fossa is formed by the frontal, ethmoid, and sphenoid bones and is separated from the middle fossa by the sphenoid ridge. The middle fossa and sella turcica, formed by the sphenoid and temporal bones, are separated from the posterior fossa by the dorsum sellae and petrous ridge. The posterior fossa is formed by the sphenoid, temporal, and occipital bones. For the purpose of discussion, the skull is separated into the three sections diagrammed. **(A)** Anterior fossa, middle fossa, and sella turcica. Most structures of interest are in the sphenoid bone: the optic canals, orbital fissures, foramina rotundum, foramina ovale, and foramina spinosum. Each contains important neural or vascular struc-

2.2   M R I : C E N T R A L N E R V O U S S Y S T E M

Normal Anatomy of the Skull Base (continued)

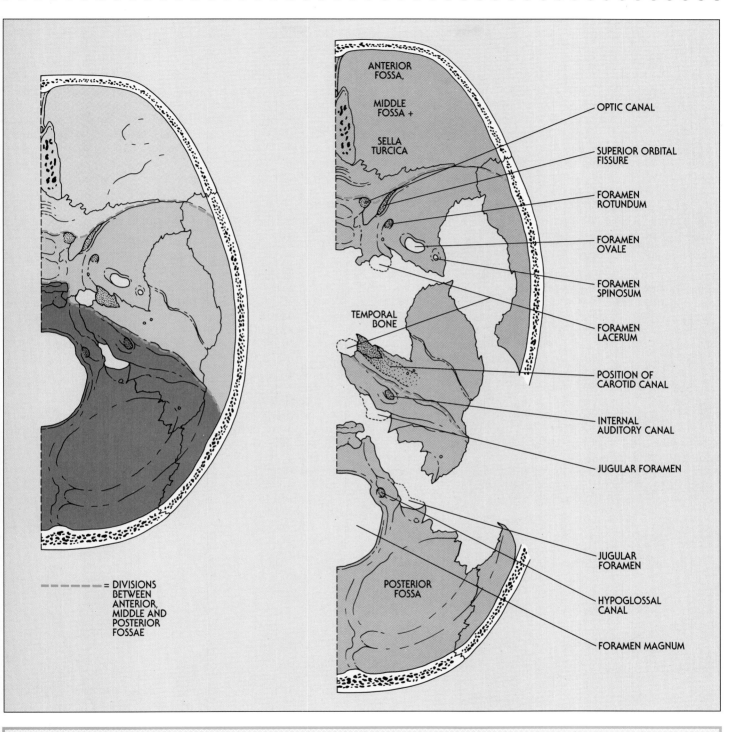

DIVISIONS BETWEEN ANTERIOR, MIDDLE AND POSTERIOR FOSSAE

ANTERIOR FOSSA,

MIDDLE FOSSA +

SELLA TURCICA

TEMPORAL BONE

POSTERIOR FOSSA

OPTIC CANAL

SUPERIOR ORBITAL FISSURE

FORAMEN ROTUNDUM

FORAMEN OVALE

FORAMEN SPINOSUM

FORAMEN LACERUM

POSITION OF CAROTID CANAL

INTERNAL AUDITORY CANAL

JUGULAR FORAMEN

JUGULAR FORAMEN

HYPOGLOSSAL CANAL

FORAMEN MAGNUM

tures. The sella turcica, also part of the sphenoid bone, contains the pituitary gland. The foramen lacerum is in the sphenotemporal suture. **(B)** Temporal bone. The temporal bone contributes to both the middle and posterior fossae. It is composed of four sections: petrous, squamous, tympanic, and mastoid. Only the petrous and squamous sections are visible intracranially. The petrous temporal bone is of greatest interest, containing the inner ear apparatus, the internal auditory canal, and the carotid canal. **(C)** Posterior fossa. The most important remaining structures of the skull base are the jugular foramen (located in the occipitotemporal suture), the hypoglossal canal, and the foramen magnum. The occipital bone forms most of the base of the posterior fossa.

INTRODUCTION

The skull base separates the brain from the face, the aerodigestive tract, and the spine. It is a complex structure that can be divided into several anatomical regions, including the sella turcica, the temporal bone, and three paired cranial fossae (anterior, middle, and posterior). The diagnosis of skull base disease requires a thorough understanding of the normal anatomy of these regions, because lesions at the skull base are often subtle—more so than in the brain, where lesions are often evident by gross abnormalities of signal. They are as much characterized by slight distortions or aberrations in the size, shape, or position of a normal structure as by abnormal signal intensity. It is, therefore, vital to recognize the normal relationships of structures at the skull base.

NORMAL ANATOMY
(Fig. 2.1)

The anatomy of the skull base is discussed in three sections. The **sella turcica** and **parasellar region** incorporates the *sella turcica*, the *cavernous sinus*, and the *suprasellar cistern*. The anterior and middle cranial fossae are included in this section because of their close anatomic relationships to the parasellar region. The **temporal bone** includes the internal auditory canal. The **posterior fossa** includes the clivus, foramen magnum, the jugular foramen, and the lower cranial nerves, but excludes the brainstem and cerebellum, which have been previously discussed in Chapter 1.

TECHNIQUE

The technique for examination of the skull base varies according to the specific region being examined; however, certain generalizations are valid. Sagittal T1-weighted images are the initial images obtained, followed by images in the coronal plane (either T1- or T2-weighted, or both). Coronal images are the mainstays of diagnosis; they provide a means of assessing bilateral symmetry and a view perpendicular to the skull base. Axial images are occasionally useful, particularly for evaluating the contents of the internal auditory canal. The field of view, slice thickness, and matrix size are chosen to achieve the spatial resolution desired. The use of flow-compensating gradients or cardiac gating is required to eliminate cerebrospinal fluid (CSF) pulsation artifacts whenever T2-weighted images are acquired (Fig. 2.2).

PATHOLOGY

Disorders of the skull base are common and varied in location. The intrinsic imaging characteristics of any one particular disease are more or less constant regardless of location, but the specific anatomic details differ. The intrinsic features of these lesions are discussed presently, and the specific anatomical details follow in the relevant sections.

NEOPLASMS
MENINGIOMA   Approximately one third of meningiomas occur along the skull base. Meningiomas may be found anywhere along the skull base but are situated most commonly in the subfrontal region, along the sphenoid wing, in the parasellar region, in the cerebellopontine angle, or near the foramen magnum. Approximately 75% of meningiomas are isointense to gray matter on both T1- and T2-weighted images (Fig. 2.3); the remainder are isointense on T1-weighted

Fig. 2.2 MRI TECHNIQUE FOR EXAMINATION OF THE SKULL BASE

Parameter	Sequence[a]			
	No. 1 T1-Weighted	No. 2 T1-Weighted	No. 3[b] T2-Weighted	No. 4 Gradient Echo
Plane	Sagittal	Axial or coronal	Variable[c]	Axial or coronal
TR (msec)	500–800	500–800	2000–3000	100–150
TE (msec)	20	20	70–100[d]	9–15
Flip angle (degrees)	—	—	—	40–50
Slice thickness (mm)	3–5	3–5	5	5
Matrix	256	256	128	256
Field of view	20	20	20	20
No. of excitations	2–4	2–4	2	4
Presaturation	Yes	Yes	No	No
Exam time (min)	5–10	5–10	10	Variable[e]

[a]Basic sequences: spin echo, multislice, head coil. Sequence 4: optional sequence, performed to differentiate vessels from solid tissue.
[b]Use of flow-compensating gradients recommended.
[c]Plane that best displays lesion (usually coronal).
[d]Second echo of two-echo study.
[e]Dependent on number of slices.

Tumor

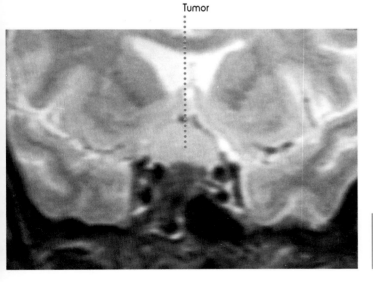

Fig. 2.3 MENINGIOMA T2-weighted coronal image. The tumor is very difficult to see. It is isointense to the adjacent cerebral cortex.

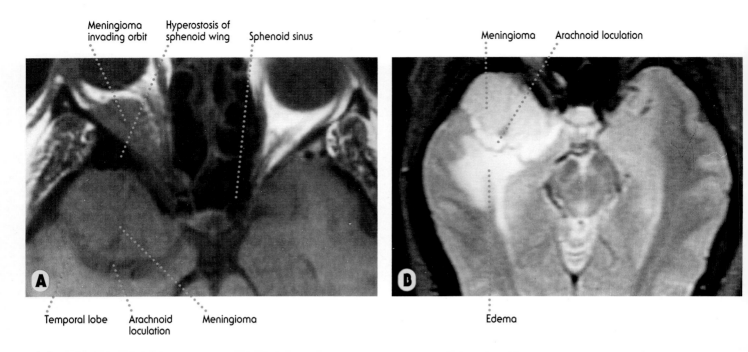

Meningioma invading orbit • Hyperostosis of sphenoid wing • Sphenoid sinus

Meningioma • Arachnoid loculation

Temporal lobe • Arachnoid loculation • Meningioma

Edema

Fig. 2.4 MENINGIOMA, SPHENOID WING (A) T1-weighted axial image. The large, isointense, extraaxial tumor occupies the anterior part of the right temporal fossa, crosses the superior orbital fissure, and infiltrates the orbit. There is hyperostosis of the sphenoid wing. **(B)** T2-weighted axial image. The tumor itself is moderately hyperintense to the brain—an occurrence that is demonstrated on T2-weighted images in approximately one quarter of meningiomas. There is a large amount of vasogenic edema in the temporal lobe, despite there being no invasion of the brain by the tumor. Cerebral edema is not an uncommon finding with extraaxial tumors, particularly large meningiomas.

Meningioma • Temporal lobe

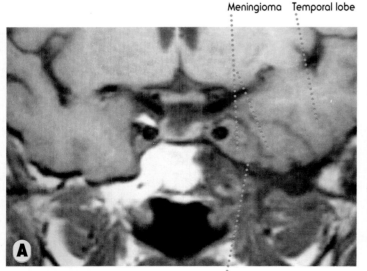

Lateral wall of cavernous sinus

Fig. 2.5 MENINGIOMA—WITHOUT AND WITH ENHANCEMENT (A) T1-weighted coronal image, unenhanced. The isointense tumor fills the left cavernous sinus and extends superiorly and laterally into the middle cranial fossa. There is no contrast between the latter component and the temporal lobe cortex. **(B)** T1-weighted coronal image, enhanced. All portions of the tumor enhance intensely and uniformly, allowing much clearer separation between the tumor and normal brain.

images and moderately hyperintense on T2-weighted images, unless calcified (Fig. 2.4). Calcified tumors are hypointense on all images. Meningiomas enhance intensely with contrast administration (Fig. 2.5).

Meningiomas demonstrate differing gross morphologic patterns: sessile, pedunculated, or flat. The latter is referred to as *meningioma en plaque* and is a common pattern at the skull base. The small en-plaque meningiomas are notoriously difficult to detect on magnetic resonance imaging (MRI) because of their small size and the lack of contrast between them and adjacent brain (Fig. 2.3).

Differential diagnosis is usually not difficult. In most cases, the extraaxial location can be clearly established and the imaging intensity is relatively characteristic. A significant differential diagnosis exists in particular locations. Along the floor of the anterior cranial fossa, meningioma must be distinguished from esthesioneuroblastoma, lymphoma, and squamous cell carcinoma. Around the sella turcica, meningiomas may resemble large pituitary adenomas. In the posterior fossa, meningiomas in the cerebellopontine angle and near the foramen magnum may be difficult to distinguish from neurinomas.

NERVE SHEATH TUMORS   Histologically, nerve sheath tumors may be divided into either schwannomas or neurofibromas. Simply stated, the schwannoma is a benign tumor of the covering Schwann cells, whereas a neurofibroma is a tumor that incorporates both the neural elements and the overlying Schwann cells. Virtually all intracranial nerve sheath tumors are schwannomas. Regardless of their histology, they have a similar MRI appearance and, for simplicity's sake, are herein referred to as neurinomas.

The most common neurinomas are those originating from cranial nerves V, VII, and VIII and from the IX, X, and XI nerve complex. The type most commonly encountered in clinical practice is the acoustic neurinoma (cranial nerve VIII).

On MR images, neurinomas are isointense to brain on T1-weighted images and hyperintense on T2-weighted studies. Internally, they tend to be heterogeneous, particularly the larger tumors. They enhance markedly with contrast administration. Neurinomas of specific cranial nerves are discussed in the subsections that follow.

ARACHNOID CYST   The arachnoid cyst is most often discovered incidentally, but occasionally it presents as a space-occupying lesion. More properly a congenital malformation than a true neoplasm, it is a CSF-filled cyst between two leaves of the arachnoid. It may also arise as an encysted CSF space secondary to postinflammatory adhesions. The most common locations are the middle fossa, the cerebellopontine angle, the cisterna magna, and the parasellar and quadrigeminal cisterns. Arachnoid cysts are of identical intensity to CSF on all conventional pulse sequences. There is usually displacement of adjacent structures (Fig. 2.6). There can be enlargement of the cyst over time, due to a ball-valve mechanism of CSF entering the cyst from the subarachnoid space.

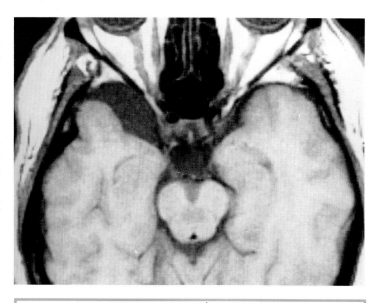

Fig. 2.6 ARACHNOID CYST   T1-weighted axial image. There is an arachnoid cyst in the anterior part of the right middle cranial fossa. It is extraaxial, well-defined, and isointense to CSF.

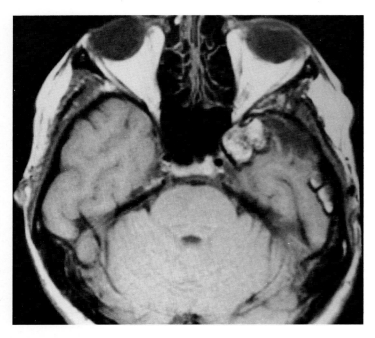

Fig. 2.7 FIBROUS DYSPLASIA T1-weighted axial image. A partial resection of an exophytic bony mass has been performed. The remaining lesion can be seen in the medial aspect of the left middle cranial fossa. It is predominantly hyperintense but inhomogeneous, with a distinct black outline of its perimeter. The internal high signal is due to marrow fat, the black line due to a cortical bone margin.

TUMORS OF BONE/CARTILAGE ORIGIN The central portion of the skull base comprises the sphenoid, temporal, and occipital bones. These can be sites of origin for primary bone tumors, the most common of which are the chondroma and chondrosarcoma. Osseous skull base masses are also seen in fibrous dysplasia (Fig. 2.7). The osseous origin of tumors arising from the bony skull base can usually be established if images in the appropriate plane are acquired. Coronal or sagittal images are generally best for this purpose. Areas of signal dropout that may be seen on these images represent calcification or ossification within the tumor. This is a useful diagnostic observation, as it identifies the tumor as having chondroid or osteoid elements. The identification of fat-containing marrow in fibrous dysplasia and some osteochondromas has similar diagnostic value.

SKULL BASE AND DURAL METASTASES Cerebral metastases are more frequent and are more easily detected than dural and skull base metastases; the latter, however, are not uncommon. Metastatic tumor spread to the skull base may occur either via the hematogenous route from anatomically remote sites (most commonly from bronchogenic or breast primaries), or by local extension, particularly from the face or nasopharynx. Careful evaluation of the skull base and meninges with T1-weighted images is required for locating small tumors. Metastases are visible as low signal intensity lesions within the normally high intensity bone marrow (Fig. 2.8), as nodularity or thickening of the meninges, or as a large, destructive soft tissue mass (Fig. 2.9).

INFECTION
Basal meningitis is caused by a wide spectrum of organisms, most commonly bacteria and fungi. Osseous involvement is much less common than meningeal infection. Meningitis may result from hematogenous seeding, either following surgery or by direct extension from the sinuses.

Acute bacterial meningitis is a rapidly progressive illness. There is little diagnostic role for imaging save excluding a space-occupying lesion. Diagnosis is readily established by CSF analysis and culture. If imaging (MRI or CT) is performed, findings are usually limited to contrast enhancement of the meninges.

As opposed to its limited role in acute meningitis, MRI is useful in the evaluation of patients with more indolent findings, e.g., unexplained hydrocephalus, cranial nerve palsy, hypothalamic dysfunction, or low grade fever. This "low-grade" type of disease pattern is typical of granulomatous, e.g., tuberculosis, or fungal infections (especially aspergillosis and candidiasis). The findings may include thickening and

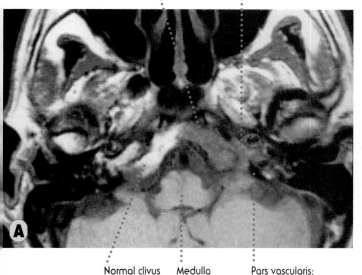

Tumor infiltrating clivus — Pars nervosa: jugular foramen

Normal clivus — Medulla — Pars vascularis: jugular foramen

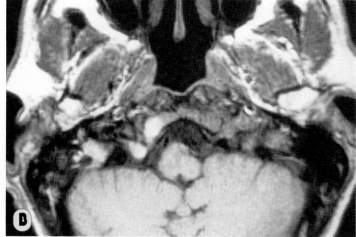

Fig. 2.8 METASTATIC LUNG CARCINOMA **(A)** T1-weighted axial image. This patient presented with palsies of nerves IX, X, XI, and XII on the left. The normal hyperintense marrow signal is present on the right side of the clivus, but is replaced by tumor on the left, with involvement of the jugular foramen. **(B)** T1-weighted axial image. The tumor extends inferiorly, involving the inferior tip of the clivus.

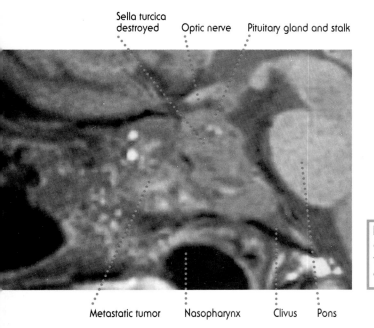

Sella turcica destroyed — Optic nerve — Pituitary gland and stalk

Metastatic tumor — Nasopharynx — Clivus — Pons

Fig. 2.9 METASTATIC BREAST CARCINOMA T1-weighted sagittal image. The ill-defined lesion is centered in the sphenoid sinus. It invades and destroys the sella turcica and clivus, and also involves the pituitary gland.

irregularity of the dura (Fig. 2.10), a mass in the subarachnoid space (Fig. 2.11), bone destruction, and occasionally, hydrocephalus. The mastoid and paranasal sinuses should be closely inspected as possible sources of infection. On MRI, chronic meningeal infection may be indistinguishable from lymphomatous or carcinomatous meningitis. Differentiation requires CSF cell analysis or biopsy.

Meningitis may be complicated by the formation of an epidural abscess or a subdural empyema. Clinically, the patient may demonstrate nonresponsiveness to antibiotic therapy or may worsen after early improvement. Magnetic resonance imaging will demonstrate an extraaxial fluid collection that is hypointense on T1-weighted images and hyperintense on T2-weighted images.

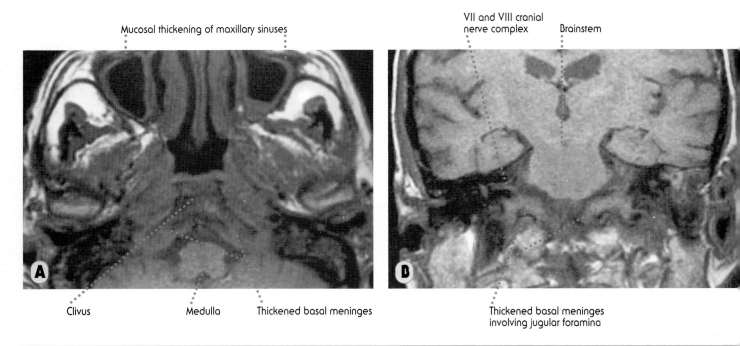

Fig. 2.10 ASPERGILLUS MENINGITIS **(A)** T1-weighted axial image. The basal meninges are thickened bilaterally alongside the clivus and extending into both jugular foramina. Normally, the meninges are imperceptible or, at most, a thin line. The mucosal thickening in both maxillary sinuses is also due to aspergillus infection. **(B)** T1-weighted coronal image. The meningeal thickening in the jugular foramen is shown to best advantage in this view.

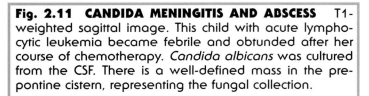

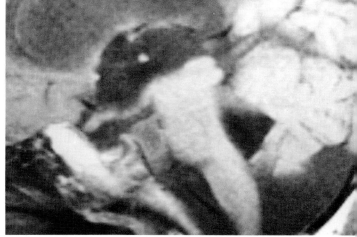

Fig. 2.11 CANDIDA MENINGITIS AND ABSCESS T1-weighted sagittal image. This child with acute lymphocytic leukemia became febrile and obtunded after her course of chemotherapy. *Candida albicans* was cultured from the CSF. There is a well-defined mass in the prepontine cistern, representing the fungal collection.

THE SELLA TURCICA AND PARASELLAR REGION

NORMAL ANATOMY (Figs. 2.12 to 2.15)

The sella turcica is a hemispherical depression in a central, bony promontory formed by the sphenoid bone. The sella is subdivided into three parts from front to back: the tuberculum sellae, the pituitary fossa, and the dorsum sellae. It measures approximately 5 to 10 mm (depth) x 10 to 15 mm (length) x 10 to 12 mm (width). It is completely enveloped by dura. The roof of the sella is formed by a dural leaf, the diaphragma sella, which is pierced by the pituitary stalk and portal vessels. The pituitary gland is the only structure within the sella turcica. It consists of the anterior and posterior lobes. A third, tiny lobe, the intermediate lobe, is occasionally present but it is not of any significance. The anterior lobe is the largest, occupying the anterior three quarters of the sella. It has two lateral wings that extend posteriorly on either side of the small, centrally positioned posterior lobe. On T1-weighted images the posterior lobe is high signal intensity and the anterior lobe isointense relative to white matter. The size of the normal gland is variable, particularly its height which varies from 3 to 9 mm. Usually it fills the sella turcica in all directions.

The pituitary stalk consists of the axons of cells lying in the hypothalamus and terminating in the posterior lobe and an investing sheath of portal veins. The stalk extends from the inferior hypothalamus (tuber cinereum), through the suprasellar cistern, passing caudal to the optic chiasm and through the diaphragmatic hiatus into the pituitary gland. It slopes anteriorly and inferiorly.

The inferior border of the sella is formed by a thin layer of cortical bone and periosteum separating the pituitary gland from the air-containing sphenoid sinus. In most cases the thin, bony floor is imperceptible on MRI.

The cavernous sinuses form the lateral sellar boundaries. These are complex venous sinuses enveloped by dura on all sides. They contain the "cavernous" portion of the internal carotid artery, cranial nerves III, IV, V_1, V_2, and VI, and multiple venous spaces of different sizes. The medial wall of the cavernous sinus is exceedingly thin and difficult to see by MRI. The lateral wall is thicker and usually clearly seen. Cranial nerves III, IV, and V_1 are in the lateral wall and are positioned, respectively, above, at the same level as, and below the internal carotid artery. These nerves can occasionally be observed as areas of thickening of the lateral wall. Cranial nerve VI lies freely in the sinus and is too small to see. The internal carotid artery is the most prominent structure within the sinus. It is seen distinctly as a dark, round vessel in coronal sections. The venous spaces within the cavernous sinus are a complex maze of vascular channels, some large, some small. The larg-er channels have high rates of flow and, as expected, appear dark. Flow in the smaller spaces is slower. By and large, these do not cause a signal void. The net result is a heterogeneous appearance to the cavernous sinuses.

Meckel's cave, within the leaves of the tentorial insertion, is the posterolateral border of the cavernous sinus. It contains CSF and the gasserian ganglion (cranial nerve V). Cranial nerve V_3 branches inferolaterally, traversing the foramen ovale, and never entering the cavernous sinus. Cranial nerve V_2 branches anteriorly, coursing along the inferior margin of the sinus, and traversing the foramen rotundum. Both V_3 and V_2 are consistently visible on coronal MRI sections.

The suprasellar cistern is a CSF space above the sella and below the floor of the third ventricle. It contains the supraclinoid carotid arteries and their terminal branches (visible as dark structures), as well as the optic nerves and optic chiasm. The optic nerves enter the cranium through the optic canals, which are transversely oriented foramina in the sphenoid bone immediately lateral to the tuberculum sella. The optic nerves join above the sella to form the optic chiasm, then separate posteriorly to become the optic tracts. The chiasm resembles a horizontal figure eight, approximately 4 mm high and 12 mm wide.

The anterior clinoid processes, together with the tuberculum sellae, form the anterior border of the sella turcica. The anterior clinoids are larger and more laterally placed than their posterior counterparts. They are extensions of the lesser sphenoid wing and form the superomedial margin of the superior orbital fissure. The greater sphenoid wing is lateral to the superior orbital fissure. The two sphenoid wings together divide the anterior from the middle cranial fossa.

The floor of the anterior cranial fossa is formed by the orbital plates of the frontal bones laterally, by the cribriform plate of the ethmoid bone in the midline, and by the sphenoid bone posteriorly. The only significant structures traversing the floor of the anterior cranial fossa are the multiple rootlets of the olfactory nerve passing from the olfactory bulbs to the nasal epithelium, through multiple, tiny foramina in the cribriform plate. The olfactory bulbs, unlike the small rootlets, are normally visible on MRI (particularly on T1-weighted coronal images).

The middle cranial fossae are posterior and inferior to the sphenoid wings and lateral to the cavernous sinuses. They are rather featureless except for several foramina—the most important being the carotid canal, foramen ovale, foramen rotundum, and foramen spinosum. These transmit the internal carotid artery, the mandibular and maxillary branches of the trigeminal nerve, and the middle meningeal artery, respectively. The first three can be identified on coronal MRI; the middle meningeal artery usually cannot.

The Sella Turcica and Parasellar Region

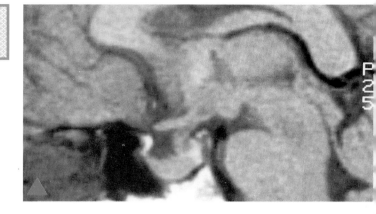

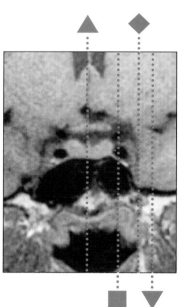

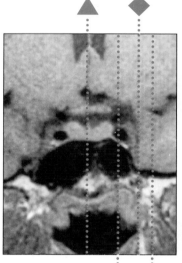

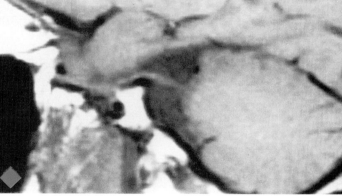

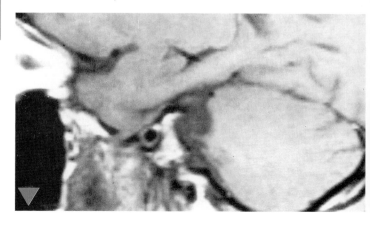

Fig. 2.12 Localizer: T1-Weighted Coronal Image Through the Anterior Pituitary Lobe The planes of section of four sagittal images are indicated: through the midline, the carotid artery, the lateral wall of the cavernous sinus, and the foramen ovale.

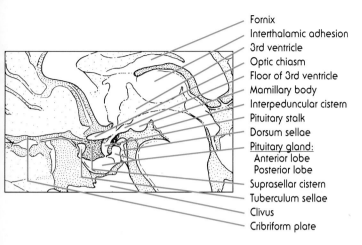

Fornix
Interthalamic adhesion
3rd ventricle
Optic chiasm
Floor of 3rd ventricle
Mamillary body
Interpeduncular cistern
Pituitary stalk
Dorsum sellae
Pituitary gland:
  Anterior lobe
  Posterior lobe
Suprasellar cistern
Tuberculum sellae
Clivus
Cribriform plate

Fig. 2.13A Midline T1-Weighted Sagittal Image
The normal midline anatomy is exquisitely defined. The most important landmarks are the anterior and posterior lobes of the pituitary gland, the pituitary stalk, and the optic chiasm. The pituitary stalk slopes anteroinferiorly and is wider superiorly than inferiorly.

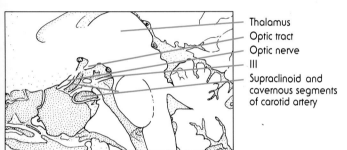

Thalamus
Optic tract
Optic nerve
III
Supraclinoid and cavernous segments of carotid artery

Fig. 2.13B T1-Weighted Sagittal Image Through the Carotid Artery The cavernous and supraclinoid portions of the internal carotid artery are visible in this plane just lateral to the pituitary gland. The optic tract and nerve traverse the suprasellar cistern, and cranial nerve III exits the interpeduncular cistern to enter the lateral wall of the cavernous sinus.

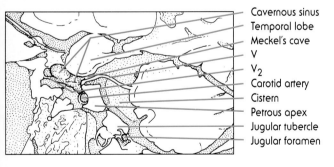

Cavernous sinus
Temporal lobe
Meckel's cave
V
V_2
Carotid artery
Cistern
Petrous apex
Jugular tubercle
Jugular foramen

Fig. 2.13C T1-Weighted Sagittal Image Through the Lateral Wall of the Cavernous Sinus Cranial nerve V traverses the prepontine cistern to enter Meckel's cave. The horizontal portion of the carotid canal is contained in the petrous temporal bone immediately below, and the cavernous sinus is immediately anterior.

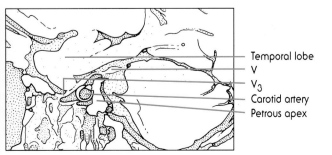

Temporal lobe
V
V_3
Carotid artery
Petrous apex

Fig. 2.13D T1-Weighted Sagittal Image Through the Foramen Ovale Cranial nerve V_3 exits anteroinferiorly through the foramen ovale. The petrous segment of the carotid artery is directly below.

The Sella Turcica and Parasellar Region

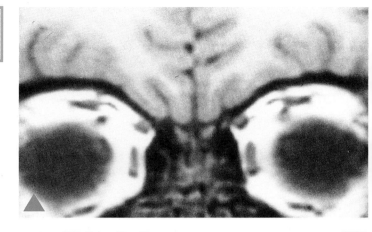

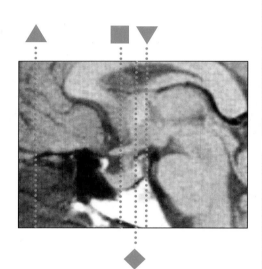

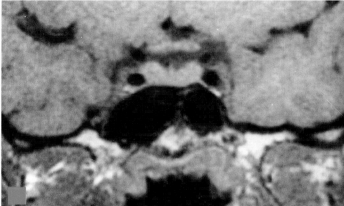

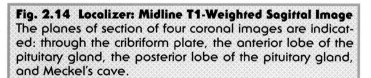

Fig. 2.14 Localizer: Midline T1-Weighted Sagittal Image
The planes of section of four coronal images are indicated: through the cribriform plate, the anterior lobe of the pituitary gland, the posterior lobe of the pituitary gland, and Meckel's cave.

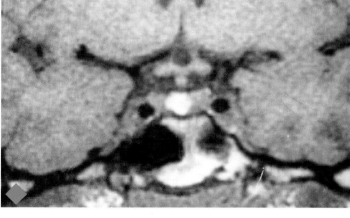

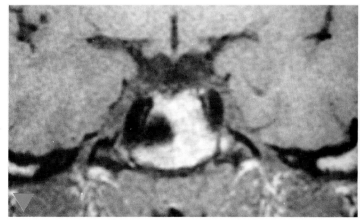

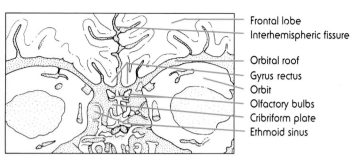

Frontal lobe
Interhemispheric fissure

Orbital roof
Gyrus rectus
Orbit
Olfactory bulbs
Cribriform plate
Ethmoid sinus

Fig. 2.15A T1-Weighted Coronal Image Through the Cribriform Plate The cribriform plate is in the midline, forming the roof of the ethmoid air cells. The olfactory bulbs run along the plate with numerous nerve rootlets (not visible) extending inferiorly through the plate to the nasal mucosa.

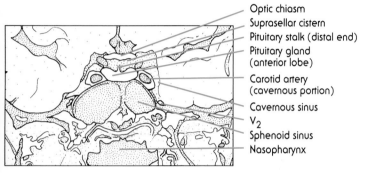

Optic chiasm
Suprasellar cistern
Pituitary stalk (distal end)
Pituitary gland (anterior lobe)
Carotid artery (cavernous portion)
Cavernous sinus
V_2
Sphenoid sinus
Nasopharynx

Fig. 2.15B T1-Weighted Coronal Image Through the Anterior Pituitary Gland The anterior lobe of the pituitary gland is of intermediate intensity and is symmetric about the midline. Above it lies the suprasellar cistern and optic chiasm, below it the sphenoid sinus. Laterally, the cavernous sinus contains the carotid artery. The medial cavernous sinus wall is imperceptibly thin, whereas the lateral wall, containing cranial nerves III, IV, V_1, and V_2, is thicker and consistently well seen.

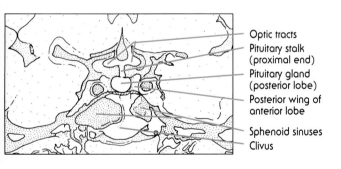

Optic tracts
Pituitary stalk (proximal end)
Pituitary gland (posterior lobe)
Posterior wing of anterior lobe

Sphenoid sinuses
Clivus

Fig. 2.15C T1-Weighted Coronal Image Through the Posterior Pituitary Gland The posterior lobe is considerably smaller than the anterior lobe; yet, it is very prominent because of its hyperintensity. It is surrounded on either side by the posterolateral wings of the anterior lobe. The stalk is directly above it.

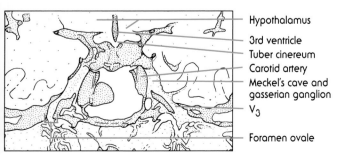

Hypothalamus

3rd ventricle
Tuber cinereum
Carotid artery
Meckel's cave and gasserian ganglion
V_3

Foramen ovale

Fig. 2.15D T1-Weighted Coronal Image Through Meckel's Cave Meckel's cave is the posterolateral portion of the cavernous sinus. It contains the gasserian ganglion. Cranial nerve V_3 exits through the foramen ovale inferolaterally. The carotid arteries are medial to it, vertically oriented at this level.

TECHNIQUE

High resolution images (thin sections, small pixels) are of the utmost importance. T1-weighted images provide the best contrast within the pituitary gland, and between that gland, the cavernous sinus, the suprasellar cistern, and the optic chiasm. Sagittal images are useful for gross anatomical display and for localization. Coronal images are the best for evaluating the pituitary gland itself with the greatest freedom from partial averaging effects of the parasellar structures. Therefore, the routine protocol is T1-weighted images (3 mm thick), 256 x 256 matrix, and a 16- to 20-mm field of view with four signal excitations (NEX) in both the sagittal and coronal planes. Two NEX may be used instead of four to reduce the examination time but the images will be perceptibly grainy. Supplementary T2-weighted images are added if there is a suprasellar lesion or if the brain itself needs to be evaluated in addition to the sella turcica.

PATHOLOGY

CONGENITAL LESIONS

PITUITARY HYPOPLASIA AND PITUITARY DWARFISM
The pituitary gland develops from two embryologically and functionally distinct sources. The anterior lobe originates from the epithelium of Rathke's pouch (or craniopharyngeal duct), an upward extension of the epithelial roof of the oral cavity. The embryologic duct involutes completely, leaving the anterior lobe as an isolated island of epithelial tissue in the sella turcica. The posterior lobe is neural tissue; it originates as a downward extension of the hypothalamus and remains connected to it by the pituitary stalk.

Interference with the migration of the embryologic precursors of either the anterior or posterior lobes can result in hypoplasia of the pituitary gland. Although small, the hypoplastic pituitary gland looks otherwise normal. The individual so affected may be clinically normal or may manifest relative deficiency of one or more pituitary hormones. Because of tremendous individual variance in the size of the pituitary gland (3 to 9 mm in height, 8 to 14 mm in width), the diagnosis of hypoplasia should not be considered unless the gland is distinctly small in all dimensions (Fig. 2.16).

Growth hormone deficiency is an interesting and special case of pituitary hypoplasia. Although the lesion responsible for growth hormone deficiency has long been assumed to be in the hypothalamus, no hypothalamic lesion has ever been demonstrated. However, using MRI, a remarkably consistent combination of complex, developmental abnormalities has been observed on MRI in the pituitary gland and pituitary stalk of these affected patients. These abnormalities consist of a small sella turcica and a small anterior lobe, absence (or extreme atrophy) of the distal stalk, and absence of the high intensity of the posterior lobe from its normal location. Instead, there is a small high intensity nodule at the tip of the truncated stalk (Fig. 2.17). This nodule is thought to represent an ectopically situated posterior lobe, which has been arrested in its migration downwards toward the sella. A full explanation for these observations has not been proven. The hypothesis is that in

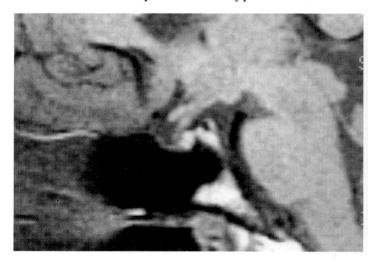

Fig. 2.16 PITUITARY HYPOPLASIA T1-weighted sagittal image. The sella turcica and anterior lobe of the pituitary gland are very small. The stalk is normal. The posterior lobe is normal in size and position.

the perinatal period there is disruption of the vascular supply to the pituitary gland and distal stalk, resulting in both ischemic damage to the gland and arrested development of the stalk. Following vascular disruption, the anterior lobe becomes ischemic, resulting in variable degrees of anterior lobe hormone deficiency. Growth hormone-secreting cells, the somatotrophs, are the most ischemically sensitive cells and are the first to clinically manifest their dysfunction (growth retardation). If carefully tested, deficiencies of other anterior lobe hormones can be demonstrated in these patients, and if followed long enough, such deficiencies will become clinically evident. Posterior lobe hormone deficiency does not occur, because these hormones are made in the hypothalamus and are still released, not from the posterior lobe but from the truncated stalk. Thus, the high intensity nodule in the stalk functionally represents an ectopic posterior lobe.

NEOPLASMS

PITUITARY ADENOMA   Pituitary adenomas are benign, epithelial neoplasms that arise from the anterior lobe of the gland. The peak incidence of clinical presentation is between the ages of 20 to 50, although several unselected autopsy series have noted a high incidence of tiny adenomas in the elderly as incidental findings. In clinical practice, young adult women are the largest group affected, usually presenting with galactorrhea or menstrual disturbances. Other relatively common presentations are acromegaly and Cushing's syndrome. The only known association with pituitary adenomas is the syndrome of multiple endocrine neoplasms. There are no known predisposing factors.

The clinical classification of pituitary adenomas is conventionally based on the functional activity of the tumor. Adenomas are broadly divided into two groups: functioning (those that secrete a hormone) and nonfunctioning (those that do not). Functioning adenomas are most commonly prolactinomas, followed in incidence by growth hormone and ACTH-secreting adenomas. Other types occur but are rare. The clinical presentation of functioning adenomas is dependent on the type and amount of hormone secreted. Patients with functioning adenomas present with either a systemic endocrinologic disorder or with compression of a parasellar structure by the tumor. The tumor may be very small when the endocrinopathy becomes manifest. Nonfunctioning adenomas are clinically silent, until they compress or involve the gland or surrounding structures sufficiently to cause clinically apparent problems, e.g., hypopituitarism, visual loss, ophthalmoplegia, or hypothalamic disturbances.

There are no imaging features that reliably distinguish between secreting and nonsecreting adenomas or between the various secreting types. Whereas, on average, nonsecreting adenomas are larger and usually have extended outside the sella turcica by the time they are discovered, this is not a reliable distinguishing feature in the individual case; many prolactinomas and growth hormone-secreting adenomas may grow to a similar size. It is rare to see a large ACTH-secreting adenoma.

Radiologically, it is convenient to separate adenomas into microadenomas (smaller than 1 cm) and macroadenomas (larger than 1 cm). On T1-weighted images, pituitary microadenomas are moderately hypointense with respect to the normal anterior lobe.

Optic nerve   Ectopic posterior lobe   Proximal stalk

Anterior lobe of pituitary   Absent hyperintensity   Distal stalk absent

Fig. 2.17 GROWTH HORMONE-DEFICIENT DWARF T1-weighted sagittal image. The anteroposterior diameter of the sella turcica and pituitary gland is slightly reduced. The posterior lobe hyperintensity is absent. The distal stalk is absent, and the proximal two thirds of the stalk is hyperintense (presumed to be functionally an ectopic posterior lobe).

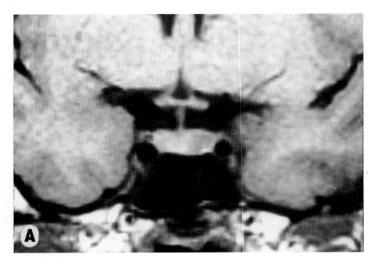

Posteror lobe
of pituitary gland

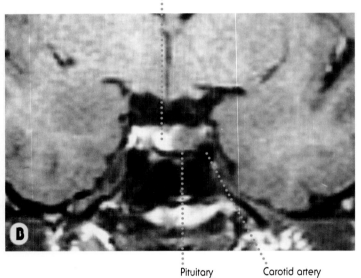

Pituitary   Carotid artery
microadenoma

Fig. 2.18 PITUITARY MICROADENOMA **(A)** T1-weighted coronal image (through middle of sella). The 5-mm adenoma is a distinct hypointense lesion on the left side of the pituitary gland. The stalk is midline, and there is no distortion of the shape of the gland. This is a common appearance of a small adenoma. **(B)** T1-weighted coronal image (through posterior sella). The adenoma extends posteriorly, displacing the hyperintense posterior lobe to the right. It is a common error to interpret the hyperintense area as being the adenoma.

The majority are laterally situated in the sella turcica and have well-defined margins (Fig. 2.18). They may be associated with contralateral displacement of the pituitary stalk and ipsilateral enlargement of the gland, but such findings are less reliable than a finding of focal hypointensity. Cystic degeneration or necrosis in the tumor may cause profound reduction in signal on the T1-weighted image. Although cystic and necrotic adenomas typically are hyperintense on T2-weighted images, pituitary adenomas tend to be poorly depicted on the T2-weighted images. Macroadenomas cause enlargement or focal erosion of the sella turcica and/or extend superiorly into the suprasellar cistern. The remaining normal gland is usually compressed to the extent that it is not identifiable (Fig. 2.19). Occasionally, there is a line of demarcation between normal tissue and an adenoma (Fig. 2.20). The signal intensity of macroadenomas does not differ substantially from smaller adenomas except that there is a higher incidence of cystic degeneration, necrosis, and intratumoral hemorrhage. Hemorrhage is readily apparent as a focal area of high signal on the T1-weighted image (Fig. 2.21).

Magnetic resonance imaging best demonstrates important anatomical relationships of large tumors that have extended superiorly beyond the confines of sella turcica to involve such vital parasellar structures as the optic chiasm, the hypothalamus, and the vessels of the circle of Willis (Figs. 2.19 and 2.21). Similarly, inferior extension into the sphenoid sinus can be precisely delineated. However, it is difficult to determine the integrity of the medial cavernous sinus wall and, therefore, difficult to accurately determine cavernous sinus invasion. The only reliable diagnostic signs of cavernous sinus invasion is deflection of the lateral cavernous sinus wall or interposition of soft tissue between the cavernous carotid artery and the lateral wall (Figs. 2.20 and 2.22).

Contrast-enhanced MRI has been shown to improve the detection rate of small adenomas. The normal pituitary gland enhances early upon contrast administration and also begins to wash out early. Adenomas enhance later and washout is similarly delayed. Immediate postcontrast scanning,

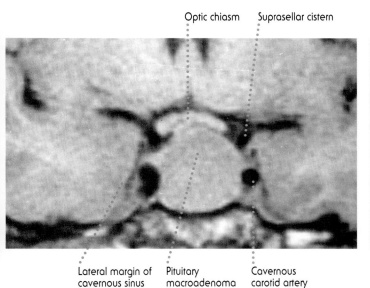

Optic chiasm   Suprasellar cistern

Lateral margin of   Pituitary   Cavernous
cavernous sinus   macroadenoma   carotid artery

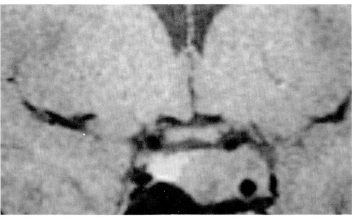

Fig. 2.19 PITUITARY MACROADENOMA T1-weighted coronal image. This patient presented with acromegaly and bitemporal hemianopsia. The large adenoma completely fills the enlarged sella turcica and extends into the suprasellar cistern, compressing and elevating the optic chiasm. The intensity of the tumor is approximately the same as that of the cerebral cortex.

Fig. 2.20 PITUITARY MACROADENOMA T1-weighted coronal image. The hypointense left-sided adenoma is clearly distinguished from the normal pituitary gland on the right side. There is involvement of the left cavernous sinus.

Suprasellar   Hemorrhagic
cistern   components to tumor   Optic chiasm

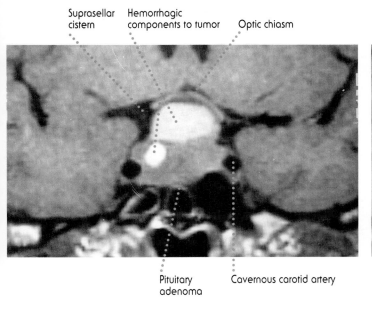

Pituitary   Cavernous carotid artery
adenoma

Tumor center,
right side of gland 3rd ventricle Optic chiasm Pituitary stalk

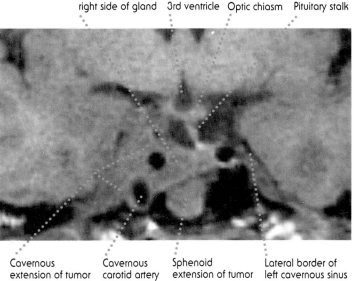

Cavernous   Cavernous   Sphenoid   Lateral border of
extension of tumor   carotid artery   extension of tumor   left cavernous sinus

Fig. 2.21 PITUITARY ADENOMA WITH HEMORRHAGE
T1-weighted coronal image. This patient suffered from amenorrhea, galactorrhea, and progressive visual loss. There are two components to the tumor, intrasellar and suprasellar. The intrasellar component has a focal area of hemorrhage on the right side but the tumor is predominantly isointense. At the point where the tumor extends into the suprasellar cistern, there is a constriction around the tumor, due to the diaphragma sellae. The suprasellar portion is hemorrhagic. The chiasm is markedly compressed.

Fig. 2.22 PITUITARY ADENOMA WITH CAVERNOUS SINUS EXTENSION T1-weighted coronal image. The adenoma originates on the right side of the pituitary gland, with displacement of the stalk to the left. There is invasion of the sphenoid and right cavernous sinuses. The right carotid artery is completely encircled by tumor. The cavernous sinus is filled with tumor, which obliterates the normal internal structure and boundaries of the sinus (compare this with normal left side).

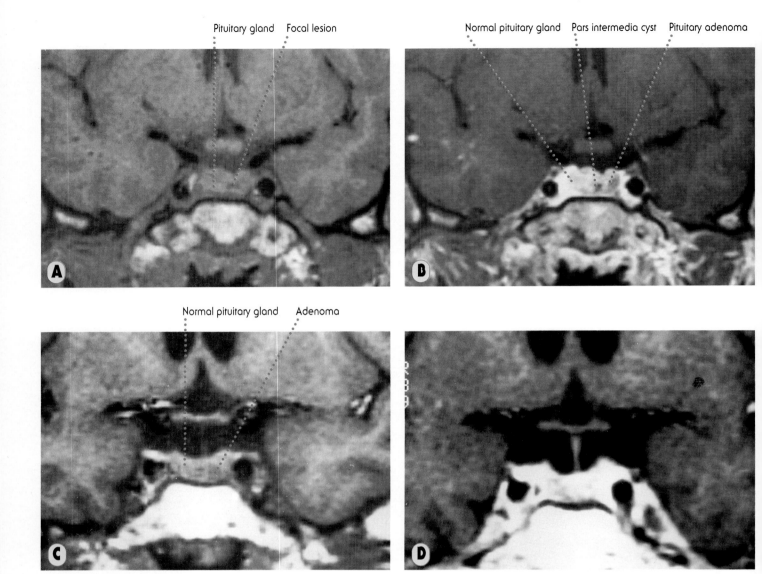

Pituitary gland   Focal lesion

Normal pituitary gland   Pars intermedia cyst   Pituitary adenoma

Normal pituitary gland   Adenoma

Fig. 2.23 CUSHING'S DISEASE **Case 1.** **(A)** T1-weighted coronal image. The pituitary gland is asymmetric. The right side is larger and has a convex superior surface; however, there is a lesion on the left side—a focal hypointensity just to the left of the midline. The appearance of this lesion is identical to that of most microadenomas. **(B)** Contrast-enhanced, T1-weighted coronal image. This image was obtained immediately after the injection of gadolinium-DTPA. Two hypointense lesions are evident. The small, left paracentral lesion proved to be a pars intermedia cyst at surgery. The larger left lateral lesion was an adenoma. Both lesions are much more evident on the postcontrast scan due to the greater hypointensity relative to the normal gland, yet they are indistinguishable from one another. **Case 2.** **(C)** T1-weighted coronal image. The adenoma is evident as a hypointense area immediately to the left of the midline. **(D)** Contrast-enhanced, T1-weighted coronal image. There was a delay of 40 min between the administration of gadolinium-DTPA and the acquisition of this image. The adenoma is now hyperintense relative to the normal gland. Using both immediate and delayed postcontrast images can improve the detection yield for small adenomas, as is illustrated in these two cases. (A and B courtesy of Dr. D. Newton, University of California, San Francisco)

therefore, can show the tumor with a greater degree of hypointensity than is possible on the noncontrast scan (Fig. 2.23). Delayed scanning occasionally will display the tumor as hyperintense (Fig. 2.23). In most cases, however, the adenoma is well-described on the noncontrast scan and contrast injection is not required. ACTH-secreting adenomas are an exception. In most series, less than half of this particular type of tumor can be seen on unenhanced studies. Contrast agents will play an important diagnostic role for such tumors.

Many patients with prolactinomas undergo medical therapy with bromocriptine. In those cases that respond to treatment (60% to 80%), the tumor shrinks and the intensity of the tumor becomes more like that of the normal gland (Fig. 2.24). These changes are usually evident within a week or two of initiating treatment.

CRANIOPHARYNGIOMA   Craniopharyngiomas originate from epithelial remnants of Rathke's pouch normally found at the junction of the pituitary stalk and pituitary gland. Half occur in childhood, the other half are spread throughout adulthood. The tumor is usually found in the suprasellar cistern but may extend into the sella turcica, up into the hypothalamus, or into the anterior, middle, or posterior cranial fossae. A small fraction are entirely intrasellar or entirely within the third ventricle.

Craniopharyngiomas are well-defined tumors that are histologically benign but can be locally invasive, making complete surgical resection difficult. They are either cystic, or partially solid and cystic. The cyst most often contains dark, machine-oil-like fluid. Occasionally, keratin is the dominant content of the cyst. Calcification, which is frequent, is finely dispersed or globular. This complex histology is reflected in a complex MRI appearance.

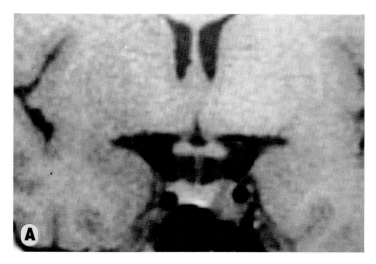

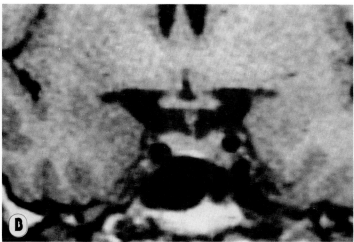

Fig. 2.24 PROLACTINOMA—BEFORE AND AFTER MEDICAL TREATMENT   (A) T1-weighted coronal image before treatment. There is a distinct hypointense lesion on the left side of the pituitary gland that is clearly distinguished from the normal pituitary gland and associated with the remodeling of the sella floor downwards. **(B)** T1-weighted coronal image after 3 months of bromocriptine treatment. The adenoma is smaller, less well-differentiated from normal pituitary gland and closer in signal intensity to that of a normal pituitary gland.

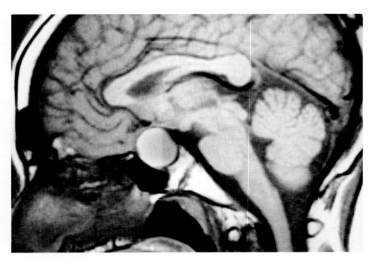

Fig. 2.25 CRANIOPHARYNGIOMA T1-weighted sagittal image. Craniopharyngiomas have several MRI appearances, this being one of the two most common types. The tumor is hyperintense with a fluid/fluid level—indicating that it is a cyst. The hyperintensity is probably due to hemoglobin breakdown products, which also account for the gross pathologic appearance of "machine-oil-like" fluid in these cysts.

In most cases the cystic component is hyperintense on the T1-weighted image (Fig. 2.25); however, when the cyst is filled only with keratin, it is usually dark on the T1-weighted image (Fig. 2.26). The solid portion of the tumor is of intermediate signal (Fig. 2.27). Globular calcification is evident as a focal region of signal dropout (Figs. 2.27 and 2.28), but very often, calcification cannot be appreciated on the MR scan, particularly if it either has a finely dispersed quality throughout the tumor or manifests itself as a thin, egg-shell capsular type. Often, the tumor is very heterogeneous, reflecting a complex combination of solid tumor, cyst, and calcification (Fig. 2.27).

RATHKE'S CLEFT CYSTS   Cysts of this type are simple epithelial cysts originating from the cleft between the anterior and intermediate lobes. They are usually incidental findings but may on occasion enlarge to cause symptoms by compression of the pituitary gland. If they extend into the suprasellar cistern, compression of the optic chiasm may occur. They usually contain a simple serous fluid but may contain mucin or cellular debris. In the former case, the diagnosis of a simple cyst is readily established, as it appears similar to CSF on all sequences. In the latter case, the lesion is hyperintense on the T1-weighted image and may be indistinguishable from a craniopharyngioma or hemorrhagic pituitary adenoma (Fig. 2.29). In those rare instances where the cyst is filled with cellular debris, it may be indistinguishable from a solid tumor.

Displaced optic nerve   Suprasellar craniopharyngioma

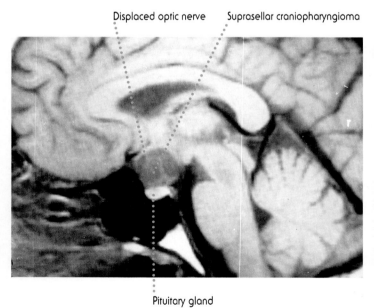

Pituitary gland

Soft tissue component   Hyperintense cyst

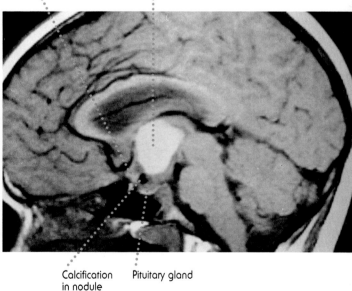

Calcification in nodule   Pituitary gland

Fig. 2.26 CRANIOPHARYNGIOMA T1-weighted sagittal image. This well-defined suprasellar tumor is very hypointense, almost as dark as CSF. The internal septation indicates that it is not a simple arachnoid cyst. This is one of the more unusual appearances of a craniopharyngioma. This type of tumor consists predominantly of keratin. The differential diagnosis for this case is an epidermoidoma.

Fig. 2.27 CRANIOPHARYNGIOMA T1-weighted sagittal image. Another common craniopharyngioma appearance. The tumor is heterogeneous, with three distinct components: a large hyperintense cyst superiorly, isointense solid soft tissue inferiorly, and a dense calcified nodule within the solid portion. This combination of findings in a suprasellar mass is specific for craniopharyngioma.

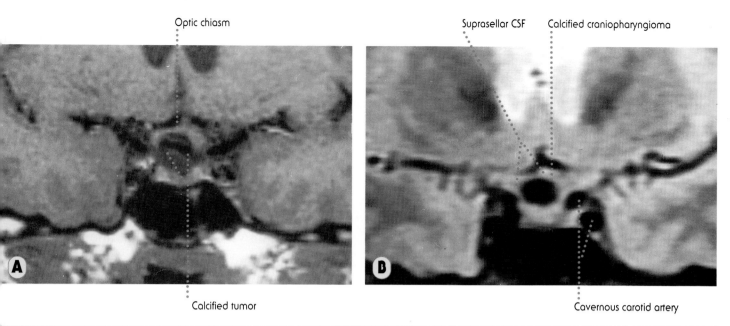

Optic chiasm

Suprasellar CSF   Calcified craniopharyngioma

A

B

Calcified tumor

Cavernous carotid artery

Fig. 2.28 CRANIOPHARYNGIOMA (A) T1-weighted coronal image. The right side of the optic chiasm is elevated and compressed, but the suprasellar tumor is difficult to see. The nodule is calcified and there is little contrast between it and the fluid in the suprasellar cistern.

(B) T2-weighted coronal image. Suprasellar CSF is hyperintense on T2-weighted images. As a result, the dark, calcified tumor is highlighted and made much more readily apparent.

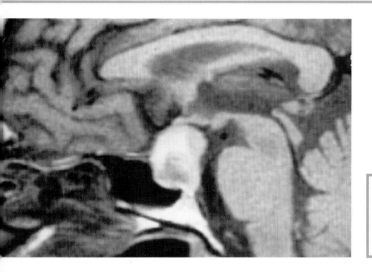

Fig. 2.29 RATHKE'S CLEFT CYST T1-weighted sagittal image. This simple cyst is indistinguishable from a craniopharyngioma or hemorrhagic pituitary adenoma. The internal inhomogeneity is accounted for by the presence of mucin and cellular debris in the cyst.

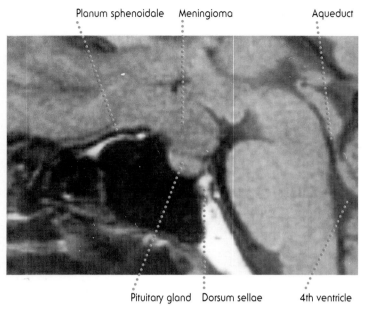

Planum sphenoidale   Meningioma   Aqueduct

Pituitary gland   Dorsum sellae   4th ventricle

Fig. 2.30 MENINGIOMA, PLANUM SPHENOIDALE T1-weighted sagittal image. This patient presented with bitemporal hemianopsia. An extraaxial tumor extends along the planum, over the tuberculum, and into the sella. However, there is a distinct plane of separation between the tumor and the pituitary gland—evidence that this is not a pituitary adenoma.

PARASELLAR MENINGIOMAS   Parasellar meningiomas account for less than 10% of all intracranial meningiomas. The histology and MRI characteristics have previously been discussed. The most important differential features vis-a-vis adenomas are a wide dural base (usually on the tuberculum sellae), a plane of separation from the pituitary gland (Fig. 2.30), and, if a contrast agent is administered, intense, early, uniform contrast enhancement. Hyperostosis of the clinoid process or tuberculum sellae is a useful differential point for meningioma but is more clearly seen on CT.

HYPOTHALAMIC AND OPTIC GLIOMAS   These two tumors are considered together for several reasons: (a) They are histologically similar, (b) they tend to affect similar age groups, and (c) they are often indistinguishable from one another on CT and MRI and even at surgery. Children are primarily affected. There is a strong association between optic gliomas and neurofibromatosis.

Hypothalamic tumors are intimately related to the third ventricle and suprasellar cistern (the hypothalamus forming the walls and floor of the inferior third ventricle). Hypothalamic tumors may remain entirely parenchymal but may fill the third ventricle or grow into the suprasellar cistern incorporating the optic chiasm. They are not associated with enlargement of the optic nerves (Fig. 2.31). Optic gliomas may involve any part of the optic nerve or chiasm. They cause fusiform enlargement or tortuosity of the nerve or chiasm (Fig. 2.32). Occasionally, an exophytic compo-

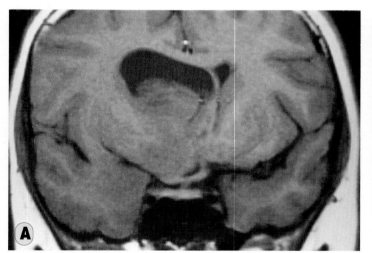

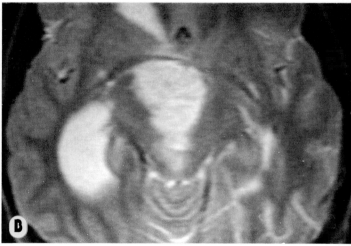

Fig. 2.31 HYPOTHALAMIC GLIOMA **(A)** T1-weighted coronal image. There is a large tumor centered in the right hypothalamus. It extends inferiorly into the suprasellar cistern, depressing the optic chiasm. Medially, it compresses and displaces the third ventricle. Superiorly, it invaginates the right lateral ventricle. **(B)** T2-weighted axial image. This image more clearly distinguishes the hyperintense tumor from the normal brain. Typical of most intraaxial tumors, it is hyperintense on T2-weighted images. The temporal horn and frontal horns are dilated due to obstructive hydrocephalus. The hydrocephalus is caused by the tumor compressing the third ventricle.

nent develops with invasion of the hypothalamus or there may be extension posteriorly along the optic tract into the optic radiations. Because of their overlapping characteristics, hypothalamic and optic gliomas are frequently confused.

The diagnosis of hypothalamic/optic glioma can usually be established with MRI on anatomical grounds. Coronal images and oblique images oriented along the axis of the optic nerve are particularly useful in defining the anatomy. If there is a significant suprasellar component, the main differential diagnosis is craniopharyngioma. In contrast to the craniopharyngioma, these tumors are rarely cystic and rarely calcify.

SUPRASELLAR GERMINOMAS   These tumors have a striking male preponderance and are most common in the late teens. Diabetes insipidus is the most common clinical presentation. Histologically, these tumors are identical to testicular seminomas and, like the testicular tumor, are very radiosensitive. The most common intracranial sites are the pineal gland and the suprasellar cistern. They have a tendency to disseminate via CSF pathways. On MR images, the suprasellar tumors are seen as nodularity or enlargement of the inferior hypothalamus or pituitary stalk; or as masses in the suprasellar cistern. They are hyperintense relative to normal brain on T2-weighted images. The differential diagnosis includes craniopharyngioma, hypothalamic glioma, and hypothalamic hamartoma.

OLFACTORY NEUROBLASTOMA (ESTHESIONEUROBLASTOMA)   This is an uncommon tumor that is thought to arise from the neural elements of the olfactory epithelium. Histologically, it is composed of collections of small neuroblastic cells separated by hyalinized stroma. Grossly, it appears as a friable red mass in the upper nose. The tumor occurs exclusively in the anterior fossa. The tumor is situated in the midline and most frequently bridges the cribriform plate with intracranial and intranasal components. The tumor is locally invasive and can involve the dura and brain. Invasion of the brain may be accompanied by significant intracerebral edema.

The tumor is best displayed on coronal images. A slightly lobulated mass is typically seen in the upper nasal cavity and above the floor of the anterior cranial fossa (Fig. 2.33). With larger tumors, the brain is elevated from the floor of the anterior cranial fossa. If the dura is breached, there is obliteration of the tissue plane between the tumor and the inferior surface of the frontal lobe. Dural involvement is commonly accompanied by cerebral edema, which is best visualized on T2-weighted images. The differential diagnosis is subfrontal meningioma, lymphoma, and squamous cell carcinoma. The latter two tumors invade the anterior cranial fossa by extension through the cribriform plate.

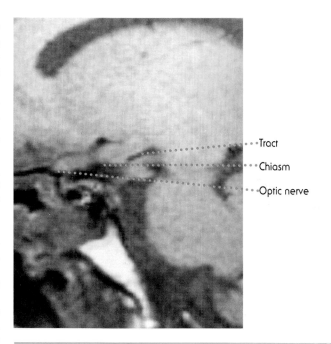

Fig. 2.32 OPTIC CHIASM GLIOMA   T1-weighted sagittal image. There is marked thickening of the optic nerve, chiasm, and tract. There is a clear plane of separation between the tumor and the hypothalamus.

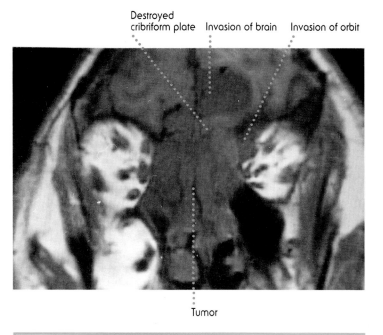

Fig. 2.33 ESTHESIONEUROBLASTOMA   T1-weighted coronal image. This man presented with a friable red mass in the nose. The tumor fills the upper nasal cavity, crosses the cribriform plate, and invades the brain. There is also invasion of the left orbit.

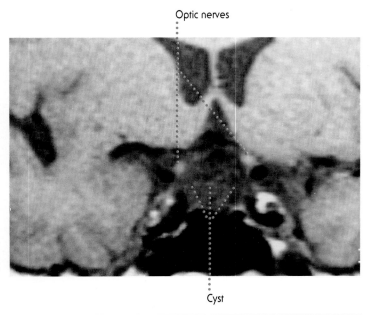

Optic nerves

Cyst

Fig. 2.34 SUPRASELLAR ARACHNOID CYST T1-weighted coronal image. The cyst is not directly evident because its fluid contents are isointense to CSF in the suprasellar cistern. The cyst's presence is indicated by the upward displacement of the optic nerves and the nonvisualization of the pituitary stalk.

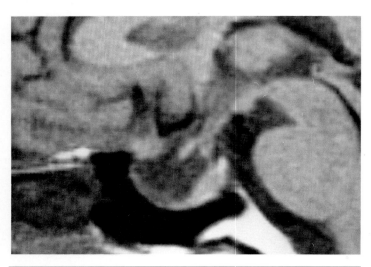

Fig. 2.35 EMPTY SELLA TURCICA T1-weighted sagittal image. The sella turcica is enlarged and filled predominantly with CSF (continuous with the suprasellar cistern). The pituitary gland is flattened inferiorly and posteriorly. The stalk is clearly seen traversing the cistern to the gland.

TUMOR-LIKE CONDITIONS

TUBER CINEREUM HAMARTOMAS   Hamartomas are not true neoplasms but rather are malformations characterized by disorganized tissue, in this case, an excess of gray matter in the inferior hypothalamus. Male children are the group predominantly affected. With MRI, enlargement of the tuber cinereum is seen with mild hyperintensity on T2-weighted images.

HISTIOCYTOSIS X   Also a disease of childhood, histiocytosis X may be primarily osseous or parenchymal. In the osseous form there may be either secondary invasion of the sellar region from local skull base lesions or localized masses in the hypothalamus without bone involvement. Nodularity and/or thickening of the stalk are the typical MRI features. T2-weighted images show hyperintensity in affected areas. The lesions are often radioresponsive and diminish considerably in size after treatment.

ARACHNOID CYST   This entity has been described earlier. It is important to consider the arachnoid cyst in the differential diagnosis of suprasellar lesions; in particular, it must be distinguished from an empty sella. The walls of this cyst are thin and the intensity of the fluid contents is identical to that of CSF in the basal cisterns; therefore, separation from the surrounding suprasellar cistern is difficult. Subtle evidence of mass effect may be the only evidence of a space-occupying lesion (Fig. 2.34). Large suprasellar arachnoid cysts may cause hydrocephalus by compression of the third ventricle.

EMPTY SELLA TURCICA   The empty sella turcica may be discovered either as an incidental finding on MRI performed for an unrelated reason or when the patient is referred to MRI because of radiographic findings of an enlarged sella turcica. The entity is common and is of no clinical significance except in rare circumstances. It is due to a deficiency in the diaphragma sella. Magnetic resonance imaging clearly shows the fluid-filled sella turcica in direct communication with the suprasellar cistern. The pituitary gland is flattened into a semilunar shape along the floor of the sella turcica (Fig. 2.35). The sella turcica may be of normal size or enlarged. The pituitary stalk must be closely scrutinized and should have a straight course from the tuber cinereum to the gland. If the stalk cannot be identified or is significantly deviated from its expected course, an intrasellar cyst should be suspected.

INFLAMMATION

As in other areas, inflammatory lesions in and around the sella turcica can be considered in two groups: infectious and noninfectious. In the sella turcica, however, neither form is particularly common. Also similar to other areas, inflammatory lesions in the sella turcica can be categorized by the structure involved—the pituitary gland, the basal meninges, or the cavernous sinus.

Infection of the pituitary gland is extremely uncommon. Pituitary abscess usually occurs coincident with another intrasellar mass, in association with other local infection (e.g., sphenoid sinusitis) or in the postoperative setting. An intrasellar mass is evident if MRI is performed, but, short of surgical exploration, the diagnosis is rarely made.

Lymphocytic adenohypophysis is an unusual noninfectious inflammatory condition involving the pituitary gland. It is thought to be due to a type of autoimmune reaction against the gland and is almost exclusively seen in postpartum women. The gland is enlarged without evidence of any focal abnormality.

The basal meninges can be involved with purulent or granulomatous inflammation, the former entity having been previously discussed.

Tuberculous and fungal infection and sarcoidosis are the most common types of granulomatous meningitis, the latter not being a true infection but sharing similar histologic and imaging findings. In each of these types, the meninges may be thickened; there may also be associated lesions at the base, or in the parenchyma, of the brain (Fig. 2.36), or there may be obstructive hydrocephalus due to interference with normal CSF absorption.

Granulomatous inflammation in the cavernous sinus results in a painful ophthalmoplegia and venous distention in the ipsilateral eye. The pathology is identical to that seen with orbital pseudotumor. Magnetic resonance imaging shows an enlarged cavernous sinus that is usually slightly hypointense on T2-weighted images.

PARASELLAR ANEURYSMS

Intracranial aneurysms have been previously discussed (Chapter 1). It is important to consider them at this point for one main reason, namely, to ensure consideration of them in the differential diagnosis of intrasellar and parasellar masses. As discussed earlier, the appearance of aneurysms depends on their size and their status as patent or thrombosed. In either case, the aneurysm can, more often than not, be readily differentiated from solid lesions—the patent aneurysm, by the presence of the signal void within the vessel lumen (Fig. 2.37), and the throm-

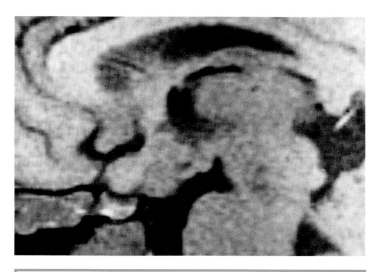

Fig. 2.36 SARCOIDOSIS T1-weighted sagittal image. A lobulated mass envelopes the optic chiasm. The appearance is more that of a neoplasm than an inflammatory process. A biopsy demonstrated the typical noncaseating granulomas of sarcoidosis. All cultures were negative.

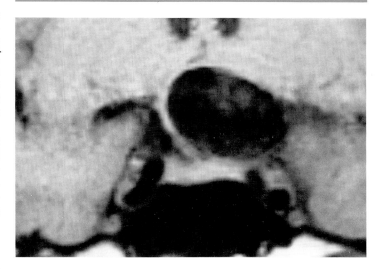

Fig. 2.37 SUPRASELLAR ANEURYSM T1-weighted coronal image. There is a large aneurysm on the left side of the suprasellar cistern, originating from the left internal carotid artery (supraclinoid portion). The signal void in the aneurysm indicates that it is patent. (The gray signal in the aneurysm is due to motion-induced artifact.)

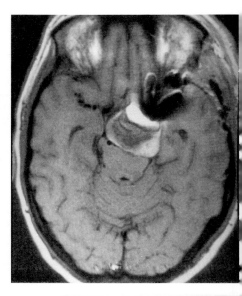

Fig. 2.38 THROMBOSED CAROTID ARTERY ANEURYSM T1-weighted axial image. A left, internal carotid artery aneurysm has been surgically clipped. Artifact from the clip is present at the carotid artery termination, but it does not obscure visualization of the aneurysm. The aneurysm lumen is filled with clot of different ages. There is no suggestion of flow that would indicate incomplete surgical occlusion of the aneurysm neck.

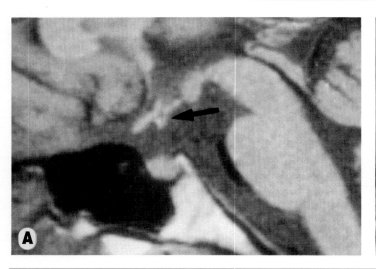

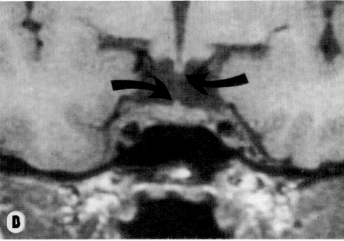

Fig. 2.39 TRAUMATIC DISRUPTION OF THE PITUITARY STALK (A) T1-weighted sagittal image. This teen-aged male developed diabetes insipidus after a motor vehicle accident. The distance between the tuber cinereum and the pituitary gland is increased, and only the proximal stalk is seen. The hyperintensity normally seen in the posterior lobe is absent. **(B)** T1-weighted coronal image. The discontinuity between the proximal and distal stumps of the pituitary stalk is obvious (arrows).

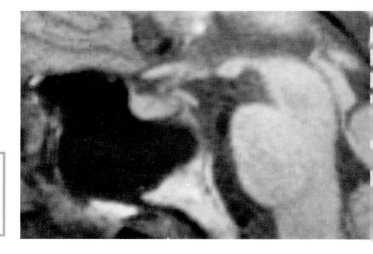

Fig. 2.40 CENTRAL DIABETES INSIPIDUS T1-weighted sagittal image. The sella turcica and pituitary gland are normal in size and shape. The hyperintensity normally found in the posterior lobe is absent. The stalk is normal.

bosed aneurysm, by the high signal of the clot on the T1-weighted image (Fig. 2.38). A small aneurysm, however, may be difficult or impossible to detect, or the scan appearance may be incorrectly attributed to a vascular loop. Close scrutiny of the intrasellar contents and surrounding vessels is required to prevent a serious error in interpretation.

TRAUMA

Skull base fractures involving the sella turcica and sphenoid bone are best evaluated with thin section CT. The use of MRI for this purpose is clearly limited. However, interesting observations on the appearance of the pituitary gland and stalk have been made. Generally, damage to the pituitary gland and stalk only occurs with severe head trauma, usually so severe that most patients die or remain in a permanent vegetative state and the pituitary damage incurred remains an unappreciated event. In a few instances, disruption of the pituitary stalk has been documented, due to shear forces at the level of the diaphragma resulting from rapid deceleration (Fig. 2.39). The pituitary gland may infarct, but this has not been observed in patients, presumably because those so affected do not survive the trauma.

DIABETES INSIPIDUS

There are two forms of diabetes insipidus. The central form is due to a disturbance of vasopressin production or release. The nephrogenic form is due to end-organ (the collecting tubule of the kidney) unresponsiveness. The latter is not discussed here. The central form of diabetes insipidus may be due either to primary failure of the hypothalamic nuclei to produce vasopressin or to interruption or destruction of part of the transport pathway from the hypothalamus to the posterior lobe of the pituitary gland. Whichever cause is attributed in a given case, the normal high signal intensity present on the T1-weighted images of the posterior lobe of the pituitary gland is absent (Fig. 2.40). One might conclude that the posterior lobe high signal represents either vasopressin or material related to it, e.g., a carrier protein or a membrane-bound lipid.

In the idiopathic, central form there are no other findings and, interestingly, no lesions of the hypothalamus have been observed. In the cases of diabetes insipidus due to tumor, histiocytosis, inflammation, or trauma, there is usually some evidence of the primary disease.

● ●

THE TEMPORAL BONE

NORMAL ANATOMY (Figs. 2.41 and 2.42)

The temporal bone has four major parts: squamous, mastoid, tympanic, and petrous. The squamous portion is a large, flat bone that forms part of the floor of the middle cranial fossa. It is relatively featureless and is of little radiologic interest. The mastoid portion, composed of tiny air cells, extends posteroinferiorly from the external auditory canal, the tympanic cavity, and the pinna. The tympanic and petrous portions are the most complex and interesting. Together, they resemble a horizontal pyramid, with the base of the pyramid forming part of the lateral skull and its apex pointing medially. They contain the internal and external auditory canals, tympanic cavity, the ossicles, the vestibule, the cochlea, the semicircular canals, the facial nerve, the geniculate ganglion, and portions of the eustachian tube and carotid canal. With the exception of the ossicles, all of these structures by virtue of MRI are visible to a greater or lesser degree. The most identifiable landmarks are the horizontally oriented internal and external auditory canals. At the lateral end of the internal auditory canal, several small structures are present, apparent because of the fluid they contain. The vestibule, the largest of these structures, forms the anchor for the three semicircular canals. The semicircular canals are all oriented orthogonally with respect to one another. Only a portion of any of the canals is seen on any one image, due to their oblique orientation to conventional scan planes. The cochlea is immediately anterior to the vestibule. Lateral to the vestibule is the tympanic cavity.

Of particular importance are the vestibulocochlear and facial nerves (cranial nerves VIII and VII, respectively). Together, they emerge from the internal auditory canal, traverse the cerebellopontine angle cistern, and course medially to the pontomedullary junction. In most cases, the nerves are distinctly seen in the cistern and well into the internal auditory canal. The eighth nerve consists of three divisions—the cochlear nerve and the inferior and superior vestibular nerves—all terminating with small branches at the vestibule and cochlea. The facial nerve follows a more complex route, divided into four segments: intracanalicular (in the internal auditory canal), labyrinthine (between the internal auditory canal and geniculate ganglion), tympanic (between the geniculate ganglion and the posterior genu), and mastoid (between the posterior genu and the stylomastoid foramen). The labyrinthine segment is in the true transverse plane and is angled about 45° anteriorly. The geniculate ganglion, visible as a slight enlargement of the nerve, gives origin to the greater petrosal nerve. At the ganglion, the course of the nerve turns abruptly posteriorly (the anterior genu) and runs in the same transverse plane, but posteriorly. Just posterior to the vestibule, the nerve again turns suddenly, but this time downwards (the posterior genu). It then travels in the vertical plane and exits in the stylomastoid foramen. An understanding of the facial nerve's complex path is necessary to select the optimal image plane for demonstrating facial nerve pathology.

The Temporal Bone

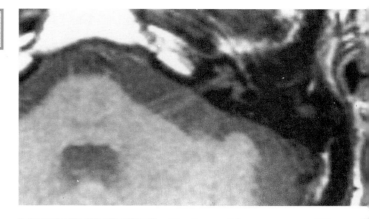

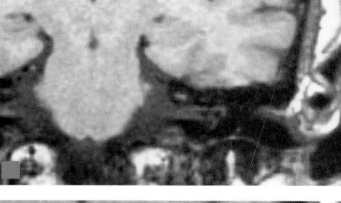

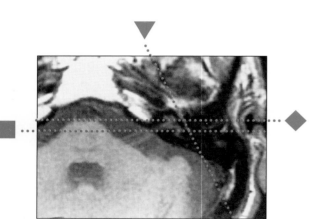

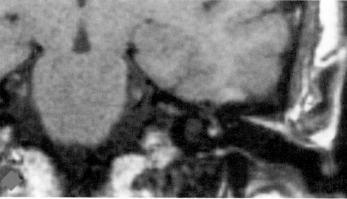

Fig. 2.41 Localizer: T1-Weighted Axial Image Through the Internal Auditory Canal The planes of section of three images are indicated: coronal images through the internal and external auditory canals, and an oblique sagittal view of the facial nerve. The axial image through the internal auditory canal is labeled in figure 2.42A.

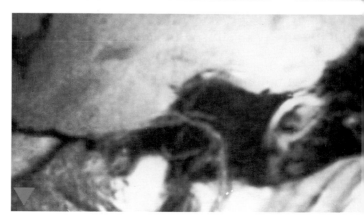

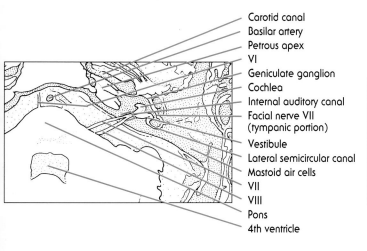

Carotid canal
Basilar artery
Petrous apex
VI
Geniculate ganglion
Cochlea
Internal auditory canal
Facial nerve VII
(tympanic portion)
Vestibule
Lateral semicircular canal
Mastoid air cells
VII
VIII
Pons
4th ventricle

Fig. 2.42A T1-Weighted Axial Image Through the Internal Auditory Canal Cranial nerves VII and VIII are clearly visualized in the cerebellopontine angle cistern as they enter the internal auditory canal. Their separation is not as distinct within the canal. The lateral margin of the canal is delineated by the cochlea and vestibule. Lateral to these structures is the tympanic portion of the facial nerve canal.

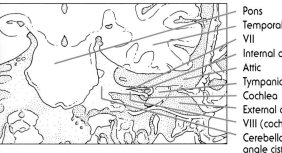

Pons
Temporal lobe
VII
Internal auditory canal
Attic
Tympanic cavity
Cochlea
External auditory canal
VIII (cochlear division)
Cerebellopontine angle cistern

Fig. 2.42B T1-Weighted Coronal Image Through the Internal Auditory Canal The individual nerves within the internal auditory canal are visible. The facial nerve is superior, the cochlear division of cranial nerve VIII is inferior. A portion of the external auditory canal is also visible.

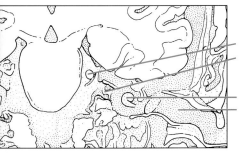

V
Opening of internal auditory canal (porus acusticus)
Cochlea
External auditory canal

Fig. 2.42C T1-Weighted Coronal Image of the External Auditory Canal The external canal is visualized in its full length. Medially, it is delineated by the tympanic cavity. Medial to the tympanic cavity is the cochlea.

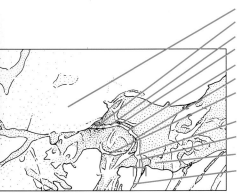

Temporal lobe
Tensor tympani muscle
Geniculate ganglion
Anterior genu
Tympanic segment
Posterior genu
Floor of external auditory canal
Mastoid segment
Stylomastoid foramen
Mastoid air cells
Facial nerve VII (extracranial segment)

Fig. 2.42D T1-Weighted Oblique Sagittal View of the Facial Nerve This view is obtained by aligning the image plane along the course of the tympanic portion of the facial nerve (as seen on the axial image). It demonstrates the entire horizontal and descending portions of the facial nerve canal in one plane. The nerve exits through the stylomastoid foramen.

TECHNIQUE

In most cases, the thinnest possible sections are used; usually, T1-weighted images suffice. Axial sections are the standard, with coronals serving as a frequent supplement, particularly where there is concern that the lesion extends upwards into the cranial cavity or downwards through the skull base. An especially useful image plane for evaluation of facial nerve dysfunction is an oblique sagittal image that is oriented in the axis of the horizontal portion of the facial nerve canal. This plane allows the entire facial nerve—an area from the geniculate ganglion to its exit from the skull at the stylomastoid foramen—to be visualized in one image.

The cerebellopontine angle and internal auditory canal are also best examined with a T1-weighted technique. Personal preference dictates whether axial or coronal sections are used but it is not necessary to use both. T2-weighted images are added in the event that the tumor is atypical or large. T2-weighted images are necessary as well, where the examination is normal

and the brainstem needs to be scrutinized, because some intrinsic brainstem pathology can clinically mimic an acoustic neuroma.

PATHOLOGY

CONGENITAL MALFORMATIONS   Most congenital malformations of the temporal bone are best characterized by analysis of the osseous anatomy, thus, thin-section CT, with its superb fine bone detail, is the mainstay of diagnosis. Magnetic resonance imaging has no significant diagnostic role for these types of disorders.

NEOPLASMS
THE PINNA AND EXTERNAL AUDITORY CANAL There are many histologic variants of tumors affecting the external ear. The benign tumors are most commonly hemangiomas, adenomas, osteomas, and exostoses. These tumors are accessible to direct visu-

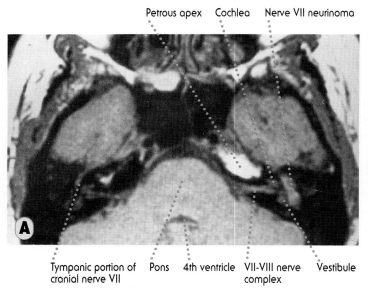

Petrous apex   Cochlea   Nerve VII neurinoma

Tympanic portion of cranial nerve VII   Pons   4th ventricle   VII-VIII nerve complex   Vestibule

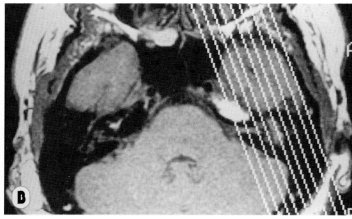

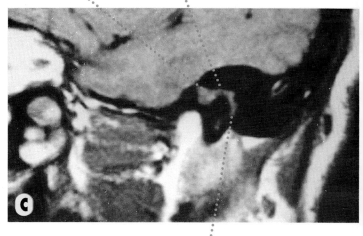

Geniculate ganglion   Nerve VII neurinoma (tympanic portion)

Nerve VII tumor (mastoid portion)

Fig. 2.43 FACIAL NERVE NEURINOMA   (A) T1-weighted axial image. This patient presented with conductive hearing loss on the left side. There is an oblong mass in the horizontal (tympanic) portion of the left facial nerve canal. **(B)** T1-weighted axial image. The axial section is used as a scout view for determining the obliquity of the next set of images of the facial nerve. **(C)** T1-weighted oblique image. This plane of section demonstrates the horizontal and vertical segments of the facial nerve tumor in a single image. The tumor extends from the geniculate ganglion to the midportion of the vertical segment of the facial nerve.

al inspection. The only function of MRI (or CT) is to determine the deep extension of the tumor, and, even then, usually only if surgery is planned. Squamous cell carcinoma and basal cell carcinoma of the skin are the most common malignant tumors of the external ear. Diagnosis is usually by biopsy; in the case of benign tumors, imaging is reserved for staging.

THE MIDDLE EAR (TYMPANIC CAVITY) AND FACIAL NERVE CANAL Hemangioma, glomus tympanicum, and facial nerve schwannoma are the most common benign tumors that occur in or near to the tympanic cavity. Clinical presentations include tinnitus, conductive hearing loss, and facial paralysis. Otoscopic examination may demonstrate a nodule or mass behind the tympanic membrane. Magnetic resonance imaging has an important diagnostic function, not only in confirming the clinical diagnosis of tumor but occasionally allowing for a specific diagnosis, particularly in the case of glomus tympanicum and facial neurinoma. The former is discussed in the general context of glomus tumors (see section on Posterior Fossa).

Neurinomas may involve any part of the facial nerve, with some predilection to the region of the geniculate ganglion. Patients present with facial paralysis, hearing loss, or disturbances of taste, tearing, or salivation. On CT images, these conditions are characterized by benign expansion of the facial nerve canal. Magnetic resonance imaging shows the bony canal poorly, but the nerve is superbly demonstrated. Therefore, any tumorous enlargement is also well-seen. The tumor can extend along the facial nerve canal or possibly break out of this thin bony canal into the adjacent tympanic cavity or mastoid air cells. Facial neurinomas are indistinguishable from acoustic neurinomas if located in the internal auditory canal; the diagnosis is straightforward, though, if the tumor is in the facial nerve canal. Neurinomas are isointense on the T1-weighted sections and hyperintense on the T2-weighted sections. A combination of images in both the axial plane and the oblique sagittal plane along the axis of the nerve is the optimal means for displaying the full extent of the tumor (Fig. 2.43).

Malignant tumors of the middle ear are rare. In adults, such tumors are usually manifested as squamous cell or adenocarcinoma; in children, rhabdomyosarcoma.

THE PETROUS PYRAMID (APEX) The petrous portion of the temporal bone is an uncommon site for neoplasms. Those that do occur are tumors of osseous or cartilaginous origin or tumors that arise from embryonic rests (e.g., epidermoidoma). The most common of these are the chondroma, osteochondroma, and chondrosarcoma. These tumors present because of compression of either the adjacent brainstem or the cranial nerves. The diagnosis is confirmed by the appearance of a primarily bony tumor originating from the skull base.

THE INTERNAL AUDITORY CANAL
ACOUSTIC NEURINOMAS These neurinomas constitute 5% to 10% of all intracranial tumors and occur predominantly in middle-aged and older patients, females outnumbering males two to one. Such tumors usually originate from the peripheral portion of the vestibular nerve. They are schwannomas histologically. They are always located at the porus acusticus and may either grow preferentially into the cerebellopontine angle cistern or laterally into the internal auditory canal. A valuable differential feature is enlargement of the bony internal auditory canal, which is not usually seen with other types of tumors.

The acoustic neurinoma is typically a well-circumscribed tumor, usually 1 to 4 cm in size. It is best seen on a T1-weighted image, because the contrast is better on this particular sequence between the tumor and surrounding CSF in the cistern (Fig. 2.44). On T2-weighted images, the tumor is typi-

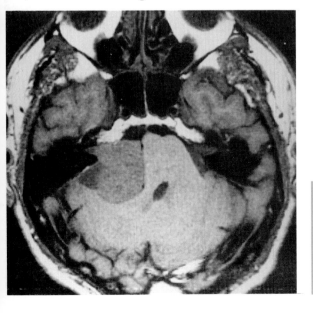

Fig. 2.44 ACOUSTIC NEURINOMA T1-weighted axial image. The tumor has two components—one in the right cerebellopontine angle cistern and the other in the right internal auditory canal. The tumor's extension into the internal auditory canal is the most diagnostically useful finding, as it distinguishes the acoustic neurinoma from other cerebellopontine angle tumors.

cally brighter than nearby brain but may be isointense with CSF. These tumors enhance intensely with contrast agents (Fig. 2.45). Larger tumors are equally well seen on T1- and T2-weighted images. It is important to use high resolution techniques when examining the internal auditory canal. Thick sections or coarse matrix sizes may result in spatial resolution inadequate for the detection of small tumors. A contrast-enhanced form of MRI is indicated where the noncontrast study is negative or equivocal in ruling out an intracanalicular tumor (Fig. 2.45).

The most significant differential diagnosis for these tumors includes meningioma (Fig. 2.46), other neurinomas (of cranial nerve VII or V), aneurysms of the anterior-inferior cerebellar artery, dural metastases, arachnoid cysts (Fig. 2.47), and epidermoid tumors. Usually the anatomical and intensity characteristics of the lesion are sufficiently characteristic to permit an unambiguous diagnosis.

INFECTION
External otitis is a benign, self-limited illness confined to inflammation of the skin and the mucous membrane of the external canal. There are significant exceptions to this definition, particularly the entity referred to as *malignant external otitis*, an aggressive gram-negative bacterial infection (usually *Pseudomonas*) most commonly seen in diabetics. This

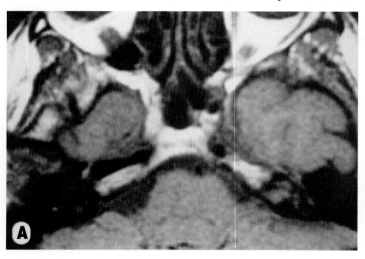
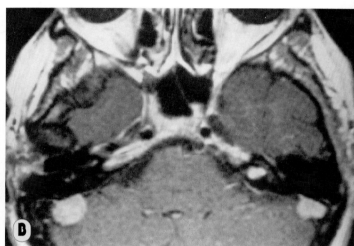

Fig. 2.45 ACOUSTIC NEURINOMA (INTRACANALICULAR) (A) T1-weighted axial image. A small isointense mass is in the left internal auditory canal. The normal nerve roots cannot be identified in the left internal auditory canal, and the right internal auditory canal is not in the plane of section because of slight head tilt. **(B)** T1-weighted axial image (post-gadolinium-DTPA).

The intracanalicular neurinoma in the left internal auditory canal enhances intensely, allowing a much more confident diagnosis of acoustic neurinoma. Two small bilateral meningiomas were incidentally discovered on the same scan, findings that led to a diagnosis of neurofibromatosis in this patient.

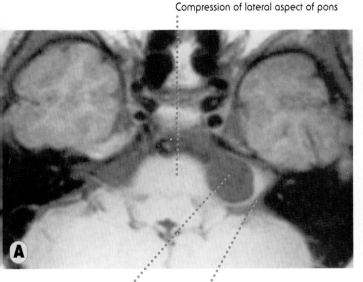

Basilar artery   Tympanic portion of nerve VII

Pons   Cranial nerve VII-VIII complex   Meningioma

Fig. 2.46 MENINGIOMA—CEREBELLOPONTINE ANGLE
T1-weighted axial image. There is an ovoid, extraaxial tumor isointense to the brain in the left cerebellopontine angle. The tumor is posterior to the internal auditory canal and can be clearly separated from cranial nerve VIII. This latter finding distinguishes this meningioma from an acoustic neurinoma.

Compression of lateral aspect of pons

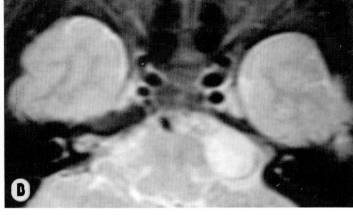

Arachnoid cyst   Displaced nerve VII-VIII complex

Fig. 2.47 ARACHNOID CYST (A) T1-weighted axial image. The cyst is isointense to CSF and has imperceptibly thin walls. It compresses the lateral aspect of the pons and displaces the cranial nerve VII–VIII complex posteriorly. **(B)** T2-weighted axial image. The cyst remains isointense to CSF on T2-weighted images, typical of a simple arachnoid cyst.

infection involves the deep soft tissues and may destroy the bone. Radiologically, it is indistinguishable from an aggressive neoplasm (Fig. 2.48).

Otitis media is characterized by fluid accumulation in the tympanic cavity. It may be associated with mastoiditis, in which case fluid may be seen in the mastoid air cells and/or the eustachian tube. There is little need to image these cases, but if fluid in the tympanic or mastoid cavities is noted during the course of an examination, the radiologist should confirm that there is no mass obstructing the middle ear or the eustachian tube (Fig. 2.49).

Cholesteatoma is the inflammatory disease most often requiring detailed investigation. It is due to benign epithelial proliferation at the margin of the tympanic membrane. They originate at the scutum in the posterior-superior quadrant of the tympanic membrane. The earliest imaging signs are erosion of the bony scutum, the ossicles, or the Korner's septum, usually accompanied by a small, soft tissue mass. These signs are all better evaluated with CT, which continues to be the method of choice (Fig. 2.50). Magnetic resonance imaging, to date, has not added any significant information in the investigation of this disease.

Infection infiltrating bony walls
of canal and tympanic cavity   Internal auditory canal

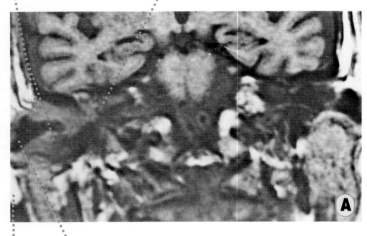

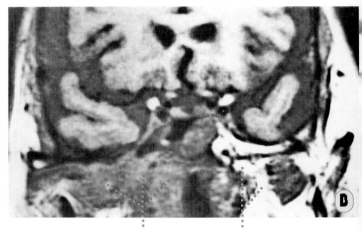

Ear   External auditory canal

Infiltrative soft
tissue infection   Normal parapharyngeal
fat planes

Fig. 2.48 "MALIGNANT" OTITIS EXTERNA T1-weighted coronal images. The infection originates in the external auditory canal but is extremely aggressive. Here it has infiltrated deep into the skull base and nasopharynx.

"Malignant" refers to the severe morbidity associated with this infection, but a more accurate term is *otogenic osteomyelitis*. (Courtesy of Dr. Anton Hasso)

Petrous apex   Glomus tympanicum

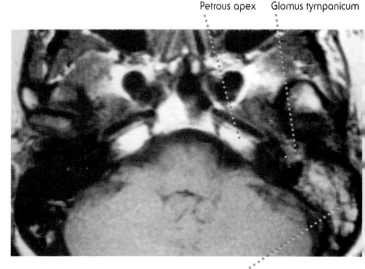

Fig. 2.49 GLOMUS TYMPANICUM AND OBSTRUCTED MASTOID CAVITY T1-weighted axial image. A small isointense mass, the glomus tumor, fills the left tympanic cavity. The mastoid air cells are filled with hemorrhagic fluid. Hemorrhage, usually of a petechial nature, is common in obstructed sinuses, whatever the cause of the obstruction.

Obstructed mastoid cavity

Cholesteatoma

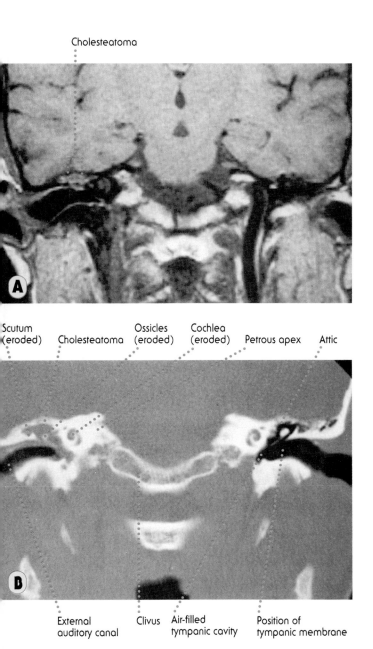

Scutum   Ossicles   Cochlea
(eroded)   Cholesteatoma   (eroded)   (eroded)   Petrous apex   Attic

External   Clivus   Air-filled   Position of
auditory canal   tympanic cavity   tympanic membrane

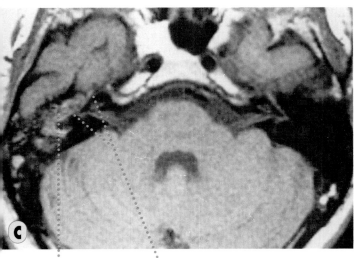

Cholesteatoma   Facial nerve

Fig. 2.50 CHOLESTEATOMA **(A)** T1-weighted coronal image. The lesion is an intermediate gray, located in the tympanic cavity, extending into the attic. Early cholesteatomas are evident only by subtle bony erosion, a finding that is impossible to visualize on MRI. Computed tomography is the preferred modality. **(B)** Coronal CT scan (1.5-mm section). This high resolution scan demonstrates the superior fine bone detail possible with CT. **(C)** T1-weighted axial image. One useful feature of MRI for the assessment of cholesteatomas is the ability to clearly define the relationship of the lesion to the facial nerve. At surgery, the lesion involved the lateral aspect of the facial nerve canal but did not encase the nerve.

An unusual tumor-like condition peculiar to the petrous apex is the cholesterol granuloma. Pathologically, it is characterized as a well-defined, expansile, intraosseous mass centered in the petrous apex. It contains an accumulation of inflammatory debris and hemosiderin-laden macrophages. It is thought to be secondary to obstruction of air cells in the petrous apex. The contralateral petrous apex is usually air-filled. The MRI appearance is almost pathognomonic: an expansile lesion, homogeneous, and hyperintense on both T1- and T2-weighted images (Fig. 2.51).

VASCULAR LESIONS AND VARIANTS

Aneurysms and aberrant vessels are the most important entities in this category. Aneurysms within the skull base are rare, but their appearance is absolutely typical—a round lesion void of signal (Fig. 2.52).

There are two significant vascular variants of normal that require recognition. One is the aberrant carotid artery and the other is the high-riding jugular bulb. The high contrast with which large blood vessels are seen with MRI facilitates the recognition of all vascular structures.

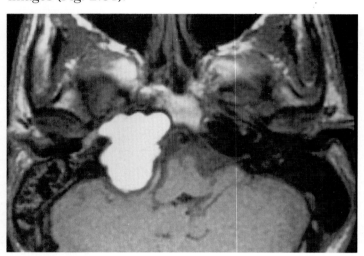

Fig. 2.51 CHOLESTEROL GRANULOMA   T1-weighted axial image. A well-defined expansile mass arises from the right petrous apex. The lesion extends anteriorly into the carotid canal and medially into the clivus; it posteriorly compresses the cerebellum. The location and marked hyperintensity are characteristic of this entity.

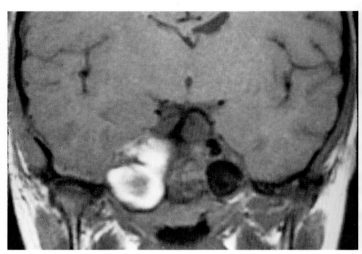

Fig. 2.52   BILATERAL CAROTID ANEURYSMS —PETROUS BONE   T1-weighted coronal image. The right petrous temporal bone was surgically explored, because a CT scan (not shown) demonstrated an enhancing intraosseous lesion, subsequently proved to be an aneurysm. Substantial bleeding was encountered during the operation as the aneurysm was approached, necessitating ligation of the internal carotid artery. The right-sided aneurysm is thrombosed, the left demonstrates the typical flow void of an arterial lesion.

THE POSTERIOR CRANIAL FOSSA

NORMAL ANATOMY (Figs. 2.53 to 2.58)

The base of the posterior fossa extends from the dorsum sellae, posteriorly down along the intracranial surface of the clivus (the basiocciput) to the foramen magnum, and then up along the squamous portion of the occipital bone to the level of the internal occipital protuberance. By and large, all of the structures of interest are in the anterior half of this fossa. They are the subject of the discussion that follows. The petrous portion of the temporal bone forms the anterolateral boundary of the posterior fossa and, along with the internal auditory canal, has been discussed in the previous section.

The clivus is a midline structure extending from the dorsum sellae to the anterior margin of the foramen magnum. It is formed by the sphenoid and occipital bones, which join at the sphenooccipital synchondrosis. This is visible as an obliquely oriented line within the clivus on sagittal sections. The clivus itself is thicker than most of the bones of the skull base as it contains a generous marrow space. On T1-weighted images in adults, the clivus appears bright due to the presence of marrow fat. In children, the marrow space is of intermediate intensity, typical of most of the immature skeleton that is still actively involved in hematopoiesis.

Meckel's cave is a CSF-filled dural invagination immediately lateral to the clivus between the dorsum sellae and the petrous tip. It houses the gasserian ganglion. Cranial nerve V can consistently be visualized crossing the lower prepontine cistern from the brainstem to this ganglion.

The internal auditory canal is a horizontally oriented canal in the temporal bone, which runs directly lateral at the level of the pontomedullary junction. It and its contents have been discussed.

Immediately inferior to the internal auditory canal, the jugular foramen is found in the temporal-occipital suture. It is separated into two parts by the bony jugular spine. The pars nervosa is the anteromedial part of the foramen transmitting cranial nerve IX and the inferior petrosal sinus. Posteriorly, the pars vascularis transmits cranial nerves X and XI and the sigmoid sinus. The inferior petrosal and the sigmoid sinuses join at the jugular foramen to form the internal jugular vein. The hypoglossal canal is inferior and medial to the jugular foramen and contains cranial nerve XII.

The foramen magnum is the largest of the basal foramina. The entire neuraxis passes through the foramen magnum. Anteriorly, the paired vertebral arteries enter the cranium through this foramen. Although the arteries are paired structures, they are usually asymmetric in size. The cervicomedullary junction should lie at the level of the foramen magnum and the entire cerebellum should be at or above this plane.

Normal Anatomy of the Skull Base (Figs. 2.53 to 2.58)

The Posterior Cranial Fossa

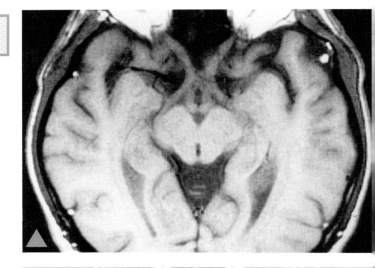

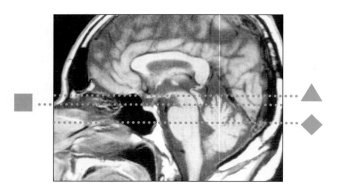

Fig. 2.53 Localizer: Midline T1-Weighted Sagittal Image
The planes of section of three axial images are indicated: through the optic nerves and tracts, cranial nerve III, and cranial nerve V.

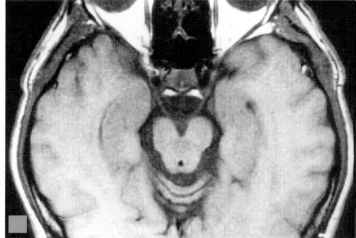

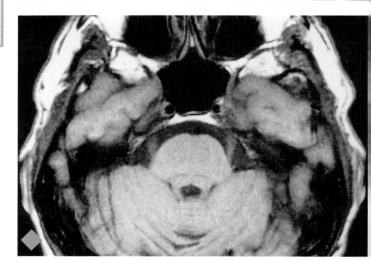

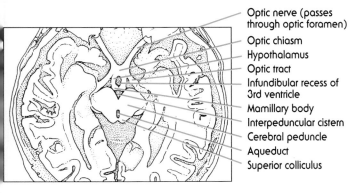

Optic nerve (passes
through optic foramen)
Optic chiasm
Hypothalamus
Optic tract
Infundibular recess of
3rd ventricle
Mamillary body
Interpeduncular cistern
Cerebral peduncle
Aqueduct
Superior colliculus

Fig. 2.54A T1-Weighted Axial Image Through the Optic Nerves and Tracts The optic nerves, chiasm, and tracts are displayed in their full length. Immediately posterior to the optic chiasm lies the infundibular recess of the third ventricle, its walls being formed by the inferior hypothalamus. Posterior to this (in succession) are the mamillary bodies, the interpeduncular cistern, and the upper midbrain.

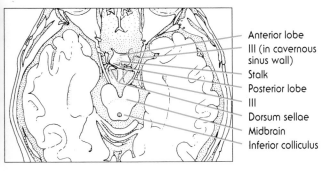

Anterior lobe
III (in cavernous
sinus wall)
Stalk
Posterior lobe
III
Dorsum sellae
Midbrain
Inferior colliculus

Fig. 2.54B T1-Weighted Axial Image Through the Level of Cranial Nerve III Cranial nerve III exits the midbrain through the interpeduncular cistern and enters the lateral wall of the cavernous sinus. The full intracranial courses is visualized herein. Marrow within the dorsum sellae is visible as a hyperintense area demarcating the posterior margin of the sella turcica. The inferior portion of the pituitary stalk is seen as it attaches to the superior surface of the pituitary gland.

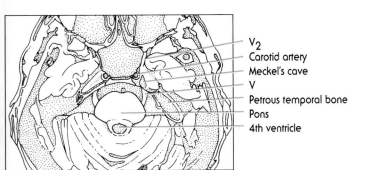

V₂
Carotid artery
Meckel's cave
V
Petrous temporal bone
Pons
4th ventricle

Fig. 2.54C T1-Weighted Axial Image Through Cranial Nerve V Cranial nerve V is one of the largest cranial nerves and has a course from the lateral aspect of the midpons, across the pontine cistern, and into Meckel's cave. At Meckel's cave, the third branch turns inferolaterally, whereas the first two branches are incorporated into the lateral wall of the cavernous sinus and extended anteriorly. The carotid arteries are seen at the point they enter the inferior aspect of the cavernous sinus.

The Posterior Cranial Fossa

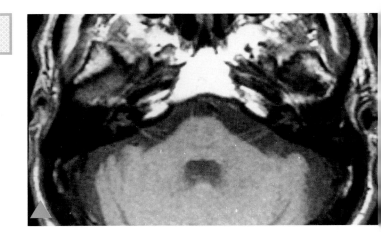

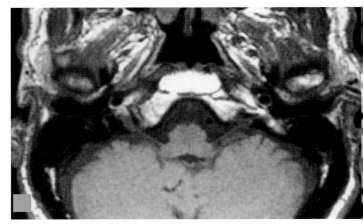

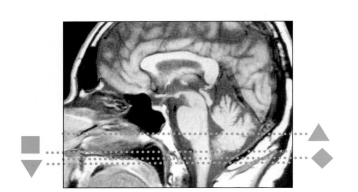

Fig. 2.55 Localizer: Midline T1-Weighted Sagittal Image
The planes of section of four axial sections are indicated: through the internal auditory canal, the jugular foramen, the hypoglossal canal, and the foramen magnum.

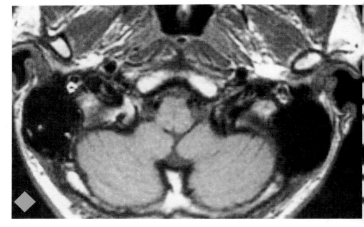

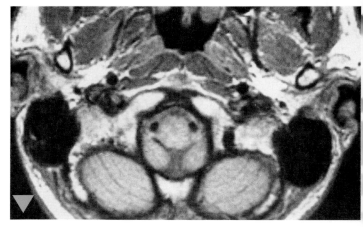

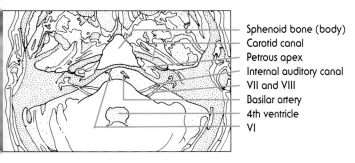

Sphenoid bone (body)
Carotid canal
Petrous apex
Internal auditory canal
VII and VIII
Basilar artery
4th ventricle
VI

Fig. 2.56A T1-Weighted Axial Image Through the Internal Auditory Canal   The basal skull anatomy at this level is complex. Cranial nerves VII and VIII are distinct structures traversing the cerebellopontine angle cistern to enter the internal auditory canal. At the lateral margin of the canal, the cochlea and vestibule are evident. Immediately lateral to this is the tympanic portion of the facial nerve canal. Just to the left of the midline is cranial nerve VI. The petrous temporal bones and the clivus form the anterior bony skull base at this level. Immediately anterior to the petrous apex is the horizontal portion of the carotid artery.

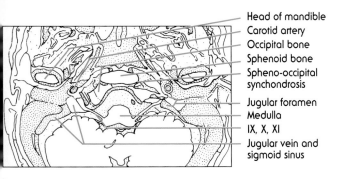

Head of mandible
Carotid artery
Occipital bone
Sphenoid bone
Spheno-occipital synchondrosis
Jugular foramen
Medulla
IX, X, XI
Jugular vein and sigmoid sinus

Fig. 2.56B T1-Weighted Axial Image Through the Jugular Foramen   Cranial nerves IX, X, and XI run as a conglomerate from the upper medulla anterolaterally into the anterior portion of the jugular foramen. The posterior half of the jugular foramen is occupied by the sigmoid sinus as it empties into the jugular vein. Immediately anterior to this is the carotid artery. The anteromedial border of the jugular foramen is formed by the jugular tubercle. The left vertebral artery is apparent in the medullary cistern. The right vertebral artery is hypoplastic.

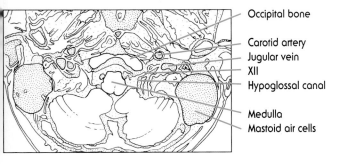

Occipital bone

Carotid artery
Jugular vein
XII
Hypoglossal canal

Medulla
Mastoid air cells

Fig. 2.56C T1-Weighted Axial Image Through the Hypoglossal Canal   The hypoglossal canal transmits cranial nerve XII. It is oriented anterolaterally.

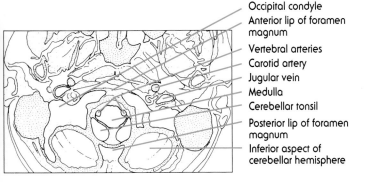

Occipital condyle
Anterior lip of foramen magnum
Vertebral arteries
Carotid artery
Jugular vein
Medulla
Cerebellar tonsil
Posterior lip of foramen magnum
Inferior aspect of cerebellar hemisphere

Fig. 2.56D T1-Weighted Axial Image Through the Foramen Magnum   The inferior aspect of the cerebellar tonsils are located at the level of the foramen magnum. The paired vertebral arteries are situated on either side of the medulla. The occipital condyles form the lateral border of the foramen magnum.

The Posterior Cranial Fossa

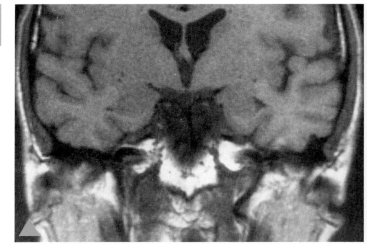

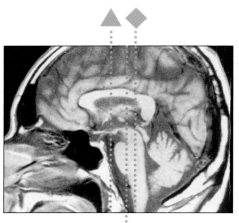

Fig. 2.57 Localizer: Midline T1-Weighted Sagittal Image
The planes of section of three coronal images are indicated: through the plane of the basilar artery, the belly of the pons, and the internal auditory canal.

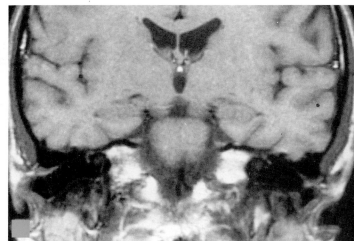

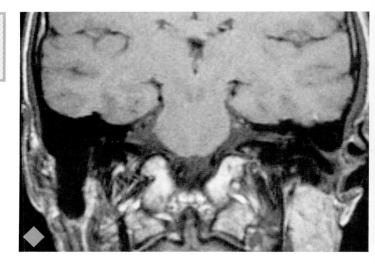

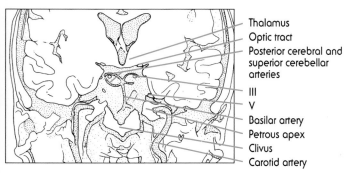

Thalamus
Optic tract
Posterior cerebral and superior cerebellar arteries
III
V
Basilar artery
Petrous apex
Clivus
Carotid artery

Fig. 2.58A T1-Weighted Coronal Image Through the Basilar Artery   The basilar artery terminates by bifurcating into the posterior cerebral arteries. Note the relationship of cranial nerve III to the terminal branches of the basilar artery—the nerve is interposed between the posterior cerebral artery and the superior cerebellar artery.

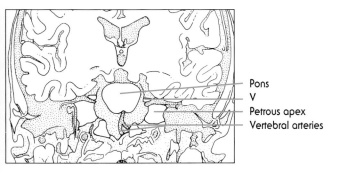

Pons
V
Petrous apex
Vertebral arteries

Fig. 2.58B T1-Weighted Coronal Image Through the Belly of the Pons   The confluence of the vertebral arteries is directly below the belly of the pons. Lateral to the pons, the large cranial nerve V is seen just posterior to Meckel's cave. The hyperintense signal beneath cranial nerve V is the marrow in the bone of the petrous apex.

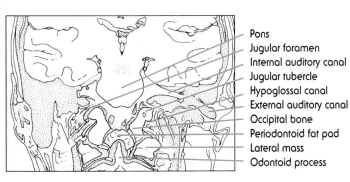

Pons
Jugular foramen
Internal auditory canal
Jugular tubercle
Hypoglossal canal
External auditory canal
Occipital bone
Periodontoid fat pad
Lateral mass
Odontoid process

Fig. 2.58C T1-Weighted Coronal Image Through the Internal Auditory Canal   The head is slightly turned such that the internal auditory canal is visualized on the left side, whereas the jugular foramen and the hypoglossal canal are visualized on the right side. The contents of the auditory canal are not well-visualized. However, the relationship of the jugular foramen and the hypoglossal canal to the jugular tubercle is demonstrated. Generally, these three structures—the internal auditory canal, the jugular foramen, and the hypoglossal canal—are all in the same coronal plane.

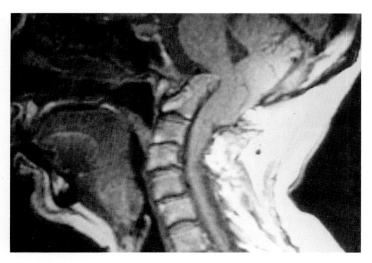

Fig. 2.59 BASILAR INVAGINATION (WITH CHIARI MALFORMATION) T1-weighted sagittal image. The foramen magnum is large and the cerebellar tonsils and brainstem are positioned below it. The odontoid process protrudes through the foramen, compressing the upper medulla. This bony deformity was readily apparent on plain radiography but the extent of brainstem compression could not be assessed.

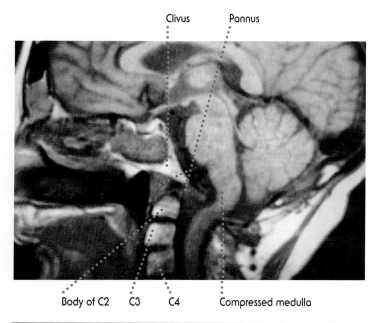

Clivus   Pannus

Body of C2   C3   C4   Compressed medulla

Fig. 2.60 RHEUMATOID ARTHRITIS T1-weighted sagittal image. The odontoid process and anterior arch of atlas are eroded by a soft tissue mass, presumed to be pannus. This results in craniocervical subluxation and compression of the brainstem.

TECHNIQUE

The clinical findings are very important in directing and individualizing the design of each examination. Generally, T1-weighted images are the principal sequences used, and extensive use is made of the thinnest possible sections targeted to the specific area of interest.

The clivus and foramen magnum are best examined with closely spaced, 3-mm-thick sagittal sections, supplemented with either axial or coronal sections through the level of the suspected pathology.

The jugular foramen is the most difficult area to examine properly, due to the venous structures in the foramen. Flow-related effects from these veins can mimic small tumors. T1-weighted axial and coronal sections should be performed in every case and should be done with presaturation pulses to ensure that the vessels remain free of flow-related enhancement effects. If an area is questionable, gradient-echo sequences can highlight vessels and separate them from solid structures. T2-weighted images are occasionally added.

T1-weighted sagittal images are the single most useful images for evaluation of the foramen magnum. They can be supplemented with either axial or coronal sections (using either a T1- or T2-weighted technique) to further define or lateralize any lesion discovered.

PATHOLOGY

BONY DEFORMITIES
BASILAR INVAGINATION By definition, this term refers to invagination of the margins of the foramen magnum into the skull base; however, in its more usual context, it is taken to mean invagination of the odontoid process above the level of the foramen magnum. It may be due to developmental bone anomalies or to acquired disorders that result in bone softening (osteomalacia, Paget's disease, fibrodysplasia, osteogenesis imperfecta), or bone destruction (tumor, infection). Basilar invagination occasionally results from trauma. In some diseases it is caused by multiple factors. For example, in rheumatoid arthritis it is caused

by bone softening, ligamentous instability, and erosive changes in the synovial joints. Basilar invagination may be associated with brainstem dysfunction due to compression of the medulla by the invaginated odontoid process.

The diagnosis is readily established by a routine lateral radiograph of the cervical spine, demonstrating the odontoid process that extends above the level of the foramen magnum. These same bone abnormalities can be visualized using MRI, due to the high intensity signal from the marrow of the bone (Fig. 2.59). Magnetic resonance imaging has the added benefit of being able to document the extent of compression of the brainstem and the nature of any associated pathologic processes, e.g., tumors or the pannus formation seen in rheumatoid arthritis (Fig. 2.60).

PLATYBASIA This term refers to the flattening of the skull base. It may be associated with basilar invagination, but as an isolated finding, it is insignificant.

NEOPLASMS

CHORDOMAS Chordomas originate from intraosseous remnants of the primitive notochord. They are located in the sacrum (50% of all cases), the clivus (40%), or the spinal column (10%). They are almost always midline and are frequently lobulated. Sacral and spinal chordomas are discussed in the chapter given to the spine. The current discussion is confined to clival chordomas.

Young adults are the age group most commonly affected. Patients usually present with cranial nerve palsies. Clival chordomas may extend posteriorly into the posterior fossa (with resultant brainstem compression), anteriorly into the sphenoid sinus or nasopharynx, or superiorly into the sella turcica. Magnetic resonance images demonstrate destruction of the marrow space of the clivus by tumor. This is best seen on T1-weighted sagittal images as an area of reduced signal in the normally high signal intensity marrow. Most have a lobulated contour and are bright on T2-weighted images (Fig. 2.61). Internally, the tumor tends to be nonhomogeneous. Calcification, which is common, appears as regions of signal dropout. Adjacent structures may be involved, as the tumor is locally invasive.

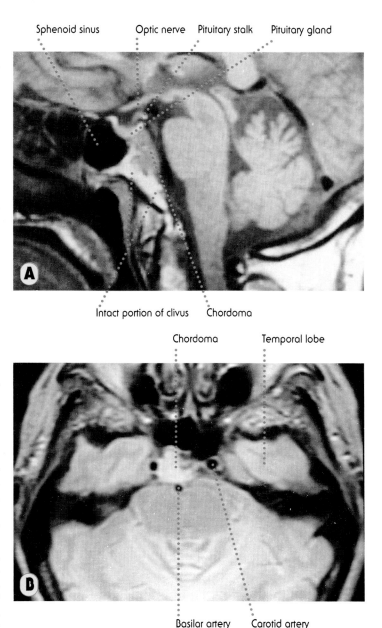

Fig. 2.61 CHORDOMA (A) T1-weighted sagittal image. The tumor causes irregular destruction of the normally uniform hyperintensity of the clivus. There is slight dorsal extension into the prepontine cistern. **(B)** T2-weighted axial image. Typical of most chordomas, this tumor is located at the midline and is hyperintense on T2-weighted images.

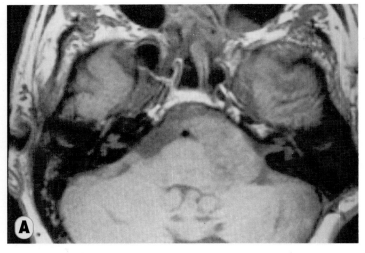

Basilar artery   Epidermoid tumor

Surface irregularities

Fig. 2.62 EPIDERMOID TUMOR (A) T1-weighted axial image. There is a large tumor in the left cerebellopontine angle cistern. It is hypointense to the brain but considerably brighter than the CSF. There is a wide differential—in particular, meningioma and neurinoma. **(B)** T2-weighted axial image. Now almost isointense to CSF, some surface irregularities are apparent on the tumor, evidencing an epidermoid tumor.

EPIDERMOID TUMOR   Epidermoid tumors are benign extraaxial tumors with an irregular, external surface. They have a thin epithelial lining and contain desquamated material usually rich in cholesterol crystals and keratin. Most intracranial epidermoid tumors are located in the cerebellopontine angle, temporal fossa, or parasellar region. They are most common in the fifth decade of life. Most epidermoidomas are distinctly hypointense on T1-weighted images and hyperintense on T2-weighted images (Fig. 2.62). Their irregular outline can occasionally be appreciated on MR images; they can be better defined with CT scanning, though, following subarachnoid injection of a contrast agent that fills the surface interstices of the tumor.

GLOMUS JUGULARE/GLOMUS TYMPANICUM TUMORS Glomus tumors are paragangliomas histologically related to the pheochromocytoma. In the skull base, the tumor may arise anywhere along the course of Jacobson's or Arnold's nerves—branches of the ninth and tenth cranial nerves, respectively, that extend from the jugular foramen to the region of the tympanic cavity. Symptoms classically are pulsatile tinnitus, hearing loss, or a jugular foramen syndrome. Magnetic resonance images show the well-defined tumor mass in either the jugular foramen, the tympanic cavity, or anywhere in between (Fig. 2.63, see also Fig. 2.49). The tumor may extend intracranially or along the jugular vein. Coronal images are particularly useful in demonstrating the latter. These tumors tend to be hyperintense on T2-weighted images, with punctate areas of reduced signal causing a speckled appearance. This inhomogeneity is preserved on contrast-enhanced studies (Fig. 2.64).

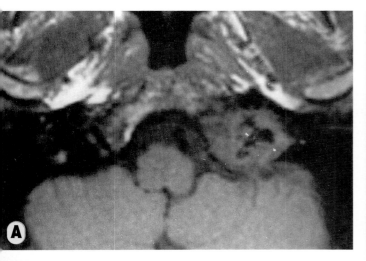

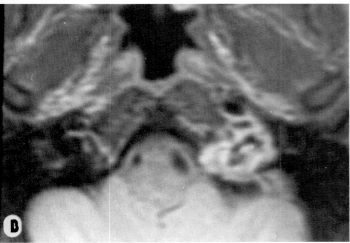

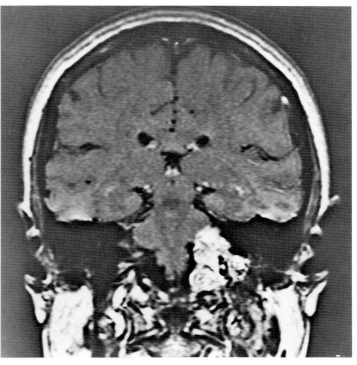

Fig. 2.64 GLOMUS JUGULARE TUMOR—CONTRAST ENHANCED T1-weighted coronal image. There is intense enhancement of the left glomus jugulare tumor. The nonuniformity of the tumor is a useful differential diagnostic feature, as it is uncommonly seen in neurinomas. (Courtesy of Dr. Anton Hasso)

Fig. 2.63 GLOMUS JUGULARE TUMOR **(A)** T1-weighted axial image. The glomus tumor is centered on the jugular foramen and extends into the basal cistern; it also invades the surrounding bone. Internally, it is coarsely inhomogeneous—a typical, but not specific, feature. **(B)** T2-weighted axial image. Hyperintensity and inhomogeneity ("speckling") are typical findings. Neurinomas can be similar in appearance but usually the speckling is much finer.

OTHER NEURINOMAS Acoustic and facial neurinomas have been discussed previously. Less common neurinomas are those originating from cranial nerves V, IX, X, XI, or XII. The fifth nerve neurinoma is the most prevalent of these; most are found in Meckel's cave or in the prepontine cistern (Fig. 2.65). The diagnosis of a neurinoma is made by establishing the relationship between the tumor and the cranial nerve. The major differential diagnosis is usually meningioma. Glomus jugulare may warrant particular consideration if the tumor is in the region of the jugular foramen (Fig. 2.66).

MENINGIOMA Meningioma must always be considered in the differential diagnosis of intracranial extraaxial tumors. The posterior fossa is no exception. The most common locations in the posterior fossa are the foramen magnum (Fig. 2.67), the cerebellopontine angle cistern, retroclival area, beneath the tentorium, and at the junction of the transverse and sigmoid sinuses.

METASTASES Metastases, like meningiomas, are ubiquitous. The bone marrow and meningeal surfaces may be involved. It is particularly important to closely examine these areas in patients with unexplained cranial nerve palsies (Fig. 2.68).

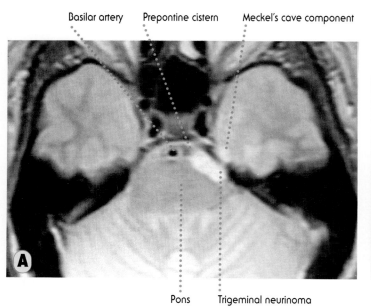

Basilar artery   Prepontine cistern   Meckel's cave component

Pons   Trigeminal neurinoma

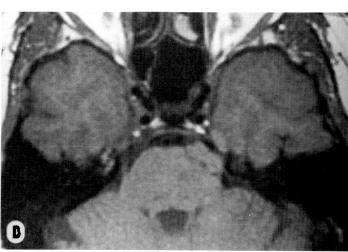

Fig. 2.65 TRIGEMINAL NEURINOMA (A) Proton density axial image. The hyperintense tumor is easily identified in the left prepontine cistern. The component extending into Meckel's cave, though more subtle, is an important diagnostic feature in that it indicates that the tumor follows the course of the trigeminal nerve. **(B)** T1-weighted axial image. The component of the tumor in Meckel's cave is more clearly demonstrated here than on the proton density image. **(C)** T1-weighted sagittal image. The tumor in the cistern is clearly evident, as is its extension into Meckel's cave.

Nerve V neurinoma

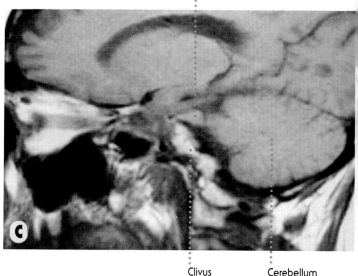

Clivus   Cerebellum

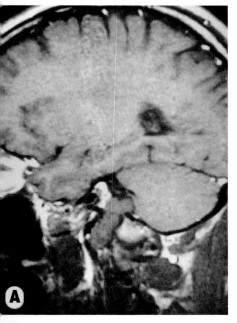

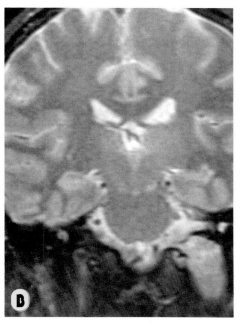

Fig. 2.66 JUGULAR FORAMEN NEURINOMA **(A)** T1-weighted sagittal image. The neurinoma is centered in the jugular foramen. It extends intracranially into the cistern and inferiorly along the neurovascular bundle. There is slight internal inhomogeneity. **(B)** T2-weighted coronal image. The tumor is moderately hyperintense and relatively uniform. Glomus tumors, the main differential, are usually much less uniform internally.

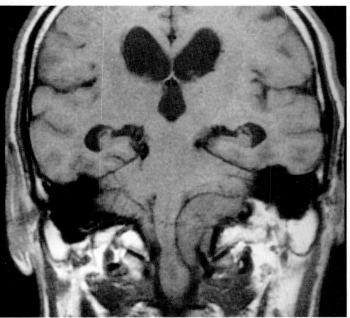

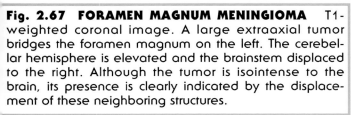

Fig. 2.67 FORAMEN MAGNUM MENINGIOMA T1-weighted coronal image. A large extraaxial tumor bridges the foramen magnum on the left. The cerebellar hemisphere is elevated and the brainstem displaced to the right. Although the tumor is isointense to the brain, its presence is clearly indicated by the displacement of these neighboring structures.

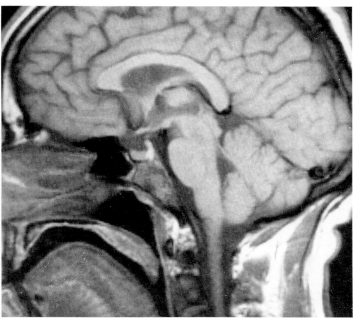

Fig. 2.68 CLIVUS METASTASIS FROM LUNG CARCINOMA T1-weighted sagittal image. The normal marrow hyperintensity of the clivus has been completely replaced by a low signal intensity tumor. This finding can be easily overlooked, because a distinct focal lesion is not evident.

BIBLIOGRAPHY

BOOKS

Mancuso AA, Hanafee WN. *Computed tomography and magnetic resonance imaging of the head and neck*, 2nd ed. Baltimore: Williams and Wilkins, 1985.
Newton TH, Hasso AN, Dillo WP, eds. *Modern neuroradiology: computed tomography of the head and neck*, vol 3. New York: Raven Press, 1988.
Wilson-Pauwels L, Akesson E, Stewart PA. *Cranial nerves: anatomy and clinical comment.* Burlington: BC Decker, 1988.

JOURNAL ARTICLES AND BOOK CHAPTERS

Atlas SW. Intracranial vascular malformations and aneurysms. Current imaging applications. *Radiol Clin North Am* 1988;26(4):821–837.
Berry I, Brant-Zawadzki M, Osaki L, et al. Gadolinium-DTPA in clinical MR of the brain: II. extra-axial lesions and normal structures. *AJNR* 1986;7:789.
Daniels DL, Czervianke LF, Pech P, et al. Gradient recalled echo MR imaging of the jugular foramen. *AJNR* 1988;9:675.
Davis PC, Friedman NC, Fry SM, et al. Leptomeningeal metastasis: MR imaging. *Radiology* 1987;163:449.
Dwyer AJ, Frank JA, Doppman JL, et al. Pituitary adenomas in patients with Cushing's disease: initial experience with gadolinium-DTPA-enhanced MR imaging. *Radiology* 1987;163:421.
Kucharczyk W, Davis DO, Kelly WM, et al. Pituitary adenomas: high resolution MR imaging at 1.5 T. *Radiology* 1986;161:761.
Kucharczyk W, Peck WW, Kelly WM, et al. Rathke cleft cysts: CT, MR imaging and pathologic features. *Radiology* 1987;165:491.
Mafee ME. Acoustic neurinoma and other acoustic nerve disorders: role of MRI and CT. *Semin US CT MR* 1987;8:256.
Pusey E, Kortman KE, Flannigan BD, et al. MR of craniopharyngiomas: tumor delineation and characterization. *AJNR* 1987;8:439.
Rhoton AL Jr. Microsurgical anatomy of the sellar region. In: Wilkins RH, Rengachany SS, eds. *Neurosurgery.* New York: McGraw Hill, 1985;811–191
Sze G, Uichanco LS, Brant-Zawadzki MN, et al. Chordomas: MR imaging. *Radiology* 1988;166:187–191.
Valvassori GE, Morales FG, Palacios E, et al. MR of the normal and abnormal internal auditory canal. *AJNR* 1988;9:115.
Yeakley JW, Kulkarni MV, McArdle CB, et al. High-resolution MR imaging of juxtasellar meningiomas with CT and angiographic correlation. *AJNR* 1988;9:279.

chapter three

the head
and neck

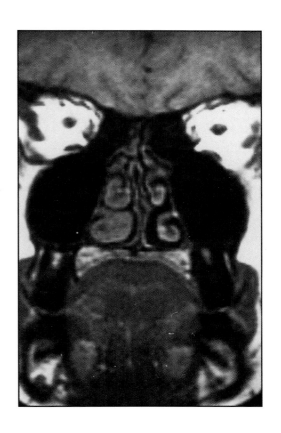

M. ANNE KELLER   ROGER M. L. SMITH

INTRODUCTION

Although the advent of computed tomography (CT) several years ago revolutionized diagnostic imaging of the head and neck, this modality has not successfully demonstrated all pathologies to full advantage. Magnetic resonance imaging (MRI) is able to provide valuable information in the diagnostic work-up of head and neck lesions, given its advantages of multiple planes, less dental artifact, and better mucosal definition. The purpose of this chapter is to provide an overview of the pathologies that MRI is most frequently called upon to evaluate in depth. These include tumors, developmental abnormalities, and deep infections. Although inflammatory lesions of the respiratory tract are those most often encountered clinically, as a rule they are self-limited and involve only mucosal surfaces and regional lymph nodes; such disorders, therefore, rarely warrant detailed investigation. On the other hand, some inflammatory processes deserve discussion because they have unique imaging characteristics or extend to deeper tissue planes, thereby mimicking aggressive malignant neoplasms.

Although trauma to the head and neck is very common, there is little or no role for MRI in the diagnosis of such trauma. If imaging is required, plain radiographs and CT are the mainstays of detection.

NORMAL ANATOMY AND LYMPHATICS (Figs. 3.1 to 3.3)

The head and neck can be regarded as a series of interrelated compartments that allow longitudinal transport of muscles, nerves, blood vessels, and lymph nodes. The head lends itself well to compartmentalization, as clear-cut margins are provided either by bone or by fat planes. The infratemporal fossa, the parapharyngeal space, the neurovascular bundle, and the nasopharynx are soft tissue spaces that are well-demarcated, but intimately related to each other. Since they are separated only by fat planes, pathologies occurring within each compartment have easy access to adjacent compartments. An understanding of each compartment's contents and corresponding pathologies provides a clear concept of the spread of disease.

The compartments in the neck are more autonomous than those in the head. The spread of disease usually occurs longitudinally within a single compartment, rather than across several of them.

The structures common to all areas of the head and neck are the lymph nodes (Fig. 3.1). The lymph node groups and the areas that they drain must be appreciated at the outset of any discussion of the head and neck, because the lymph node chains are

Normal Anatomy of the Head and Neck (Figs. 3.1 to 3.3)

●●●

FIG. 3.1 THE LYMPHATIC SYSTEM OF THE HEAD AND NECK

Chains	Groups	Area Drained
Spinal accessory	OCCIPITAL	Occipital region
Internal jugular	MASTOID	Parotid gland, parietal region of scalp, external ear
	PAROTID	Parotid gland, skin of face, forehead, temporal region
	RETROPHARYNGEAL	Nasopharynx, oropharynx, palate, paranasal sinuses, middle ear, posterior nasal cavity
	JUGULODIGASTRIC[a]	Tonsil
	SUBMANDIBULAR[a]	Nose, anterior nasal cavity, palate, anterior tongue, floor of mouth
	FACIAL[a]	Skin of midface
	SUBMENTAL[a]	Floor of mouth, anterior tongue
Transverse cervical	ANTERIOR JUGULAR	Skin of neck, upper anterior chest wall, larynx, thyroid, esophagus

[a] The submandibular, facial and submental lymph node groups in turn drain into the jugulodigastric lymph node.

the common connecting channels in the compartments of the neck. The head and neck have a rich lymphatic system of multiple groups of lymph nodes (Fig. 3.2). Although the groups are extensive, they all drain into the thorax by one of three chains. The **spinal accessory chain** in the posterior compartment closely follows the course of the spinal accessory nerve (cranial nerve XI), interconnecting with the **internal jugular chain** at the base of the neck via the **transverse cervical chain**. Spinal accessory nodes are more frequently enlarged by infection than by metastatic tumor, whereas the internal jugular chain receives lymphatic drainage from the entire head and neck, its nodes are frequently enlarged by metastatic disease. The internal jugular lymph node chain closely follows the course of the neurovascular bundle throughout the length of the neck. Although lymph node locations and drainage patterns are important in evaluating the extent of head and neck tumors, the appearance of lymphadenopathy on MR images does not allow for histologic differentiation of inflammatory versus neoplastic change (Fig. 3.3).

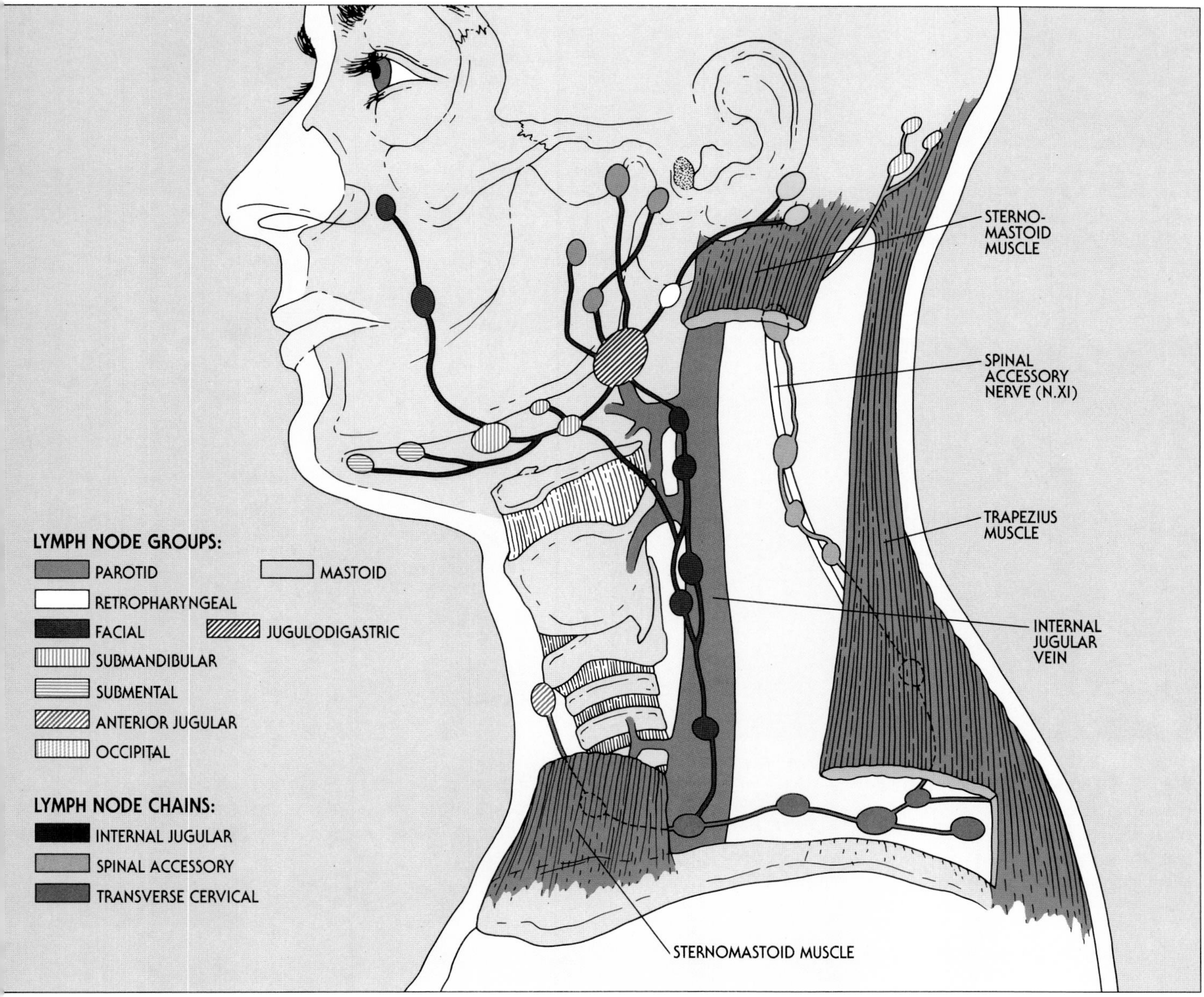

LYMPH NODE GROUPS:

- PAROTID
- RETROPHARYNGEAL
- FACIAL
- SUBMANDIBULAR
- SUBMENTAL
- ANTERIOR JUGULAR
- OCCIPITAL
- MASTOID
- JUGULODIGASTRIC

LYMPH NODE CHAINS:

- INTERNAL JUGULAR
- SPINAL ACCESSORY
- TRANSVERSE CERVICAL

STERNO-MASTOID MUSCLE

SPINAL ACCESSORY NERVE (N.XI)

TRAPEZIUS MUSCLE

INTERNAL JUGULAR VEIN

STERNOMASTOID MUSCLE

Fig. 3.2 The Major Lymph Node Groups and Chains of the Neck

The Lymphatic System

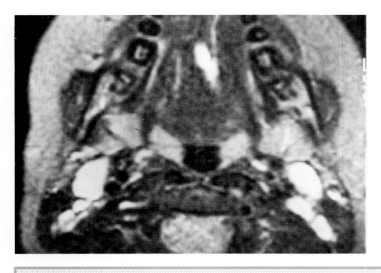

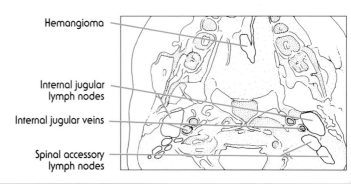

Fig. 3.3A Inflammatory Lymphadenopathy T2-weighted axial image. Enlarged, homogeneously high signal intensity lymph nodes are present bilaterally in the spinal accessory and internal jugular chains. This child had a recent upper respiratory infection. Note the high signal intensity hemangioma in the left side of the tongue.

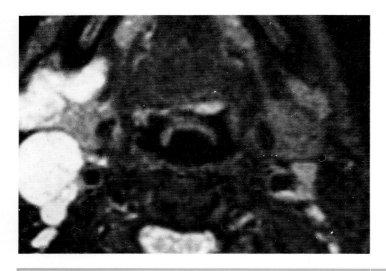

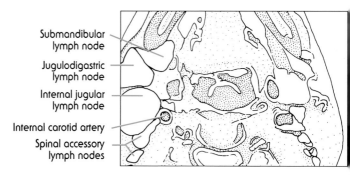

Fig. 3.3B Malignant Lymphadenopathy T2-weighted axial image. Enlarged lymph nodes of homogeneous high signal intensity are present in both the right internal jugular chain and the submandibular group of nodes, as well as in the spinal accessory chains bilaterally. The patient had a rhabdomyosarcoma of the right ethmoid sinus. Note that the internal architecture of metastatic lymph nodes is indistinguishable from that of inflammatory nodes.

TECHNIQUE

Magnetic resonance imaging examinations of head and neck regions at or above the level of the hyoid bone are performed with a circumferential head coil; regions below the level of the hyoid bone are examined with an anteriorly positioned surface coil. A variety of surface coils are commercially available. The choice is usually between a saddle-shaped coil that is contoured to the shape of the neck (Fig. 3.4) or a flat coil (Fig. 3.5). The former is strongly pre-

ferred, as it provides a greater field depth and a considerably more uniform image intensity.

In most cases a combination of T1-and T2-weighted images should be obtained. It is advisable to begin with a localizer, or scout view, usually a T1-weighted sagittal image; the anatomy is easily understood and scan times are very short. A more detailed sagittal view can be substituted, if necessary, with a small time penalty. The sagittal image is followed by the diagnostic portion of the study, consisting of axial T2-weighted images, axial T1-weighted images, and occa-

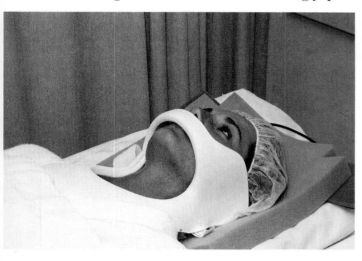

Fig. 3.4 SADDLE-SHAPED SURFACE COIL The coil is within a plastic case contoured to fit comfortably over the neck. It extends from the sternum inferiorly, to the mouth superiorly, to the posterior margin of the sternomastoid muscle posteriorly. The cut-out allows patients with tracheostomies to be examined. This is the preferred type of coil. It covers a large area and provides images of uniform intensity over a relatively deep field.

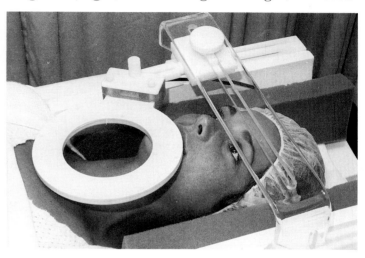

Fig. 3.5 FLAT SURFACE COIL This coil provides excellent signal intensity in the very near field. However, the depth of field is reduced, images are non-uniform in intensity, and anatomical coverage is reduced. Furthermore, patients who are unable to extend their necks compound the problem by creating "dead space" between the coil and the anterior surface of the neck.

sionally, coronal T1-weighted images. Individual (case-by-case) modifications are regularly made for optimal display of the pathology. Incremental changes in repetition time (TR) and echo time (TE) are possible without substantially changing image contrast. A 256 x 256 matrix is used throughout the study, with fields of view ranging from 16 cm to 24 cm. Two excitations are used for all T1-weighted studies, one excitation for T2-weighted studies.

Phase-encoding artifacts from blood flow in the major vessels cause artifactual ghosting, which is potentially very troublesome. These artifacts can mask true abnormalities or mimic lesions that do not exist. Presaturation pulses should be applied on both sides of the imaged volume in the Z axis (the long axis of the magnet bore). This pulse application substantially reduces the artifacts but may not entirely eliminate them. In most cases, the phase-encoding direction should be assigned to the anterior/posterior axis to avoid casting any remaining artifacts across the regions of interest. The technique is summarized in Fig. 3.6.

FIG. 3.6 STANDARD MRI TECHNIQUE FOR THE EXAMINATION OF THE HEAD AND NECK

	Sequence[a]				
Parameter	No. 1A[b] T1-Weighted	No. 1B[b] T1-Weighted	No. 2 T2-Weighted	No. 3 T1-Weighted	No. 4 T1-Weighted
Plane	Sagittal	Sagittal	Axial	Axial	Coronal
TR (msec)	200	500-800	2000-3000	500-800	500-800
TE (msec)	20	20	70-100[c]	20	20
Slice thickness (mm)	5	5	5	5	5
Slice gap (mm)	1	1	2.5	1	1
Matrix	128	256	256	256	256
Field of view (cm)	24	20-24	16-24	16-24	20-24
No. of excitations	1	2	1	1	1
Presaturation	No	Yes	Yes	Yes	Yes
Exam time (min)	<1	5	10	5	5

[a] All sequences: spin echo, multislice.
[b] Use 1A if only localizer needed, 1B if diagnostic quality needed.
[c] Second echo of two-echo study.

THE NASAL CAVITY AND PARANASAL SINUSES

NORMAL ANATOMY (Figs. 3.7 to 3.9)

The nasal cavity extends from the nostrils to the posterior end of the nasal septum, a midline partition that separates the passage into two halves. Posteriorly, it ends in the nasopharynx. The floor of the nasal cavity, formed by the hard palate, is the roof of the mouth. The lateral wall is formed superiorly by ethmoidal air cells and inferiorly by the medial wall of the maxillary antrum. Three turbinate bones project from the lateral wall. Beneath the free edge of each are the ostia, which drain the paranasal sinuses. The inferior turbinate also covers the opening of the nasolacrimal duct.

The lymphatic drainage of the anterior half of the nasal cavity follows the venous pathways, draining across the face to the submandibular lymph nodes. The posterior half of the nose and nasopharynx drain to the retropharyngeal nodes and to the anterosuperior nodes of the internal jugular chain.

There are four paired paranasal sinuses—**maxillary, ethmoid, frontal**, and **sphenoid**. The maxillary and ethmoid sinuses form the lateral wall of the nasal cavity. The frontal sinus forms part of the roof of the orbit, and the sphenoid sinus forms the roof of the nasopharynx. The frontal, ethmoid, and sphenoid sinuses abut in the midline and are often asymmetric. The sinuses are rudimentary or absent at birth. They enlarge at the eruption of the second dentition (at age six or seven) and, again, at puberty.

The **maxillary sinus**, the largest of the sinuses, is pyramidal, the base being the lateral wall of the nose and the apex being the zygomatic process. The roof forms the orbital floor, ridged by the passage of the infraorbital nerve. The floor is the superior alveolar ridge. The posterior bony wall and its most important relation, the infratemporal fossa, are separated by a fat plane. The ostium of the maxillary antrum opens below the middle turbinate in the nasal cavity (at the posterior end of the hiatus semilunaris).

The **ethmoid sinus**, a collection of numerous small air cells, lies between the orbit and the nose. It forms the medial wall of the orbit. The sinus cavity has multiple, incomplete septa. It is divided into posterior, middle, and anterior parts. The ostium of the posterior ethmoids drains below the superior turbinate. The anterior and middle ethmoids drain to the anterior end of the hiatus semilunaris. Lymph drainage from the posterior ethmoid is to the retropharyngeal nodes. The anterior and middle ethmoid lymphatic drainage is to the submandibular group of nodes.

The sphenoid sinus lies posterior to the ethmoid sinus and forms the floor and anterior wall of the pituitary fossa. Posteriorly, it is bordered by the clivus. Prominent lateral wings may extend into the sphenoid bone.

The **frontal sinus**, situated within the frontal bone, is extremely variable in its size and degree of aeration. Its medial margin forms the anteromedial part of the roof of the orbit. The frontal sinus also drains through the hiatus semilunaris. The lymphatic drainage from the frontal sinus is to the submandibular group of nodes.

Normal Anatomy of the Head and Neck (Figs. 3.7 to 3.9)

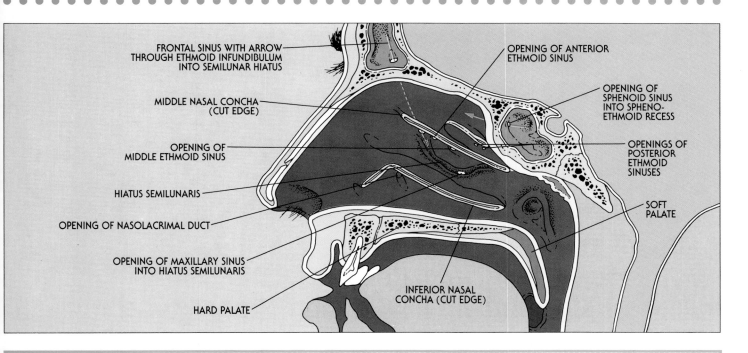

Fig. 3.7 The Lateral Wall of the Nasal Cavity and Nasopharynx   (Note that the nasal conchae have been cut away.)

The Nasal Cavity and Paranasal Sinuses

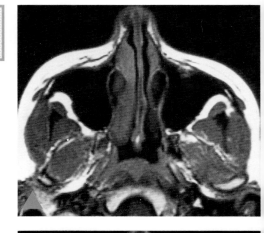

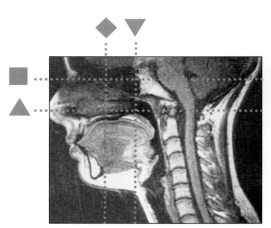

Fig. 3.8 Localizer: Midline T1-Weighted Sagittal Image
The planes of section of four images are indicated: an axial image through the maxillary sinus and nasal cavity, an axial image through the ethmoid and sphenoid sinuses, a coronal image through the ethmoid and maxillary sinuses and nasal cavity, and a coronal image through the sphenoid sinus and posterior nasal cavity.

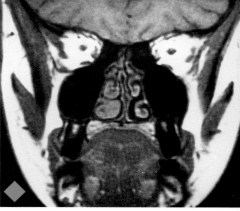

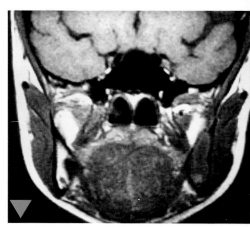

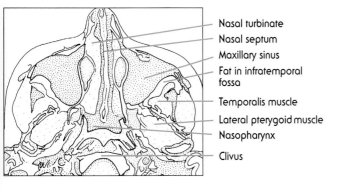

Nasal turbinate
Nasal septum
Maxillary sinus
Fat in infratemporal fossa
Temporalis muscle
Lateral pterygoid muscle
Nasopharynx
Clivus

Fig. 3.9A T1-Weighted Axial Image Through the Maxillary Sinus, Nasal Cavity, and Base of the Skull The fat planes of the infratemporal fossa separate the maxillary sinus from the temporalis muscle and the lateral pterygoid muscle.

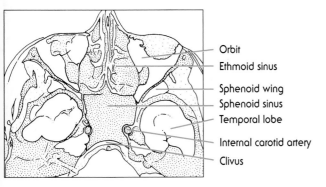

Orbit
Ethmoid sinus
Sphenoid wing
Sphenoid sinus
Temporal lobe
Internal carotid artery
Clivus

Fig. 3.9B T1-Weighted Axial Image Through the Ethmoid and Sphenoid Sinuses The high intensity signal from the sphenoid wing and lateral clivus indicates the marrow space. The signal void from the internal carotid artery lies immediately adjacent to the lateral sphenoid sinus wall.

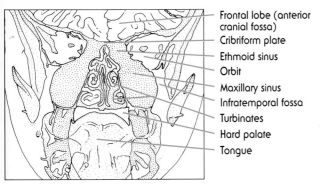

Frontal lobe (anterior cranial fossa)
Cribriform plate
Ethmoid sinus
Orbit
Maxillary sinus
Infratemporal fossa
Turbinates
Hard palate
Tongue

Fig. 3.9C T1-Weighted Coronal Image Through the Ethmoid and Maxillary Sinuses and Nasal Cavity The dorsal aspect of the tongue is closely applied to the hard palate. Note the fat plane separating the lateral aspect of the maxillary sinus from the infratemporal fossa.

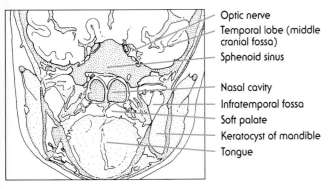

Optic nerve
Temporal lobe (middle cranial fossa)
Sphenoid sinus
Nasal cavity
Infratemporal fossa
Soft palate
Keratocyst of mandible
Tongue

Fig. 3.9D T1-Weighted Coronal Image Through the Sphenoid Sinus and Posterior Nasal Cavity The optic nerves can be seen immediately lateral to the superior aspect of the sphenoid sinus. There is an incidental keratocyst in the left mandible, obliterating the fatty marrow.

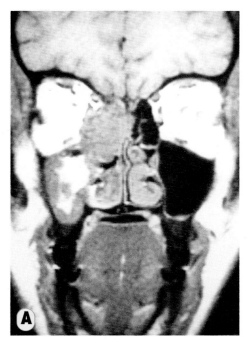

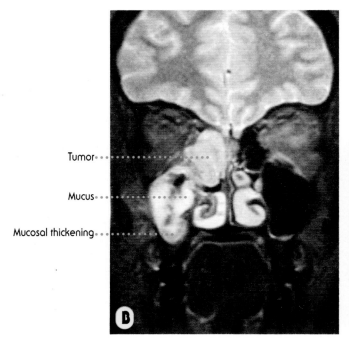

Tumor · · · · ·

Mucus · · · · ·

Mucosal thickening · · · · ·

TECHNIQUE

The MRI technique employed to examine the nasal cavity and the paranasal sinuses does not differ significantly from the standard head and neck examination protocol (see Fig. 3.6) except that T2-weighted coronal images are usually substituted for the T2-weighted axial images.

PATHOLOGY

The nose and paranasal sinuses are affected by similar disease processes, the most common of these being sinusitis and viral and allergic rhinitis. In most cases, these disorders are self-limited and rarely require detailed evaluation. Mucosal thickening or fluid accumulation may be noted, but usually as only incidental findings on examinations performed for other reasons.

THE NASAL CAVITY
Developmental anomalies, trauma, bacterial and fungal infections, noninfectious granulomatous processes, inflammatory masses, and neoplasms are all known to occur with various degrees of frequency in the nasal cavity. Most of the more common disorders of the nasal cavity do not warrant MRI. Small polyps

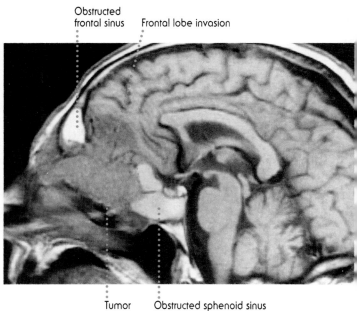

Obstructed frontal sinus   Frontal lobe invasion

Tumor   Obstructed sphenoid sinus

Fig. 3.10 NASOETHMOID RHABDOMYOSARCOMA (A) T1-weighted coronal image. This 18-year-old girl presented with nasal congestion. Extending into the nasal cavity and the right orbit extraconally is a homogeneous, destructive lesion with an isointense signal to muscle centered in the right ethmoid air cells. **(B)** T2-weighted coronal image. The tumor is hyperintense on this sequence. The lower signal stromal pattern within the tumor is due to fibrous tissue strands. The high T2 signal intensity appearance differs from that seen in most squamous cell carcinomas. Note the mucosal thickening and retained high signal mucus within the right maxillary sinus resulting from obstruction of the sinus by tumor.

Fig. 3.11 ESTHESIONEUROBLASTOMA T1-weighted sagittal image. There is a large mass in the superior nasal cavity extending across the cribriform plate into the brain. It is similar to the case of squamous cell carcinoma of the ethmoid sinus (see Fig. 3.19B). There is also extension of the tumor to an extracranial subcutaneous location anterior to the frontal sinus. The frontal and sphenoid sinuses are obstructed.

and other inflammatory masses are accessible by direct (visual) inspection. Traumatic lesions and developmental anomalies are ideally suited for CT studies because of the fine bony detail that this modality can provide. Assessments of neoplasms and complicated inflammatory processes (infectious or otherwise) generally warrant use of MRI.

In the nasal cavity, aggressive inflammatory lesions occur with fungal infections (mucormycosis, aspergillosis) and granulomatous diseases (leprosy, tuberculosis, sarcoid, Wegener's granulomatosis). They are accompanied by soft tissue thickening and bone destruction. Involvement of cortical bone is often difficult to detect on MR images, whereas involvement of the marrow space is easily appreciated. However, the appearance of marrow space involvement is nonspecific, in that aggressive tumors present the identical picture.

Hemangioma, neurofibroma, and lipoma are the most common benign neoplasms of the nasal cavity. Antrochoanal polyps are common inflammatory masses. Malignant neoplasms in the adult are usually of epithelial origin. It is more usual for the nose to be involved secondarily by carcinoma arising in the maxillary or ethmoid sinus than it is for it to be primarily affected.

Rhabdomyosarcoma (Fig. 3.10) is the most common nasal malignancy in children. It is a disease that primarily occurs in the first decade of life—more than three quarters of those affected presenting by the time they are 12 years old. Forty percent of the cases arise in the region of the head and neck, e.g., the orbit, the middle ear, the nasopharynx, the nasal cavity, the paranasal sinuses, and the soft tissues of the neck. The majority arise from unsegmented and undifferentiated mesoderm and only a small number from myotome-derived skeletal muscle. Almost all rhabdomyosarcomas present as a mass, and as many as 50% have lymph node or distant metastases at the time of diagnosis. Other sarcomas are angiosarcoma and chondrosarcoma, which usually involve the nasal septum.

Olfactory neuroblastoma is a rare tumor that arises from olfactory mucosa and occurs in the upper nasal fossa. As a mass in the nasal fossa, it does not have any unique features; but its propensity to cross the cribriform plate into the cranium may suggest the diagnosis (Fig. 3.11). It may be indistinguishable from ethmoid sinus squamous cell carcinoma, although squamous cell carcinoma has a greater tendency to extend laterally into the orbits.

THE PARANASAL SINUSES

INFLAMMATION AND INFECTION   The paranasal sinuses, like the nasal cavity, are commonly affected by inflammatory lesions (Fig. 3.12). An untreated sinusitis may progress to a local osteomyelitis. Subsequent extension into the epidural space, coupled with formation of an epidural abscess, is a well-recognized complication.

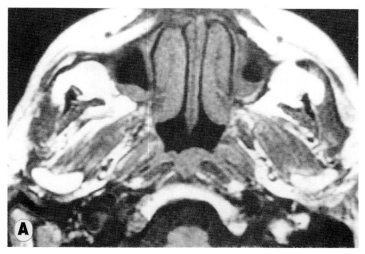
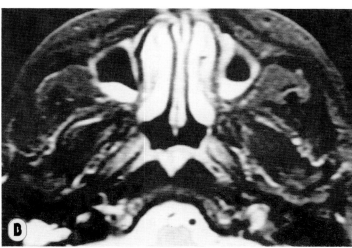

Fig. 3.12 ACUTE ON CHRONIC SINUSITIS   T1-weighted **(A)** and T2-weighted **(B)** axial images. There is generalized thickening of the maxillary sinus mucosa. An air-fluid level is present in the left maxillary sinus, indicating active disease. The fluid and the mucosa are of similar intensity on the T1-weighted image, and both are hyperintense on the T2-weighted image.

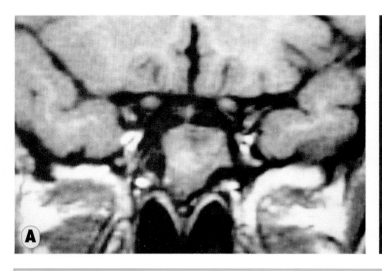 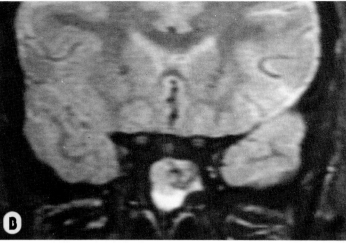

Fig. 3.13 *ASPERGILLUS* SINUS INFECTION   T1-weighted **(A)** and T2-weighted **(B)** coronal images. A mixed intensity mass is present in the sphenoid sinus, the walls of which are intact. On the T2-weighted image, the high signal portion is typical of mucus in an obstructed sinus. The low signal intensity in the remainder of the sinus is classically seen in fungal infection, although it is not completely diagnostic of this disease. The dark signal is thought to be due to a fungus ball. (Courtesy of Dr. W. Dillon, University of California at San Francisco)

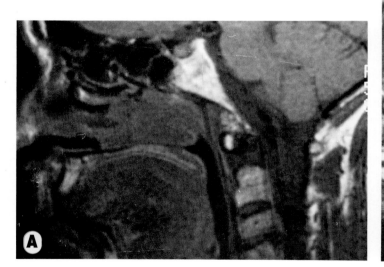 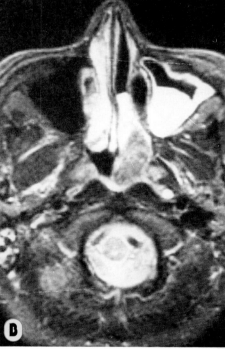

Fig. 3.14 CHOANAL POLYP AND MAXILLARY SINUS MUCUS RETENTION CYST   (A) T1-weighted sagittal image. The patient presented with left nasal obstruction. There is a homogeneous soft tissue mass in the posterior aspect of the nasal cavity with an intermediate signal intensity. **(B)** T2-weighted axial image. A moderately high signal intensity mass obstructs the left nasal passage. Its intensity is lower than the surrounding nasal mucosa and thickened mucosa of the left maxillary antrum. A mucus retention cyst occupies the posterior portion of the sinus.

The appearance of fungal sinus infection on T2-weighted images differs from that of other inflammatory sinus conditions. Most inflammatory sinus conditions are hyperintense on T2-weighted images, whereas fungal infections are usually hypointense (see Fig. 3.13). To date, there has not been an adequate explanation for this hypointense appearance.

BENIGN MASSES   The most common masses involving the paranasal sinuses are mucus retention cysts and polyps (Fig. 3.14). Mucus retention cysts are caused by obstruction of seromucous glands. The majority of polyps are associated with topical hypersensitivity and can produce nasal or sinus obstruction (Fig. 3.15). They may predispose a patient to the development of malignancy.

Mucoceles are unique to the paranasal sinuses. Where either an ostium becomes obstructed by chronic inflammation or the mucosa is damaged secondary to trauma or surgery, a mucocele or mucopyocele may develop; its resultant enlargement may lead to an expansion of the sinus walls. Mucoceles/mucopyoceles occur most frequently in the frontal sinus (Fig. 3.16), followed in frequency by the ethmoid, sphenoid, and maxillary sinuses, respectively. The maxillary sinus, however, is rarely involved.

Although it accounts for only 4% of nasal and sinus tumors, inverting papilloma is important because of its locally aggressive tendencies and its potential for undergoing malignant change (Fig. 3.17). The tumor arises from epithelial hyperplasia, which inverts into the underlying stroma, most commonly occurring at the junction of the antrum and the ethmoid sinuses on the lateral nasal wall (see Fig. 3.16). Although slow-growing, the tumor aggressively causes bone

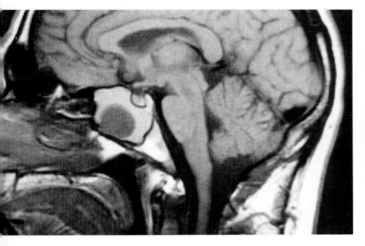

Fig. 3.15 MUCOSAL POLYP WITH SPHENOID SINUS OBSTRUCTION   T1-weighted sagittal image. The ostium of the sphenoid sinus is obstructed by an intermediate signal intensity mucosal polyp. The retained mucus within the obstructed sinus is of characteristically high signal intensity.

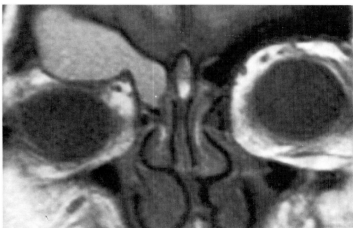

Fig. 3.16 FRONTAL MUCOCELE   T1-weighted coronal image. There is homogeneous fluid filling the right frontal sinus. The sinus is enlarged with displacement of the orbital roof inferiorly. The mucus-filled sinus is hyperintense on T1-weighted images relative to muscle. This is a common observation with respect to mucoceles; it is thought to be due to either recurrent bleeding or a high protein concentration in the retained mucus.

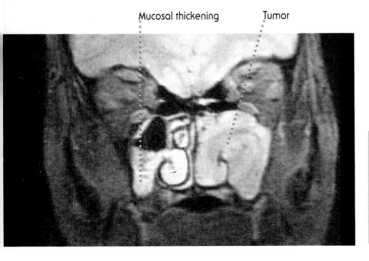

Mucosal thickening   Tumor

Fig. 3.17 INVERTING PAPILLOMA   T2-weighted coronal scan. A well-defined mass fills the left maxillary sinus and the left nasal cavity. The mass is predominantly hyperintense with strands of low intensity within it: this finding is in contrast to most polyps, which are more uniform in intensity. Note the mucosal thickening. (Courtesy of Dr. W. Dillon, University of California at San Francisco)

Tumor in infratemporal fossa   Tumor

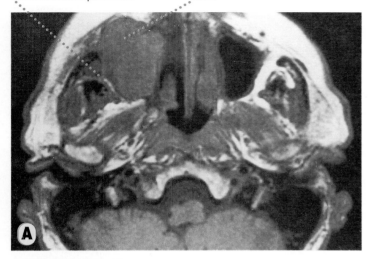

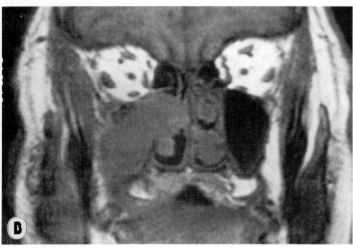

Fig. 3.18 SQUAMOUS CELL CARCINOMA OF THE MAXIL-LARY SINUS **(A)** T1-weighted axial image. This patient had a history of chronic sinusitis. The right antrum is filled with a homogeneous, intermediate signal intensity tumor. The anterior and medial walls have been eroded. The fat plane separating the anteroposterior wall of the sinus from the muscles of the infratemporal fossa has been obliterated. However, more posteriorly, the wall of the sinus is displaced; but it appears intact by virtue of the low signal intensity line separating tumor from the fat lying along the anterolateral margin of the lateral pterygoid muscle. **(B)** T1-weighted coronal image. There is extension of the tumor through the ostium below the middle turbinate into the nasal cavity. Loss of the fat signal adjacent to the lateral wall indicates extension into the infratemporal fossa. The tumor extends to the orbital floor but there is no bony displacement or erosion.

destruction, locally invading the orbit and the paranasal sinuses, and, occasionally, extending intracranially. Bone proliferation may be seen centrally and is best visualized by the use of CT.

MALIGNANT TUMORS Primary malignant tumors in the paranasal sinuses are usually of epithelial origin but may also arise from glandular elements of the mucosa (accessory salivary glands), the neuroepithelium, supporting structures (muscles, cartilages, bones, vessels), or lymphatic tissue.

Squamous cell carcinoma is the most common malignancy in the paranasal sinuses, accounting for as many as 90% of all neoplasms. Nasal polyps and chronic sinusitis preexist in 15% of the cases. Maxillary sinus carcinoma (Fig 3.18) accounts for 80% of the lesions that involve the paranasal sinuses, although only 25% of said lesions are limited to this space at the time of presentation. Discernible bone destruction occurs in 70 to 80% of the cases. Ten to 20% occur in the ethmoid sinuses (Fig 3.19), with a marked propensity for erosion through both the medial wall of the orbit and the cribriform plate into the anterior cranial fossa. Squamous cell carcinoma in this region bears a poor prognosis because of the often extremely advanced stage of the disease at presentation. Magnetic resonance imaging, with its excellent tissue detection and multiplanar characteristics, is proving to be extremely valuable in defining the tumor extension prior to surgical resection. Magnetic resonance imaging's tumor definition holds particular utility in cases where a lesion extends to the skull base, where there is perineural invasion through the foramina and fissures, or where there is obstruction of the sinus ostia. In the latter case, mucus within the obstructed sinus is hyperintense—particularly on the T2-weighted image—and is well-distinguished from the tumor that usually is isointense to muscle. This distinction is difficult to make on CT.

Adenocarcinoma accounts for 5% to 10% of carcinomas in the paranasal sinuses, the majority of which involve the ethmoid sinus. Salivary gland tumors occurring in the nose and the paranasal sinuses are very uncommon, but when detected, are usually found to be of the adenoid cystic variety. These tumors are indistinguishable from squamous cell carcinoma. They arise from the minor salivary glands in the mucosa.

Primary lymphoma of the nasal cavity and the paranasal sinuses is rare in the general population, but has a higher incidence in immunosuppressed patients. In affected individuals, the paranasal sinuses are frequently invaded by direct extension from malignancies in the oropharynx, the palate, and the infratemporal fossa. Metastatic involvement occurs through hematogenous dissemination of malignant melanoma (Fig. 3.20), hypernephroma, and carcinoma of the lung.

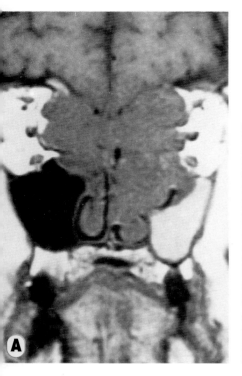

Obstructed frontal sinus   Intracranial extension of tumor

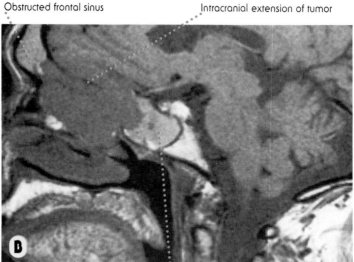

Obstructed sphenoid sinus

Fig. 3.19 ETHMOID SINUS CARCINOMA WITH ORBITAL AND INTRACRANIAL EXTENSION (A) T1-weighted coronal image. There is extension of the ethmoid tumor laterally into the orbit, superiorly into the cranium, inferiorly into the nasal passage, and inferolaterally into the left maxillary sinus. Inspissated mucus within the obstructed left maxillary antrum shows a high signal intensity. **(B)** T1-weighted sagittal image. There is extension through the cribriform plate into the anterior cranial fossa, as evidenced by the discontinuity of the thin cortical bone of the cribriform plate. Note the obstructed sphenoid and frontal sinuses.

Tumor Orbital extension

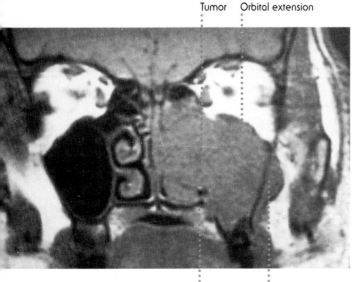

Hard palate extension Infratemporal fossa extension

Fig. 3.20 METASTATIC MELANOMA T1-weighted coronal image. This patient presented with a left facial mass. There is a homogeneous mass filling and expanding the left maxillary sinus. The tumor has extended into the infratemporal fossa laterally, the orbit and ethmoid sinus superiorly, and the nasal cavity medially. The palate is eroded adjacent to the alveolar ridge. The image indicates a very aggressive malignant tumor, but not the histologic diagnosis. The extremely short clinical history in this case suggested metastatic disease. Histology confirmed the diagnosis of metastatic melanoma. Most metastatic melanomas have been reported to have high intensity on T1-weighted images. This case is atypical, in that it lacks this usual feature.

THE NASOPHARYNX, PARAPHARYNGEAL SPACE, AND INFRATEMPORAL FOSSA

NORMAL ANATOMY (Figs. 3.21 and 3.22)

The **nasopharynx** in continuity with the posterior nasal cavity, is a tubular structure lined by respiratory epithelium and enclosed in a muscular sling suspended from the skull base. The roof of the nasopharynx is formed by the sphenoid bone superiorly and by the basiocciput, upper cervical vertebrae and prevertebral muscles posteriorly. The nasopharynx extends inferiorly to the level of the soft palate, where a narrow transversely oriented muscle (Passavant's muscle) demarcates the junction of the nasopharynx and oropharynx. The superior pharyngeal constrictor muscle, acting as a muscular sling surrounding the lateral and posterior walls of the nasopharynx, is incomplete in its superior lateral aspect. Through this deficiency in the muscular wall, the eustachian tube extends posteriorly from the lateral wall of the nasopharynx to communicate with the middle ear cavity. The anterior end of the eustachian tube projects slightly into the nasopharynx as an important anatomic landmark, the torus tubarius. The eustachian tube orifice is at the anterior margin of the torus tubarius. The lateral pharyngeal recess, or fossa of Rosenmuller, lies immediately posterior to the torus tubarius. A small vertically oriented muscle, the salpingopharyngeus muscle, extends inferiorly from the eustachian tube to insert into the lateral pharyngeal muscular wall. The mucosal fold created by the torus tubarius and salpingopharyngeus muscle is augmented by the intimately associated levator palati muscle. These superficial landmarks are best visualized in the mid- to upper nasopharynx.

The skeletal framework of the posterior nasal choanae and the adjacent medial pterygoid plates offer rigid bony support to only the most anterior aspect of the muscular sling. There is no bony support to the lateral boundaries of the nasopharynx, yet the nasopharynx must remain rigidly patent to main-tain respiratory function. A thick, very strong pharyngobasilar fascia, attached to the skull base and medial pterygoid plates, offers appropriate support for airway patency, yet mobility for deglutition when necessary. This fascial layer lies within and extends superior to the superior pharyngeal constrictor muscle with its attachment to the skull base such that the superior aspect of the pharyngobasilar fascia is not covered by the superior pharyngeal constrictor muscle. The eustachian tube passes through a small gap between the pharyngobasilar fascia and skull base. This fascial layer, besides providing important rigid support for pharyngeal muscular structures, acts as an important barrier to spread of disease from superficial or mucosal structures to the deeper tissues. This fascial layer becomes thinner and less rigid in the more inferior aspect of the nasopharynx, to allow increased mobility required for deglutition. Consequently, it also becomes a less effective barrier to spread of disease more inferiorly.

Anatomically, the pharyngobasilar fascia separates the laterally positioned parapharyngeal space from the intrapharyngeal structures (pharyngeal mucosal space). The tensor palati and superior constrictor muscles lie lateral or deep to this fascial layer; however, the levator palati and salpingopharyngeus muscles are superficial and enclosed by the fascia. Similarly, the pharyngobasilar fascia encloses the pharyngeal mucosa and surface lymphatics. Lymphoid tissues, the adenoids or nasopharyngeal tonsils, lie posterior to the lateral pharyngeal recess and are prominent in children. These lymphatic tissues tend to compress the pharyngeal recesses. With increasing age, the lymphoid tissues involute and the lateral pharyngeal and occasionally eustachian tube recesses become more apparent as larger air spaces. This superficial lymphatic tissue in the nasopharynx (adenoids), together with the palatine and lingual tonsils, forms Waldeyer's ring. A smaller amount of lymphoid tissue, the tubal tonsils, also covers the eustachian tube opening. The superficial tissues are variable in thickness and may be irregular in contour along the air space-mucosal surface. This variability tends to reflect lymphoid tissue changes rather than changes in muscular or mucosal structures.

At the posterior border to the nasopharynx, the paraspinal musculature (longus colli, rectus capitus, and longus capitus muscles) lies anterior to the cervical spine. This prevertebral musculature accounts for most of the soft tissue density seen between the spine and the nasopharyngeal airway. The prevertebral fascia, a well-developed but thin membrane, covers the prevertebral musculature. A potential retropharyngeal space lies between the pharyngobasilar and prevertebral fascial layers. The two layers of fascia and the potential retropharyngeal space allow the "mobile" pharyngeal structures to move over the relatively fixed prevertebral and vertebral structures during movement of the neck or swallowing.

The **parapharyngeal space** is bound anteriorly by the lateral pterygoid muscle, laterally by the deep lobe of the parotid gland and posteriorly by the carotid sheath and neurovascular bundle. The parapharyngeal space extends from the skull base superiorly to the submandibular space inferiorly, thereby bridging the deeper tissues of the nasopharynx and oropharynx. It is triangular in shape with its base abutting the skull and its apex directed toward the oropharynx. The parapharyngeal space contains loose fibrofatty tissue, thereby allowing free movement of the muscles of deglutition and mastication. On MR images the space is easily defined as a high signal intensity area lying between the pharyngeal and pterygoid musculature, in direct continuity superiorly with the orbit and middle cranial fossa via the inferior and superior orbital fissures. Small branches of the external carotid artery, the pharyngeal veins, and the mandibular nerve run within the parapharyngeal space.

A thin buccopharyngeal fascia outlines the limits of the parapharyngeal space. The medial part of this fascia is the epimysium of the superior pharyngeal constrictor. The lateral component of the buccopharyngeal fascia is the reflection of the deep cervical fascia covering the pterygoid musculature and the deep lobe of the parotid gland.

The carotid sheath and contained **neurovascular bundle** lie immediately posterior to the parapharyngeal space forming the posterolateral border to the retropharyngeal space. The carotid artery is anteromedial, while the jugular vein is posterolateral. The sympathetic chain and cranial nerves IX, X, XI, and XII surround the artery. The deep lymphatics of the neck are intimately associated with the course of the internal jugular vein.

The loose, thin application of buccopharyngeal fascia to the respective muscles of origin accommodates the significant pharyngeal motion during swallowing. Similarly, such sparse and thin fascial support allows displacement or compression of the parapharyngeal space. Patterns of displacement or indentation of specific borders of the fatty parapharyngeal space represent reliable, easily recognized signs to suggest specific tissue space origins (prevertebral space, carotid sheath space, masticator space, pharyngeal mucosal space, etc.) for nasopharyngeal or parapharyngeal masses, considerably limiting the diagnostic probabilities. This fascia has no important function in limiting tumors or infectious spread to adjacent structures.

The **infratemporal fossa** lies lateral to the parapharyngeal space. It is bound anteriorly by the posterior wall of the maxillary antrum and laterally by the zygomatic arch. Inferiorly, the infratemporal fossa is continuous with the spaces of the deep face external to the buccinator muscle. The skull base (squamous temporal bone and greater sphenoid wing) forms the posterior wall and roof of the infratemporal fossa. Superiorly, above the level of the zygomatic arch, the infratemporal fossa is continuous laterally with the temporal fossa. Anteromedially, the pterygomaxillary fissure and pterygopalatine fossa represent important channels of possible pathologic tissue spread to the orbit, nasopharynx, nasal cavity, skull base, and middle cranial fossa.

The contents of the infratemporal fossa include the mandibular ramus, the lateral pterygoid plate, the medial and lateral pterygoid muscles, the masseter muscle, the inferior portion of the temporalis muscle, and the deep lobe of the parotid gland. As with the parapharyngeal space, the infratemporal fossae and their contents should appear symmetrical. Specific muscular atrophy and/or fatty replacement may suggest specific cranial nerve deficits. The mandibular masticatory musculature and tensor palati are innervated by the trigeminal nerve (V). The levator palati muscle is innervated by cranial nerve IX, the glossopharyngeal nerve.

The Nasopharynx, Parapharyngeal Space, and Infratemporal Fossa

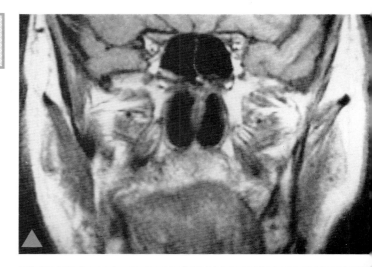

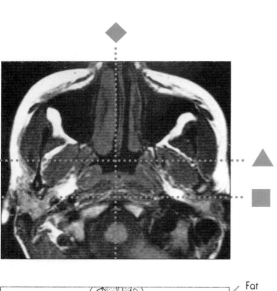

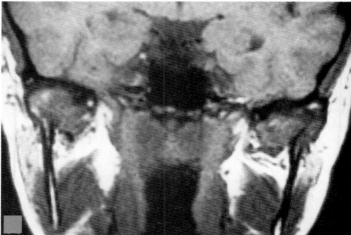

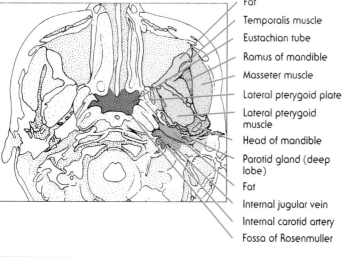

Fat
Temporalis muscle
Eustachian tube
Ramus of mandible
Masseter muscle
Lateral pterygoid plate
Lateral pterygoid muscle
Head of mandible
Parotid gland (deep lobe)
Fat
Internal jugular vein
Internal carotid artery
Fossa of Rosenmuller

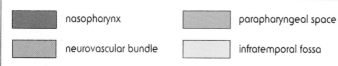

nasopharynx   parapharyngeal space

neurovascular bundle   infratemporal fossa

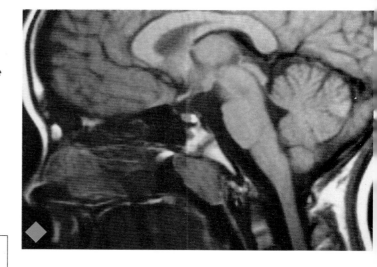

Fig. 3.21 Localizer: T1-Weighted Axial Image Through the Nasopharynx The planes of section of three images are indicated: coronal images through the inferior orbital fissure and foramen ovale, and a midline sagittal image.

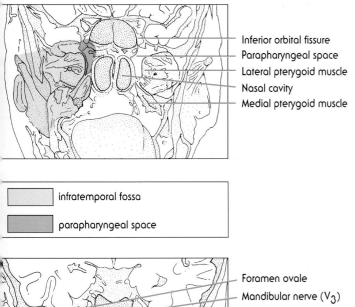

Inferior orbital fissure
Parapharyngeal space
Lateral pterygoid muscle
Nasal cavity
Medial pterygoid muscle

Fig. 3.22A T1-Weighted Coronal Image Through the Inferior Orbital Fissure The high signal intensity fat plane of the parapharyngeal space is directly continuous with the inferior orbital fissure.

infratemporal fossa

parapharyngeal space

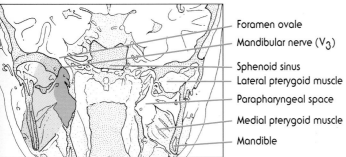

Foramen ovale
Mandibular nerve (V₃)
Sphenoid sinus
Lateral pterygoid muscle
Parapharyngeal space
Medial pterygoid muscle
Mandible

Fig. 3.22B T1-Weighted Coronal Image Through the Foramen Ovale The parapharyngeal space communicates with the base of the skull and extends to the oropharynx. The mandibular division of the trigeminal nerve passes through the foramen ovale.

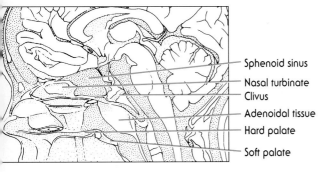

Sphenoid sinus
Nasal turbinate
Clivus
Adenoidal tissue
Hard palate
Soft palate

Fig. 3.22C Midline T1-Weighted Sagittal Image The high intensity signal of the marrow within the clivus delineates the posterosuperior extent of the nasopharynx. The intermediate intensity mass on the posterior wall is hypertrophied adenoidal tissue, which is completely normal in a child.

TECHNIQUE

The MRI technique relative to the nasopharynx, the parapharyngeal space, and the infratemporal fossa is the same as the standard for the head and neck examination protocol (see Fig. 3.6). Occasionally, individual modifications need to be made, depending on the precise site and the type of abnormality in question.

PATHOLOGY

Mass lesions of the nasopharynx, the parapharyngeal space, and the infratemporal fossa may arise from epithelial cells, accessory salivary glands, neurogenic tissue, lymphoid tissue, and various supporting structures, such as muscles, fat, bones, and blood vessels.

NASOPHARYNX

DEVELOPMENTAL LESIONS   In children it is normal to see prominent adenoidal tissue in the roof of the nasopharynx. The signal intensity is identical to lymphoid tissue elsewhere (Fig. 3.22C). The adenoids involute in late childhood and adolescence.

A common incidental finding is Thornwaldt's cyst, seen in persons of all ages, but predominantly in the young. It originates in the midline of the nasopharynx in lymphoepithelioid tissue, a remnant of the pharyngeal bursa. It is characteristically well-defined and hyperintense on both T1- and T2-weighted images (Fig. 3.23). It rarely becomes infected and is generally of no clinical significance.

Encephaloceles can present in the nasopharynx, often associated with other midline anomalies. A fluid-filled, well-circumscribed mass in communica-

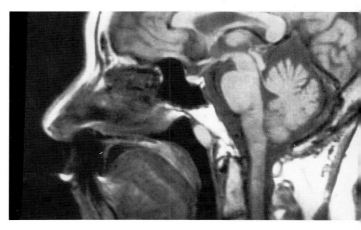

Fig. 3.23 THORNWALDT'S CYST   Midline T1-weighted sagittal image. There is a well-circumscribed, high signal intensity Thornwaldt's cyst situated in the midline on the posterior nasopharyngeal wall. This is a common incidental finding and is of no clinical significance.

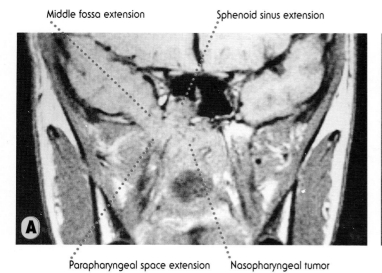

Middle fossa extension   Sphenoid sinus extension

Parapharyngeal space extension   Nasopharyngeal tumor

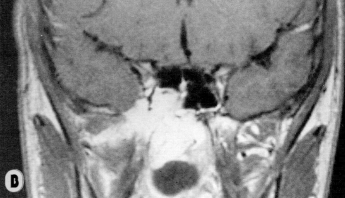

Fig. 3.24 JUVENILE ANGIOFIBROMA   (A) T1-weighted coronal image. There is a well-defined mass in the nasopharynx, extending into the parapharyngeal space and the right sphenoid sinus, and passing through the orbital fissures into the middle cranial fossa. **(B)** T1-weighted coronal image, gadolinium-DTPA enhanced.

There is homogeneous enhancement of the nasopharyngeal tumor. This enhancement is analogous to that seen on CT following the administration of iodinated contrast agents. (Courtesy of Dr. W. Dillon, University of California at San Francisco)

tion with the suprasellar cistern is diagnostic of a meningocele; herniated brain is found in an encephalocele.

INFLAMMATION AND INFECTION   Inflammatory lesions involving the nasopharyngeal mucosa and lymphoid tissue may cause airway obstruction, but they usually preserve the fat planes deep to the pharyngobasilar fascia. Although obliteration of these tissue planes can occur with infection, such destruction is more often seen with neoplasia. Differentiation between the two may be difficult; biopsy may be required. An untreated tonsillar infection, which occasionally advances to an abscess, invariably occurs in the parapharyngeal space as a well-defined, encapsulated mass. Surrounding edema results in obliteration of the fat planes. Tonsillar abscesses are rarely seen today due to early antibiotic therapy.

BENIGN NEOPLASMS   The most common benign tumor in the nasopharynx is a juvenile angiofibroma (Fig. 3.24). This characteristically arises from fibrovascular stroma in the posterior nasal cavity and nasopharynx and occurs in young males. Although the tumor is benign, it commonly behaves aggressively, extending beyond the nasopharynx into the para-

pharyngeal space and the infratemporal fossa and causing deformity of the maxillary wall. It may also extend into the nasal cavity, and occasionally into the ethmoid and sphenoid sinuses. Extension of the tumor from the infratemporal fossa into the pterygopalatine fossa allows for easy access to the medial aspect of the middle cranial fossa via the orbital fissures. Sarcomatous change occurs rarely, and usually only after radiotherapy.

MALIGNANT NEOPLASMS   Carcinoma accounts for 99% of malignant lesions of the nasopharynx, 80% of those being squamous cell. There is a particularly high geographic preponderance of carcinoma in China and an established association with smoking as well as with the Epstein–Barr virus. Adenocarcinoma and adenoid cystic carcinoma represent less than 1% of all carcinomas. Nasopharyngeal carcinoma rarely presents early and therefore is rarely confined to the mucosa at the time of diagnosis. Symptoms at presentation reflect the invasive nature of this disease. Multiple symptom complexes include (a) malignant cervical lymphadenopathy, the primary site remaining occult; (b) nasal obstruction by a mass lesion; (c) cranial nerve palsy, indicating perineural or direct skull base invasion (Fig. 3.25), and (d) serous otitis media

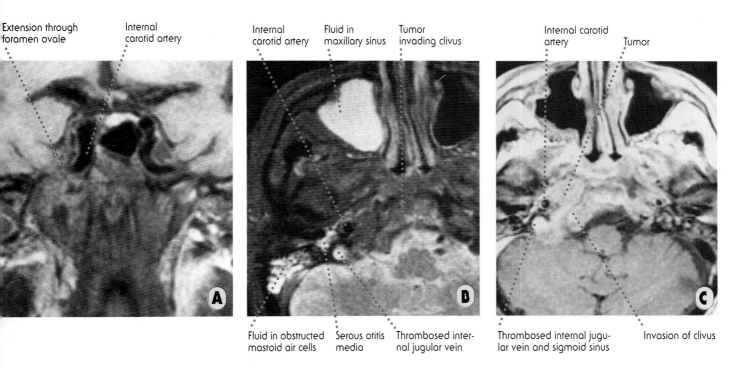

Fig. 3.25 NASOPHARYNGEAL CARCINOMA WITH SKULL BASE INVASION   **(A)** T1-weighted coronal image. This patient presented with atypical facial pain in the distribution of the mandibular nerve (cranial nerve V$_3$) on the right side. An intermediate signal intensity soft-tissue mass is seen to extend from the nasopharynx into the parapharyngeal space and through the skull base at the foramen ovale. **(B)** T2-weighted axial image. The same soft tissue mass can be identified medial to the right carotid artery. There is invasion of the clivus on the right side by the tumor. Obstruction of the eustachian tube has produced a serous otitis media evidenced by high signal intensity fluid within the middle ear and mastoid air cells on the right. The tumor extends to the internal jugular vein, which is thrombosed. Incidental note is made of fluid within the maxillary sinus. **(C)** T1-weighted axial image. Following intravenous administration of gadolinium-DTPA, the nasopharyngeal carcinoma "augments." Note the thrombus in the right internal jugular vein and sigmoid sinus.

derived from obstruction of the eustachian tube. The pharyngobasilar fascia is relatively resistant to tumor invasion; however, once it is breached, the malignancy spreads easily to the infratemporal fossa, the foramen ovale, or the cavernous sinus via the foramen lacerum or the orbital fissures. Lymphatic drainage is primarily to the retropharyngeal group of nodes, and subsequently to the internal jugular chain.

Primary lymphoma is the second most common nasopharyngeal malignancy in adulthood; it is seen with increased frequency in the immunocompromised patient. Lymphoma can arise from any of the lymphoid tissues distributed throughout the nasopharynx in Waldeyer's ring.

Rhabdomyosarcoma is the most common malignancy of the nasopharynx in children, accounting for almost 10% of malignancies in those under 15 years of age. It has a propensity for meningeal invasion and therefore carries a poor prognosis.

LESIONS OF THE NEUROVASCULAR BUNDLE AND PARAPHARYNGEAL SPACE

Paragangliomas originate from neural crest cells anywhere along the course of the sympathetic chain—from the skull base to the level of the carotid bifurcation. Bilaterality is rare, except in familial cases where up to 25% of tumors are bilateral. The typical locations where paragangliomas are found are the jugular foramen (glomus jugulare), the tympanic membrane (glomus typanicum), the cervical internal carotid artery (glomus vagale), and the carotid bifurcation (carotid body tumors) (Fig. 3.26). These tumors clinically present with a mass in the neck (carotid body, glomus vagale), pulsatile tinnitus (glomus tympanicum, glomus jugulare), or lower cranial nerve dysfunction. The typical MRI appearance is that of a well-circumscribed, nonhomogeneous mass, which bears a higher signal intensity than muscle on T1-weighted images, and a characteristic, moderately

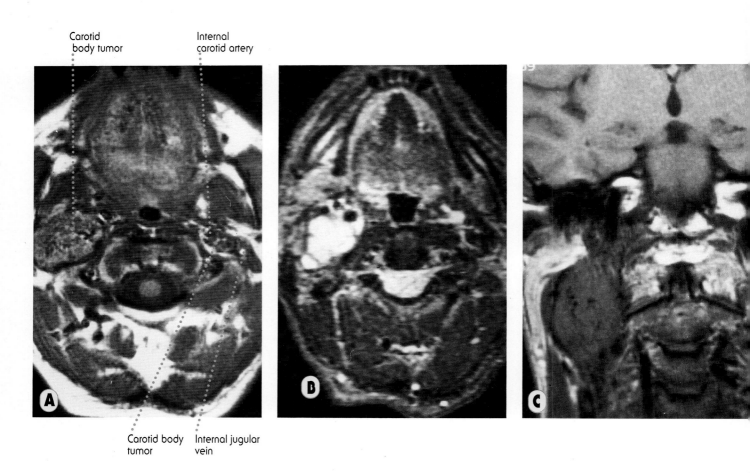

Carotid body tumor

Internal carotid artery

Carotid body tumor

Internal jugular vein

Fig. 3.26 CAROTID BODY TUMORS **(A)** T1-weighted axial image. This image, at the level of the oropharynx, reveals a typical ovoid, intermediate intensity carotid body tumor within the neurovascular bundle on the right side. The parapharyngeal fat has been obliterated and the internal carotid artery has been displaced anteromedially. Multiple low signal intensities are seen in the tumor. On the left side a small, "speckled," well-circumscribed mass is present within the carotid sheath posterior to the internal carotid artery. This was also a carotid body tumor. **(B)** T2-weighted axial image. The tumor has a bright "salt-and-pepper" appearance, characteristic of a paraganglioma. **(C)** T1-weighted coronal image. This section, through the right carotid bifurcation, reveals the typical appearance of a large carotid body tumor, displacing the carotid artery in the neck, with the tail extending to the skull base. Note the patency of the internal jugular vein.

high signal "salt-and-pepper" appearance on T2-weighted images. The larger tumors often have multiple serpiginous low signal areas that indicate their vascular nature. Smaller glomus tumors range from a relatively homogeneous appearance to a markedly speckled one. The salt-and-pepper appearance on T2-weighted sequences is relatively specific for paragangliomas.

Neurogenic tumors of the neurovascular bundle may originate from the glossopharyngeal (cranial nerve IX), the vagus (X), the spinal accessory (XI), or the hypoglossal nerve (XII). Like paragangliomas, neurofibromas are well-defined, encapsulated masses that extend along the carotid sheath, usually occurring between the angle of the mandible and the skull base (Fig. 3.27). They usually present as a mass in the neck, accompanied by pain or neurologic dys-

function. In general, neurofibromas have a much more homogeneous appearance, similar to that of muscle on T1-weighted images. On T2-weighted images, they are very bright.

The parapharyngeal space, which is composed of virtually all fat, is not noted for primary neoplasms. However, it is frequently encroached upon by neoplasms originating in the nasopharynx, the infratemporal fossa, and the neurovascular bundle.

THE INFRATEMPORAL FOSSA
Primary tumors of the infratemporal fossa are predominantly those involving salivary glands. Metastatic lesions to the infratemporal fossa are also relatively frequent. Other masses that occur in this region include chronic granulomatous inflammations, cystic hygromas, lymphangiomas, heman-

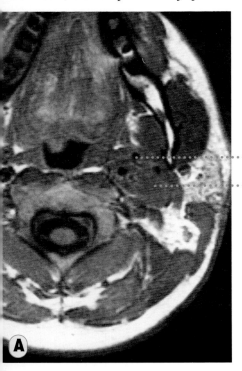
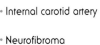

Internal carotid artery

Neurofibroma

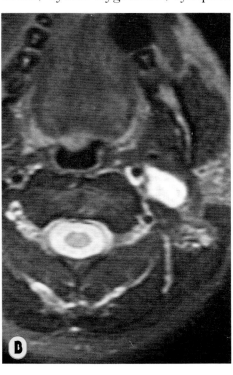

Fig. 3.27 NEUROFIBROMA **(A)** T1-weighted axial image. This young man presented with hoarseness and a neck mass. The homogeneous neurofibroma lies posterolateral to the internal carotid artery. The portion encasing the artery is slightly less homogeneous. The parapharyngeal fat is compressed and displaced but not obliterated, suggesting a benign lesion. **(D)** T2-weighted axial image. The tumor is homogeneously hyperintense. This is more characteristic of neurogenic tumors than paragangliomas. Angiography confirmed the neuroma to be avascular.

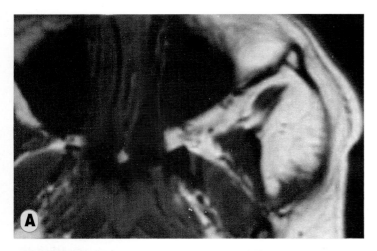

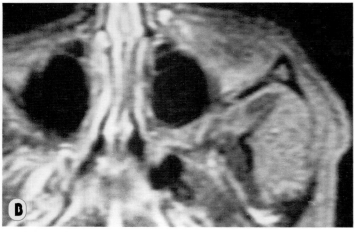

giomas (Fig. 3.28), and neuromas involving primarily branches of the trigeminal nerve.

Masses that arise outside the infratemporal fossa may extend to involve the structures within it. Lesions originating in the nasopharynx, the maxillary sinus, and the mandible can invade the infratemporal fossa (Fig. 3.29). Chordomas and sarcomas of the clivus and upper cervical spine may encroach upon the parapharyngeal space and neurovascular bundle, eventually reaching the infratemporal fossa. Superiorly, meningiomas in the middle cranial fossa can erode through the sphenoid bone into the infratemporal fossa.

SALIVARY GLAND LESIONS

Of the tumors detected in the major salivary glands, 75% to 80% involve the parotid gland and the remainder occur in the submandibular and sublingual glands. An estimated 10% to 20% of salivary gland tumors arise in minor salivary glands, in the lacrimal glands, and in the mucous glands of the palate, lips, tongue, nasopharynx, sinus, and larynx. Lesions of salivary glands in the infratemporal fossa originate in the deep lobe of the parotid gland or accessory salivary gland rests.

Inflammatory lesions of the parotid gland are relatively common, occurring secondary to viral, bacterial (Fig. 3.30), and granulomatous processes. Chronic, recurrent enlargement of the parotid gland is typical of Sjögren's syndrome (Fig. 3.31). The diagnosis is suggested by a symmetrical, lobular appearance of both parotid glands, in association with a connective tissue disease, keratoconjunctivitis sicca, and xerostomia. The MRI features are characteristic, with high signal intensity in well-differentiated acinar lobules on a T2-weighted sequence, and bilateral enlarged glands.

Tumor replacing fat in infratemporal fossa

Normal infratemporal fat

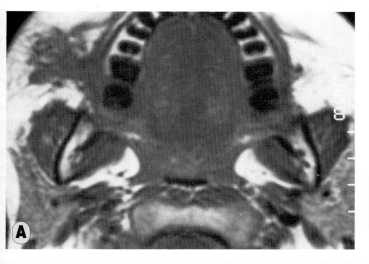

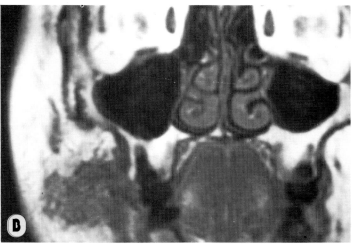

Fig. 3.30 CELLULITIS INVOLVING STENSEN'S DUCT **(A)** T1-weighted axial image. This young girl was on systemic steroids. She presented with right cheek swelling and a purulent discharge from Stensen's duct. There is an infiltrative process extending from the region of the parotid duct into the fat of the cheek. The stranding and ill-defined margination within the surrounding soft tissues is characteristic of an infective process. The remainder of the gland is normal. **(D)** T1-weighted coronal image. This image demonstrates the relationship of the infection to the buccal cavity. A similar appearance can be seen with dental sepsis.

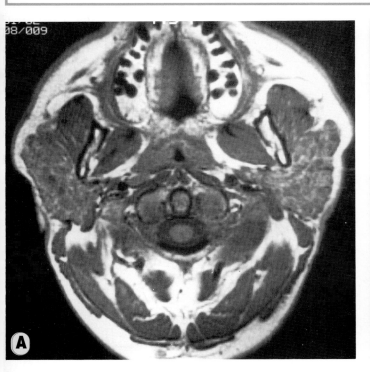

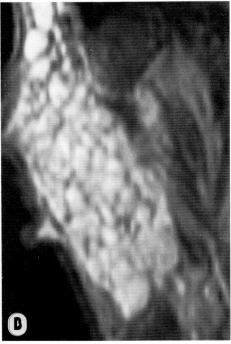

Fig. 3.31 SJÖGREN'S SYNDROME **(A)** T1-weighted axial image. The parotid glands are symmetrically enlarged with a well-defined, lobulated, acinar pattern. Their signal intensity is slightly less than that of the adjacent masseter. The glandular structure is preserved. There is a considerable degree of associated mucosal thickening within the nasopharynx. **(D)** T2-weighted coronal image (magnified view). The right parotid gland contains fluid-filled, dilated acini that are markedly hyperintense on this sequence.

The most common mass lesion is a benign mixed tumor of the parotid. It is a slow-growing, well-demarcated, smooth or lobulated tumor, with both epithelial and mesenchymal elements displacing the normal gland. It is more common in females and usually presents as a mass in the tail of the gland (Fig. 3.32).

Salivary and accessory salivary gland malignancies are subdivided into adenoid cystic carcinoma (cylindroma), mucoepidermoid carcinoma, mixed tumors, and adenocarcinoma. Adenoid cystic carcinoma is the most common, accounting for 4% of major, and 35% to 50% of minor, salivary gland malignant tumors. It occurs predominantly in males in the fourth and fifth decades of life. Histologically, it has uniform cells in a variable configuration, often containing mucus-filled pseudocysts. This probably accounts for the carcinoma's MRI appearance of high signal intensity on T2-weighted images (Fig. 3.33B). Tumors originating in the deep lobe of the parotid

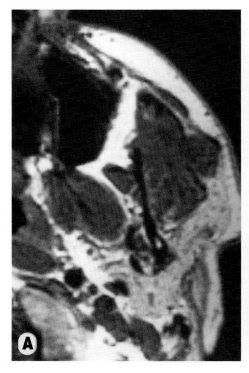

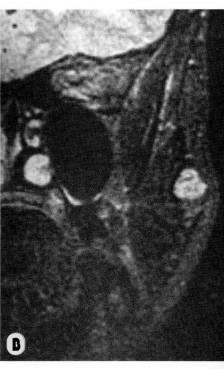

Fig. 3.32 BENIGN MIXED TUMOR OF THE PAROTID GLAND **(A)** T1-weighted axial image. A well-defined mass, isointense to muscle, is present in the tail of the parotid—the most frequent site for a benign mixed tumor. **(B)** T2-weighted coronal image. The tumor is very hyperintense compared with the normal parotid gland.

Invasion of masseter ·······

Parotid tumor ·······

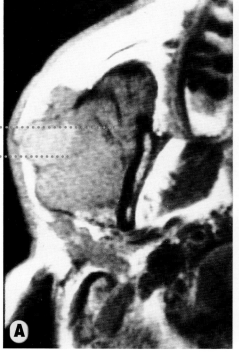

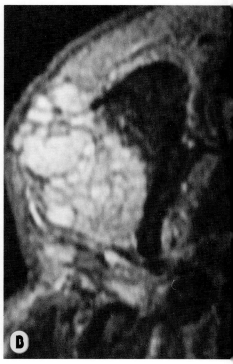

Fig. 3.33 ADENOID CYSTIC CARCINOMA T1-weighted **(A)** and T2-weighted **(B)** axial images. There is a large intraparotid mass, which invades the subcutaneous tissue and the masseter muscle. The high signal intensity in lobulated, cyst-like spaces suggests the histologic diagnosis.

gland show a distinct propensity for perineural invasion (Fig. 3.34), frequently along the facial nerve. Tumors that occur in accessory salivary glands in the infratemporal fossa may invade along the second and third divisions of the trigeminal nerve into the intracranial space. Recurrent tumors are more destructive in their behavior, often directly destroying the bone of the skull base (Fig. 3.35).

Mucoepidermoid carcinoma has a slightly higher incidence in females in the fourth to fifth decade of life. This tumor is classified as low, intermediate, or high-grade malignancy, based on the predominant cell type. Large numbers of mucous cells indicate low-grade malignancy; a large proportion of squamous cells indicates high-grade malignancy.

Adenocarcinomas account for 15% of malignant parotid gland tumors; their incidence is equal between the sexes. They are intraglandular masses, often with poorly defined borders.

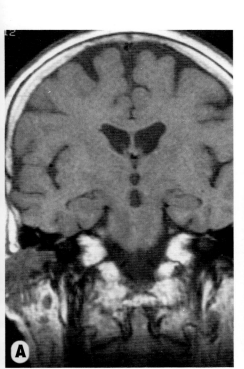
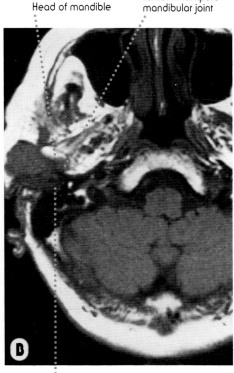

Head of mandible

Tumor in temporo-mandibular joint

Tumor in temporal bone

Fig. 3.34 ADENOID CYSTIC CARCINOMA OF THE PAROTID WITH PERINEURAL AND JOINT INVASION (A) T1-weighted coronal image. This patient presented with a right facial palsy. The low signal intensity tumor is in the superior part of the parotid gland, extending into the base of the temporal bone. **(B)** T1-weighted axial image. There is tumor involvement of the posterior aspect of the right temporomandibular joint space.

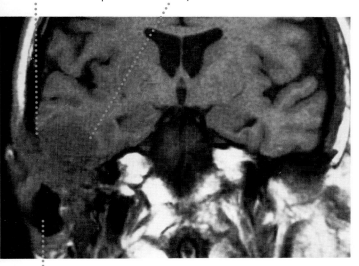

Invasion of temporal bone   Temporal lobe invasion

Surgical defect

Fig. 3.35 RECURRENT ADENOID CYSTIC CARCINOMA OF THE PAROTID WITH SKULL BASE AND BRAIN INVOLVEMENT T1-weighted coronal image. The tumor involves the temporal bone, crosses the dura and subarachnoid space, and invades the temporal lobe on the right. The old surgical defect involving the ear is visible. Following MRI assessment of this recurrence, an extensive surgical resection, including temporal bone and temporal lobe, resulted in an excellent remission.

THE OROPHARYNX AND MANDIBLE

NORMAL ANATOMY (Figs. 3.36 and 3.37)

The **oropharynx** lies below the nasopharynx, separated by Passavant's muscle and the soft palate. The posterior wall is formed by the three constrictor muscles: superior, middle, and inferior. Inferiorly, the oropharynx is separated from the hypopharynx by the epiglottis. The tongue base forms the mobile anterior wall. Laterally, there are two ridges of muscle: the palatoglossus anteriorly, and the palatopharyngeus posteriorly. Between these two is a collection of lymphatic tissue known as the palatine tonsil.

The oropharynx is separated from the mouth by the anterior pillar of palatoglossus. The oral cavity extends from this muscle to the lips and is enclosed laterally by the buccal mucosa. The hard palate forms the roof. The mylohyoid muscle forms the floor of the mouth, attached anteriorly and laterally to the mandible. It slopes downward to the midline to create a midline raphe. The midline raphe and the remaining posterior fibers of the muscle are attached to the

Normal Anatomy of the Head and Neck (Figs. 3.36 and 3.37)

The Oropharynx, Tongue, and Floor of the Mouth

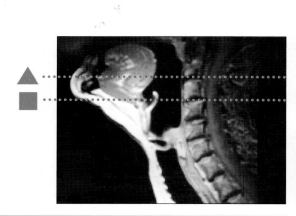

Fig. 3.36 Localizer: Midline T1-Weighted Sagittal Image
The planes of section of three images are indicated: axial section through the body of the tongue, axial section through the base of the tongue, and a coronal section through the body of the tongue. The midline sagittal section through the tongue and oropharynx is labeled in Figure 3.37D.

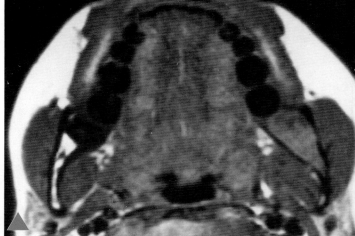

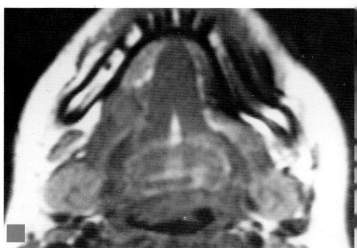

body of the hyoid bone. This structure forms a diaphragm that supports the mass of the tongue. The hyoglossus lies along the side of the tongue. It is a vertical muscle that is separated from the mylohyoid by loose fatty tissue containing the lingual nerve, the submandibular duct, and the hypoglossal nerve. The glossopharyngeal nerve, the stylohyoid muscle, and the lingual artery are situated medial to the hyoglossus muscle. The submandibular gland lies below the mylohyoid, curving around its free posterior border and ending in the duct that passes forward to open adjacent to the frenulum sublinguae. The sublingual gland lies in the midline, anterior to the hyoglossus, and separates the latter from the mylohyoid muscle.

The bulk of the tongue is made up of the genioglossus muscle. All the muscles of the tongue are supplied by the hypoglossal nerve. The lingual tonsil is a collection of lymphatic tissue on the surface of the posterior third of the tongue. Paired recesses called the valleculae lie between the tongue and the epiglottis. The retromolar trigone lies between the posterior molar, the posterior attachment of the mylohyoid, and the mandibular attachment of the medial pterygoid muscle.

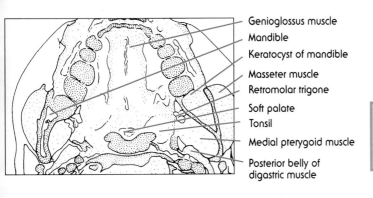

Genioglossus muscle
Mandible
Keratocyst of mandible
Masseter muscle
Retromolar trigone
Soft palate
Tonsil
Medial pterygoid muscle
Posterior belly of digastric muscle

Fig. 3.37A T1-Weighted Axial Image Through the Body of the Tongue Note the relationship of the posterior aspect of the tongue to the retromolar trigone and the tonsil.

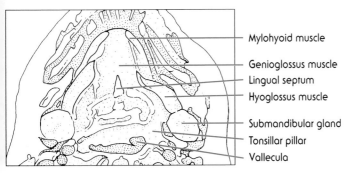

Mylohyoid muscle
Genioglossus muscle
Lingual septum
Hyoglossus muscle
Submandibular gland
Tonsillar pillar
Vallecula

Fig. 3.37B T1-Weighted Axial Image Through the Base of the Tongue The fat plane immediately lateral to the hyoglossus muscle allows the mandibular cortex to be clearly seen as a thin hypointense line. The marrow space within the mandible has high signal intensity due to fat. Note also, the close proximity of the hyoglossus muscle to the submandibular gland.

The Oropharynx, Tongue, and Floor of the Mouth

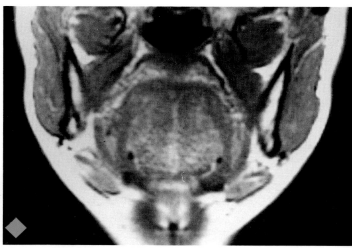

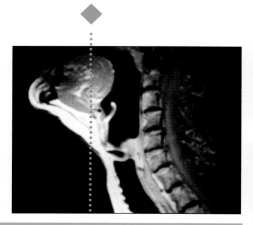

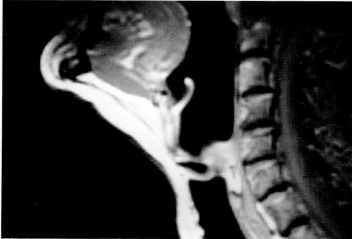

Fig. 3.36 Localizer: Midline T1-Weighted Sagittal Image
The planes of section of three images are indicated: axial section through the body of the tongue, axial section through the base of the tongue, and a coronal section through the body of the tongue. The midline sagittal section through the tongue and oropharynx is labeled in Figure 3.37D.

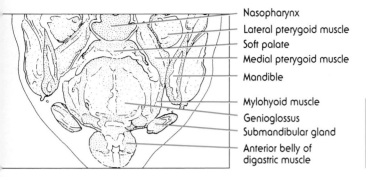

Nasopharynx
Lateral pterygoid muscle
Soft palate
Medial pterygoid muscle
Mandible

Mylohyoid muscle
Genioglossus
Submandibular gland
Anterior belly of
digastric muscle

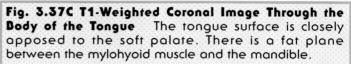

Fig. 3.37C T1-Weighted Coronal Image Through the Body of the Tongue The tongue surface is closely apposed to the soft palate. There is a fat plane between the mylohyoid muscle and the mandible.

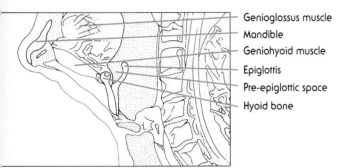

Genioglossus muscle
Mandible
Geniohyoid muscle
Epiglottis
Pre-epiglottic space
Hyoid bone

Fig. 3.37D Midline T1-Weighted Sagittal Image A midline T1-weighted image aids in evaluating the base of the tongue and the latter's relationship to the pre-epiglottic space. However, laterally placed lesions within the tongue are not well-visualized by sagittal images, due to partial volume averaging along the tongue's curved superior surface.

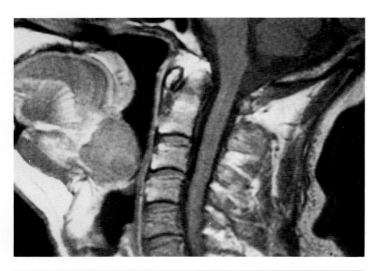

Fig. 3.38 LINGUAL THYROID Midline T1-weighted sagittal image. There is an isointense, well-circumscribed, round mass in the posterior third of the tongue. The lesion almost completely occludes the pharynx and depresses the epiglottis.

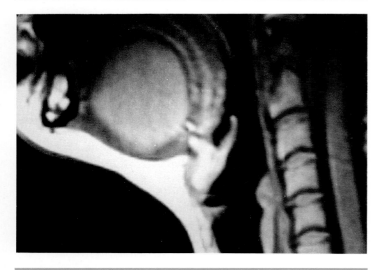

Fig. 3.39 SUBLINGUAL DERMOID CYST IN THE FLOOR OF THE MOUTH T1-weighted sagittal image. There is a uniformly hyperintense, midline lesion, which is well encapsulated; it elevates the tongue muscles. High signal intensity (relative to muscle) on T1-weighted images is characteristic of dermoids.

TECHNIQUE

The tongue, the floor of the mouth, and the oropharynx are areas that are particularly difficult to evaluate by CT scanning. Dental and motion artifact contribute to the problems involved in visualizing poorly defined infiltrative lesions. Magnetic resonance imaging provides superior soft tissue definition, relative freedom from dental artifact, and multiplanar sections. For many lesions in the floor of mouth and the mandible, it is the imaging modality of choice.

In most cases, the oropharynx can be adequately examined using a circumferential head coil. A surface coil is preferred for patients with obese, short necks, unless a head coil can be positioned sufficiently low to allow for adequate anatomical coverage. A surface coil is also used if, in addition to the primary examination of the oropharynx, the entire neck is to be evaluated for lymphadenopathy. It is often simpler to use a surface coil for the whole examination than to switch coils during the procedure.

Initially, T1-weighted sagittal images are obtained for localization and for evaluation of midline pathology. This is followed by T1-weighted axial and T1-weighted coronal images through the area of primary interest. Axial T2-weighted images complete the examination. The T2-weighted images should cover the primary area and the neck from mastoid to clavicle.

PATHOLOGY

THE OROPHARYNX
DEVELOPMENTAL LESIONS The lingual thyroid is a residual rest of thyroid tissue in the base of the tongue at the foramen cecum. It may be the only functioning thyroid tissue, and it is associated with a higher incidence of carcinoma. Any increase in the tumor's size should be viewed with suspicion of malignancy. Lingual thyroid may be either incidentally diagnosed on radionuclide scanning or clinically detected as a mass at the base of the tongue (Fig. 3.38).

Dermoid cysts in the oral cavity are usually found in the anterior portion of the floor of the mouth. They originate either from congenital tissue rests or from acquired implantation cysts, usually presenting in the second or third decade of life as a midline, sublingual (above the muscle masses of mylohyoid and digastric), or submental (beneath the mylohyoid and above the platysma) mass (Fig. 3.39). Branchial cleft cysts may occur at the level of the oral cavity; however, they are more common in the neck area.

BENIGN TUMORS   Hemangiomas and lymphangiomas are common, particularly in children. They may occur anywhere in the head and neck region and range from small, totally mucosal lesions (Fig. 3.40) to bulky masses in the floor of the mouth and base of the tongue, with infiltration apparent throughout the tissue planes. Typically, they are hyperintense on T2-weighted images (Fig. 3.41).

Neurofibromas are uncommon lesions in the head and neck region and are often associated with neurofibromatosis. There is a slight predilection for the tongue, the submandibular region, and the mandible. The morphology of these tumors can range from well-defined nodules to diffuse soft tissue involvement.

Lipomas are common throughout the body. Their appearance is exactly as expected—well-marginated, with uniformly high signal intensity on T1-weighted images.

MALIGNANT TUMORS   Squamous cell carcinomas account for 90% of all oral malignancies. There is a strong association with heavy smoking and alcohol

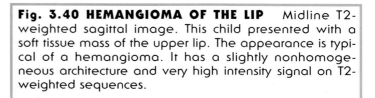

Fig. 3.40 HEMANGIOMA OF THE LIP Midline T2-weighted sagittal image. This child presented with a soft tissue mass of the upper lip. The appearance is typical of a hemangioma. It has a slightly nonhomogeneous architecture and very high intensity signal on T2-weighted sequences.

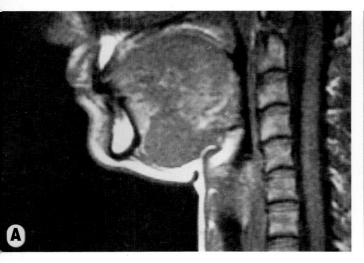

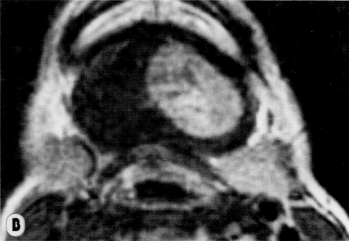

Fig. 3.41 HEMANGIOMA IN THE FLOOR OF MOUTH (A) T1-weighted sagittal image. There is a poorly defined, low signal intensity lesion in the floor of the mouth, deep to the geniohyoid muscle. **(B)** T2-weighted axial image. Typically, hemangiomas have a high signal intensity on T2-weighted images.

Tumor ·· ·· ·· ·· ·· ·· ·· ·· ·· ·· ·· ··

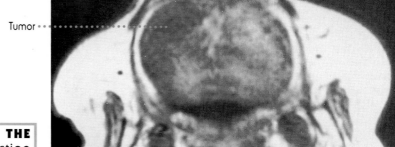

Fig. 3.42 SQUAMOUS CELL CARCINOMA OF THE TONGUE T1-weighted axial image. This section through the anterior two thirds of the tongue reveals a slightly hypointense, homogeneous, infiltrative mass that destroys the normal internal architecture of the right side of the tongue. Its malignant nature is reflected in its poorly defined margins.

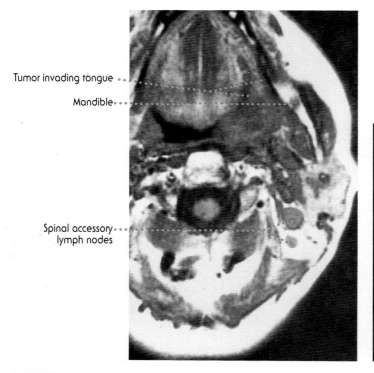

Tumor invading tongue ·· ·· ··

Mandible ·· ·· ··

Spinal accessory ·· ·· ··
lymph nodes

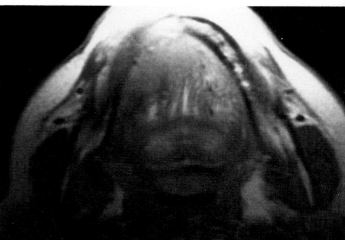

Fig. 3.43 SQUAMOUS CELL CARCINOMA OF THE TONSIL T1-weighted axial image. There is a homogeneous, intermediate intensity tumor arising from the left tonsil. The tumor is infiltrating the retromolar trigone and the base of the tongue on the left. The tumor is immediately adjacent to the mandible, but the uniform hypointense line of the cortical bone indicates that the mandible is intact. Note the enlarged lymph nodes posterior to the neurovascular bundle (spinal accessory chain).

Fig. 3.44 SQUAMOUS CELL CARCINOMA IN THE FLOOR OF THE MOUTH T1-weighted axial image. A small surface coil was used for this study, resulting in very high signal anteriorly. The tumor can be seen anteriorly on the right, distorting the internal architecture of the tongue. The cortex of the mandible has been eroded, as evidenced by the loss of the sharp, dark line representing the cortical bone.

consumption. The most common sites of involvement are the lip (where the lesion is usually ulcerated and locally confined), the floor of the mouth, and the anterior two thirds of the tongue (Fig. 3.42).

In the oropharynx, squamous cell carcinoma of the tonsil (Fig. 3.43) is more common than carcinoma of the base of the tongue and the soft palate. Of patients with tongue and floor-of-mouth neoplasms, 70% to 80% develop cervical node metastases. Tumors of the anterior and middle third of the tongue tend to have unilateral lymph node involvement; the posterior third more often has bilateral lymphatic involvement.

Cancers of the posterior tongue are often clinically silent for a long time and may present as an occult primary with malignant cervical nodes. Three quarters of all posterior tongue cancers are reported to have metastases at time of presentation.

Tumors of the floor of the mouth and base of the tongue infiltrate extensively, often eroding the mandible with invasion of the marrow space (Fig. 3.44). Squamous cell carcinomas in the region of the retromolar trigone also frequently invade the mandible, the base of the tongue, and the tonsillar pillar. Magnetic resonance imaging has proven to be extremely valuable in establishing mandibular involvement. Tumor invasion is indicated by loss of the normal high signal from the fatty marrow. The extent of mandibular resection and reconstruction can be more accurately assessed.

Lymphoma is the next most common malignancy to affect adults. Lymphomas frequently arise in the tonsillar region, presenting as a well-circumscribed mass that produces marked extrinsic compression of the pharyngeal wall. Mucosal infiltration is common, although deeper anatomy is often well-preserved (Fig. 3.45).

Carcinomas arising from the minor salivary glands are not as common as squamous cell tumors or lymphomas but they are not rare. They can be very infiltrative and aggressive. In children, rhabdomyosarcomas are the most common malignancy in this area although they are more frequently seen in the region of the paranasal sinuses and nasopharynx.

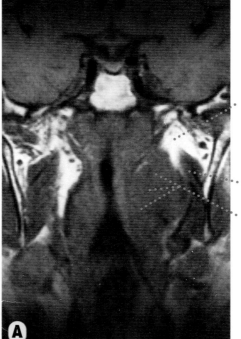

Parapharyngeal space

Medial pterygoid muscle

Tumor

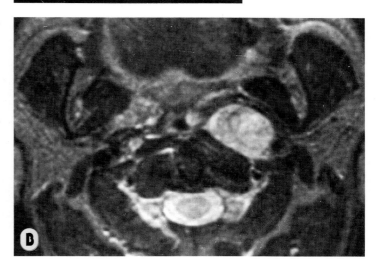

Fig. 3.45 LYMPHOMA OF THE TONSIL **(A)** T1-weighted coronal image. There is a slightly hypointense mass in the left tonsillar fossa. The tumor is obliterating the high signal intensity fat in the parapharyngeal space and displacing the medial pterygoid muscle. The smooth, well-defined outline is more characteristic of lymphoma than of carcinoma. **(B)** T2-weighted axial image. The well-encapsulated, high signal intensity tumor shows no evidence of invasion and is merely displacing the adjacent tissues.

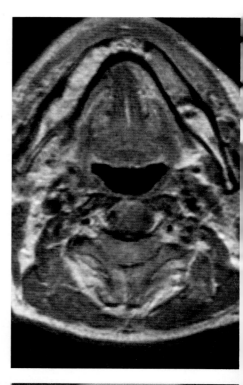

Fig. 3.46 OSTEORADIONECROSIS OF THE MANDIBLE
Proton-density axial image. The high signal intensity normally seen within the marrow space is absent on the left. The cortex is preserved.

Soft tissue component ···· of tumor

Tumor ···

Normal fatty marrow ····

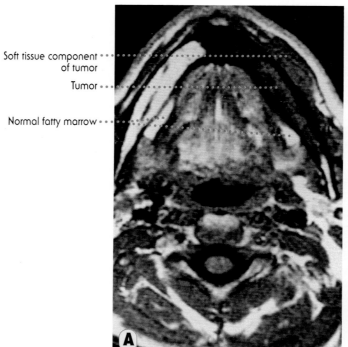

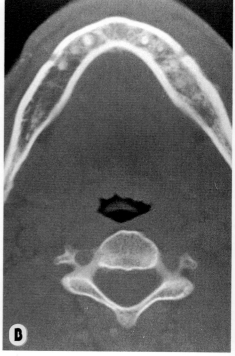

Fig. 3.47 MALIGNANT FIBROUS HISTIOCYTOMA **(A)** T1-weighted axial image. This patient presented with a soft tissue mass anterior to the mandible on the left. The lesion can be seen deep to the subcutaneous fat, which is intimately related to the mandible. The low signal intensity cortex is intact. Within the marrow space of the mandible, the loss of high signal indicates replacement by the tumor from the angle to a point beyond the symphysis on the right. This extension within the mandible was not suspected on CT. **(B)** CT axial image. Examination of bone windows fails to reveal the mandibular marrow involvement clearly shown by MRI.

THE MANDIBLE

The mandible is especially worth mentioning with regard to MRI. Pathological processes are often better evaluated by MRI than by CT, due particularly to the superior soft tissue resolution of MRI within the marrow spaces, and, to a lesser degree, to the absence of dental artifact.

Osteoradionecrosis is a rather frequent complication following radiation therapy of head and neck tumors. Clinical symptoms usually precede radiographic evidence of bone involvement. Magnetic resonance imaging is capable of demonstrating bone involvement at a much earlier stage than CT, and it clearly defines the limits of the lesion for surgical resection (Fig. 3.46). It does not, however, distinguish recurrent tumors from necrotic tissue.

Malignant lesions primarily arising from the mandible are relatively uncommon. Malignant fibrous histiocytoma may have both a soft tissue and bone component without frank bony destruction (Fig. 3.47). Squamous cell carcinoma from the oropharynx often erodes the mandible. Metastatic disease can occasionally produce a destructive mass, the characteristics of which are indistinguishable from all of the preceding malignancies.

Dental-related lesions of the mandible are relatively common. Dentigerous cysts (Fig. 3.48) are well-evaluated by MRI but no additional information is gained over CT.

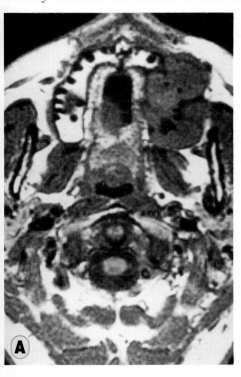 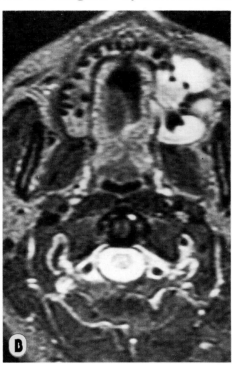 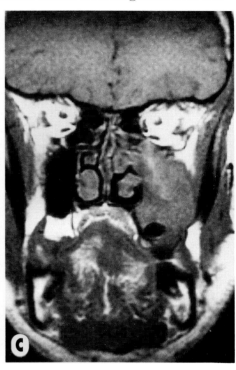

Fig. 3.48 DENTIGEROUS CYST   (A) T1-weighted axial image. The superior alveolar ridge contains a dentigerous cyst. The cyst fluid is slightly hyperintense compared with muscle. The cyst has expanded into the subcutaneous tissues and the infratemporal fossa. Posteriorly, the tooth elements are seen within it as a hypointense signal. **(B)** T2-weighted axial image. The tooth seen within the cyst is characteristic of a dentigerous cyst. The cyst fluid is very bright on the T2-weighted sequences. **(C)** T1-weighted coronal image. The cyst extends into and fills the entire maxillary antrum. There is some deformity of the hard palate on the left. The higher signal within the superior portion of the maxillary sinus represents inspissated mucus.

THE LARYNX AND HYPOPHARYNX

NORMAL ANATOMY (Figs. 3.49 and 3.50)

The larynx, hypopharynx, and the cervical esophagus are contained within the visceral compartment of the neck. They are separated from the oropharynx by the epiglottis and lateral pharyngoepiglottic folds.

The **hypopharynx** lies posterior to the epiglottis and has the piriform sinuses, which extend down laterally to the level of the false cords. At the level of the posterior cricoid cartilage, the hypopharynx becomes continuous with the esophagus.

The **larynx** extends from the epiglottis to the trachea. It is divided into three compartments: **supraglottic**, **glottic**, and the **subglottic**. The larynx is contained within a cartilaginous framework formed by the hyoid bone and the thyroid, arytenoid, and cricoid cartilages, each intimately connected by membranes.

The **supraglottic** region extends from the free edge of the epiglottis down to the level of the false cords and the ventricle. The structures contained within it are the epiglottis and the aryepiglottic folds, the false cords, and the laryngeal ventricles. The pharyngeal epithelial squamous mucosa extends down into the supraglottic region. The epiglottis, composed of elastic cartilage, rarely calcifies. The narrow base of the

Normal Anatomy of the Head and Neck (Figs. 3.49 and 3.50)

The Larynx and Hypopharynx

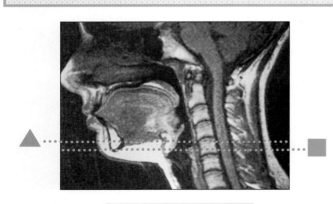

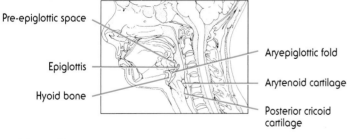

Pre-epiglottic space

Epiglottis

Hyoid bone

Aryepiglottic fold

Arytenoid cartilage

Posterior cricoid cartilage

Fig. 3.49 Localizer: Midline T1-Weighted Sagittal Image
The planes of section of five images are indicated: an axial image through the supraglottic larynx and hypopharynx, an axial image through the glottic larynx, axial image through the subglottic larynx, a coronal image through the piriform sinuses, and a coronal image through the true cords.

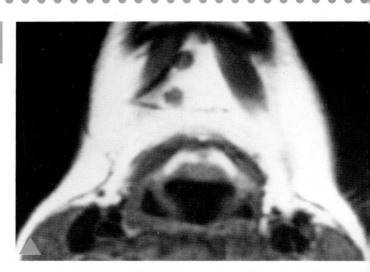

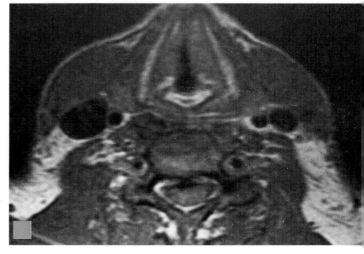

epiglottis attaches in the midline to the thyroid cartilage, just inferior to the notch. Forming the major solid structure in the supraglottis is the hyoid bone. It is suspended between the suprahyoid and the infrahyoid strap muscles. The hyoepiglottic ligament attaches the epiglottis to the hyoid bone. The thyrohyoid membrane connects the hyoid bone to the thyroid cartilage. The level of the hyoid bone marks the lower level of the jugulodigastric group of lymph nodes. Unlike the lower levels of the larynx, the supraglottic region has a rich supply of lymphatics.

The **glottis** is composed of the true vocal cords, attaching anteriorly in the midline to the thyroid cartilage at the anterior commissure. The posterior attachment of the vocal cords is to the vocalis process of the arytenoid cartilage. No lymphatics are present at the level of the glottis. Carcinoma occurring in this area must spread either supraglottically or infraglottically before metastases to lymph nodes can occur.

The **subglottis** extends from the inferior surface of the free edge of the true cords down to the tracheal cartilage. Lymphatics do occur in this area, although it is not as richly supplied as the supraglottic area.

The cartilage framework of the larynx is interconnected by a series of ligaments and synovial articulations. True synovial joints occur at the cricothyroid and cricoarytenoid joints.

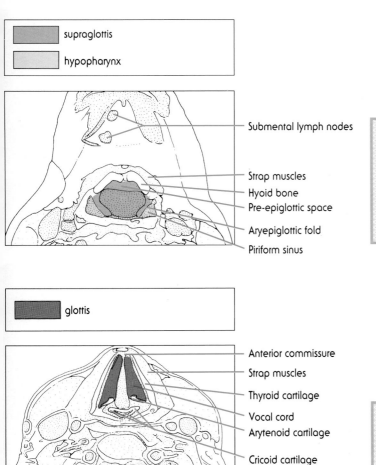

supraglottis

hypopharynx

Submental lymph nodes

Strap muscles
Hyoid bone
Pre-epiglottic space

Aryepiglottic fold

Piriform sinus

Fig. 3.50A T1-Weighted Axial Image Through the Supraglottic Larynx and Hypopharynx   The high signal intensity deep to the strap muscles is in the hyoid bone. The aryepiglottic folds separate the larynx from the hypopharynx. The mucosa of the larynx is slightly hyperintense to muscle. There are two small, incidental submental lymph nodes lying between the anterior bellies of digastric in the floor of the mouth.

glottis

Anterior commissure

Strap muscles

Thyroid cartilage

Vocal cord

Arytenoid cartilage

Cricoid cartilage
(posterior part)

Fig. 3.50B T1-Weighted Axial Image Through the Glottic Larynx   The high signal intensity within the arytenoid cartilages at their synovial articulation with the posterior cricoid are the landmarks for the true cord level. The thyroid cartilage is hyperintense centrally, layered between two black lines, representing the calcified cortex.

The Larynx and Hypopharynx

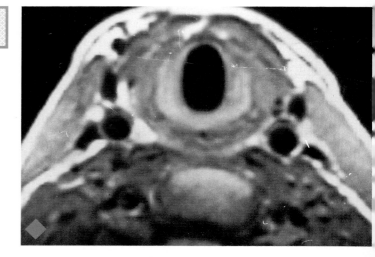

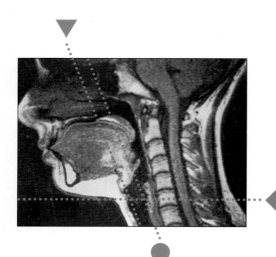

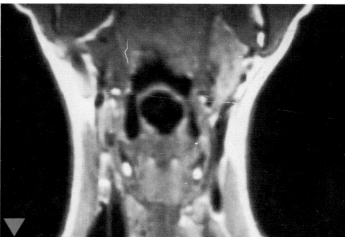

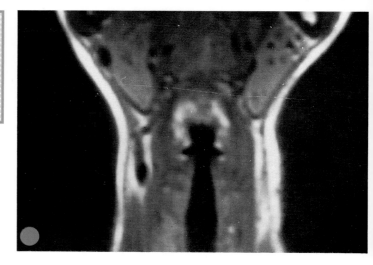

Fig. 3.49 Localizer: Midline T1-Weighted Sagittal Image
The planes of section of five images are indicated: an
axial image through the supraglottic larynx and
hypopharynx, an axial image through the glottic larynx,
axial image through the subglottic larynx, a coronal
image through the piriform sinuses, and a coronal
image through the true cords.

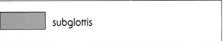
subglottis

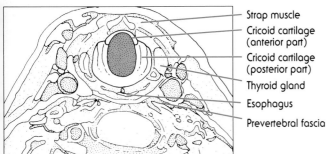

Strap muscle
Cricoid cartilage (anterior part)
Cricoid cartilage (posterior part)
Thyroid gland
Esophagus
Prevertebral fascia

Fig. 3.50C T1-Weighted Axial Image Through the Subglottic Larynx The hyperintensity in the anterior and posterior cricoid cartilages distinguishes them from the strap muscles anteriorly, the esophagus posteriorly, and the thyroid gland laterally. Only the tips of the lateral lobes of the thyroid are visible. High signal intensity fat surrounds the neurovascular bundle, separating it from the midline viscera and the posterior prevertebral fascia.

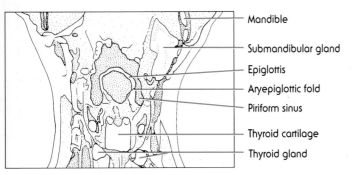

Mandible

Submandibular gland

Epiglottis

Aryepiglottic fold

Piriform sinus

Thyroid cartilage

Thyroid gland

Fig. 3.50D T1-Weighted Coronal Image Through the Piriform Sinuses The epiglottis and aryepiglottic folds are continuous structures that are attached to the anterior thyroid cartilage. The relationship of the laterally situated piriform sinuses can be appreciated.

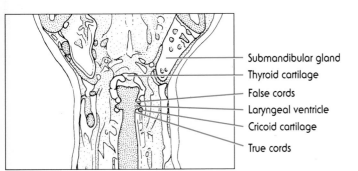

Submandibular gland
Thyroid cartilage
False cords
Laryngeal ventricle
Cricoid cartilage
True cords

Fig. 3.50E T1-Weighted Coronal Image Through the True Cords The false cords, the laryngeal ventricles, and the true cord level are identified.

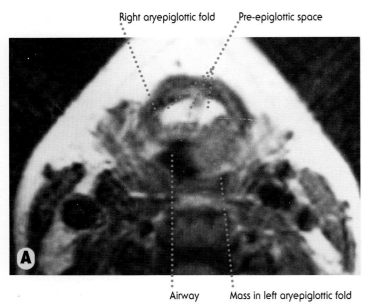

Right aryepiglottic fold   Pre-epiglottic space

Airway   Mass in left aryepiglottic fold

Mass in aryepiglottic fold   Cricoid cartilage

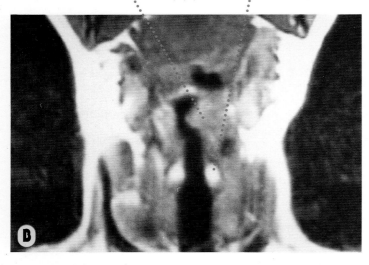

Fig. 3.51 LARYNGEAL MUCUS RETENTION CYST (A) T1-weighted axial image. The patient presented with stridor. There is a lesion related to the left aryepiglottic fold. The cyst contained inspissated mucus. **(B)** T1-weighted coronal image. The supraglottic location and its relationship to the aryepiglottic fold are demonstrated. The high signal intensity of the cricoid cartilage defines the lower limit of the larynx.

TECHNIQUE

Recommended modifications of the standard head and neck MRI protocol include the use of 3-mm-thick sections instead of the usual 5-mm on all the T1-weighted studies, as well as the practice of obliquing the coronal sections through the larynx along the long axis of the airway so as to minimize partial volume averaging effects (see Fig. 3.49). It is particularly important during the examination to prevent excessive swallowing on the patient's part. A three-part approach can serve the end of holding swallowing to a minimum: (a) guard against overextending the patient's neck, (b) make the patient as comfortable as possible, and (c) keep the scan times short. Exquisite detail is possible if motion can be entirely avoided.

PATHOLOGY

INFLAMMATION AND INFECTION   Chronic granulomatous processes in the larynx include: tuberculosis (TB), sarcoidosis, Wegener's granulomatosis and midline granulomatosis, rhinoscleroma (*Klebsiella* infection), leprosy, and syphilis. With the exception of TB, all are relatively rare. Those inflammatory processes involving synovial joints—rheumatoid arthritis, osteoarthritis, gout, and gonococcal arthritis—can affect the cricoarytenoid and cricothyroid joints. Relapsing polychondritis and perichondritis may affect the thyroid and anterior cricoid cartilages. These disorders may be idiopathic, associated with rheumatologic disorders, or may occur after radiotherapy. Magnetic resonance images are nonspecific. Findings may include an infiltrative, ill-defined soft tissue mass and destruction of involved cartilage.

CYSTS A variety of fluid-filled cysts occur in the larynx, particularly in the supraglottic area. The most common is the mucus retention cyst, which occurs secondary to obstruction of minor seromucinous glands. This cyst is most often seen in the valleculae, the epiglottis, and the aryepiglottic folds. Inspissated mucus may be difficult to distinguish from a solid lesion (Fig. 3.51).

Laryngoceles are derived from the laryngeal ventricle and are secondary to dilatation of the saccule. The cysts can be external, internal, or a combination thereof. They extend out through the thyrohyoid membrane and into the soft tissues of the neck. They may be air- or fluid-filled and can become secondarily infected. The signal intensity of the lesion will depend on its contents; air-filled cysts are black on all pulse sequences, whereas fluid-filled cysts are dark on T1-weighted images and bright on T2-weighted images.

The congenital thyroglossal duct cyst (Fig. 3.52) originates from the thyroid primordium as it descends from the foramen cecum of the tongue, in or near the midline, along the migratory path of the thyroid gland to its position in the neck. Cell remnants may persist along this line anterior or posterior to the hyoid or anterior to the thyroid and cricoid cartilages. The majority of these duct cysts (65%) are infrahyoid. The remainder occur with equal frequency either at the hyoid bone or superior to it. If the duct remains patent, it can become obstructed and secondarily infected; congenital thyroglossal duct cysts often fluctuate in size.

BENIGN TUMORS Benign tumors of the larynx are uncommon, save for papillomas, which can occur at any point in the airway, including the vocal cords. These tumors are best evaluated by laryngoscopy and rarely require diagnostic imaging. Chondromas, hemangiomas, and neurofibromas are occasionally

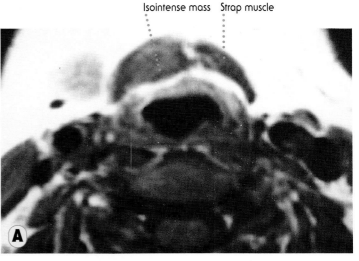

Isointense mass   Strap muscle

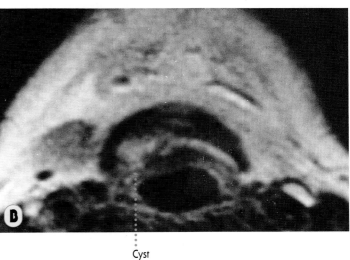

Cyst

Fig. 3.52 THYROGLOSSAL DUCT CYST T1-weighted **(A)** and T2-weighted **(B)** axial images. The T1-weighted sequence shows a small mass isointense to the strap muscles lying slightly to the right of midline, inferior to the hyoid bone. The cyst is bright on the T2-weighted image.

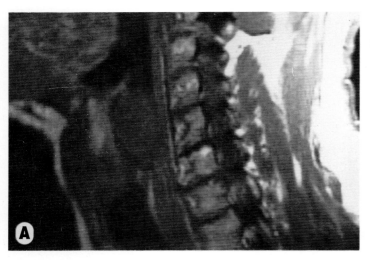

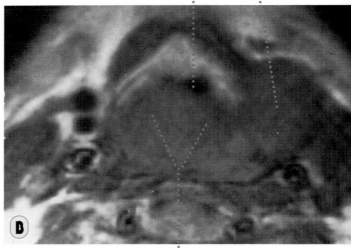

Airway   Extralaryngeal mass

Masses involving aryepiglottic folds

Fig. 3.53 NEUROFIBROMA OF THE LARYNX (A) T1-weighted sagittal image. This patient presented with dysphagia and airway obstruction. A well-circumscribed mass arises from the aryepiglottic fold, producing compression of both the larynx and the hypopharynx. Normal tissue planes are preserved. **(B)** T1-weighted axial image. Bilateral neurofibromas involving the aryepiglottic folds, which have an intermediate signal intensity, are homogeneous and well-encapsulated. A third neurofibroma is extralaryngeal on the left. T2-weighted sequences (not shown) demonstrated the tumors to be hyperintense, typical of neurofibromas.

Anterior commissure   Tumor   Thyroid cartilage

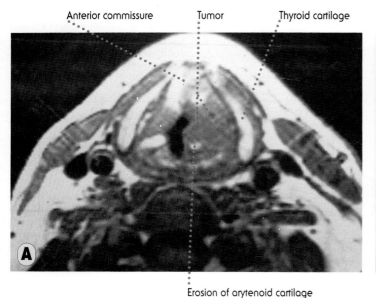

Thyroid cartilage

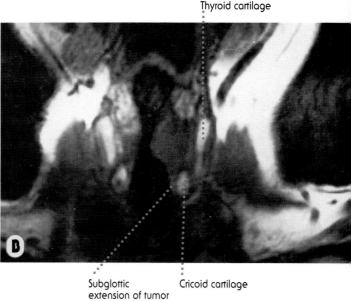

Erosion of arytenoid cartilage

Subglottic extension of tumor   Cricoid cartilage

Fig. 3.54 GLOTTIC AND UNILATERAL SQUAMOUS CELL CARCINOMA OF THE LARYNX (A) T1-weighted axial image. There is a tumor involving the left vocal cord. The high signal intensity of the cricoid, arytenoid, and thyroid cartilages clearly identifies the level of this section to be at the vocal cords. The tumor extends to the anterior commissure but does not involve it. The thyroid cartilage is intact but the left arytenoid cartilage appears eroded. **(B)** T1-weighted coronal image. The soft tissue mass has obliterated the high intensity fat signal adjacent to the thyroid cartilage (as compared with the right side). It has extended inferior to the left cricoid cartilage, into the subglottis, and superiorly into the supraglottis.

encountered. Chondromas usually originate from the lamina of the posterior cricoid cartilage, whereas neurofibromas form in the aryepiglottic folds (Fig. 3.53) or at the level of the false cords, and hemangiomas occur anywhere. Magnetic resonance imaging will demonstrate a circumscribed mass in all cases. The presence of calcium (absence of signal) suggests chondroma, but otherwise the appearance of most lesions is nonspecific.

MALIGNANT TUMORS   The most common pathology in the larynx is squamous cell carcinoma; it accounts for approximately 90% of all malignancies in this region. It occurs as either an exophytic verrucous carcinoma or as an ulceroinfiltrative lesion. Among the potential locations of origin, 60% to 70% occur in the glottis, 30% to 35% in the supraglottic region, and 4% to 6% in the subglottis. Rare forms of malignancy include pleomorphic carcinoma, adenocarcinoma, adenoid cystic carcinoma, and acinous carcinoma.

Assessment of laryngeal cancer requires detailed evaluation of the vocal cords, the cartilages, and the surrounding neck. Early disease may be confined to one vocal cord (Fig. 3.54). Magnetic resonance imaging can usually visualize tumor extension superiorly to the pre-epiglottic space (Fig. 3.55) and the piriform

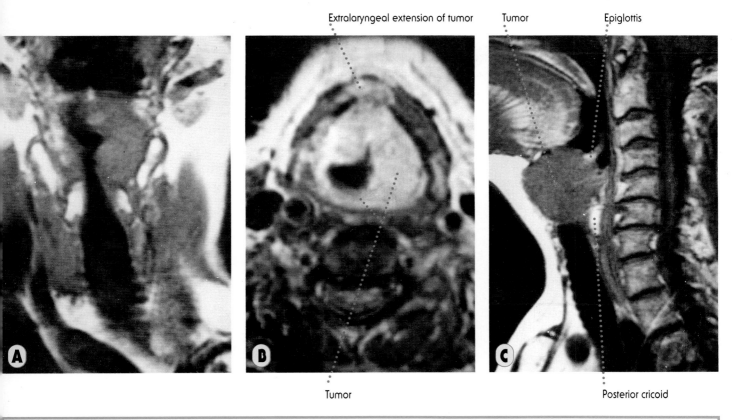

Extralaryngeal extension of tumor   Tumor   Epiglottis

Tumor

Posterior cricoid

Fig. 3.55 SUPRAGLOTTIC SQUAMOUS CELL CARCINOMA OF THE LARYNX   (A) T1-weighted coronal image. This 50-year-old female presented with hoarseness. The intermediate signal intensity tumor mass on the left originates at the level of the false cords, with superior extension along the aryepiglottic fold and inferior extension to the posterior cricoid. **(B)** T2-weighted axial image. The high signal intensity tumor extends outside the larynx through the thyroid cartilage and invades the strap muscles. It also crosses the anterior commissure to the right aryepiglottic fold. The tumor has a relatively homogeneous signal intensity. **(C)** T1-weighted sagittal image. The tumor extends into the pre-epiglottic space superiorly. The high signal intensity of the cricoid lamina can be clearly seen, defining the tumor as restricted to the supraglottis and glottis.

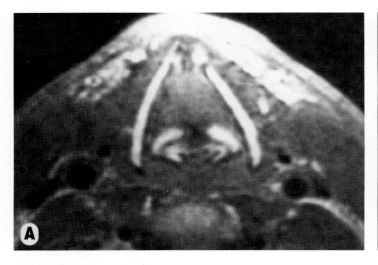

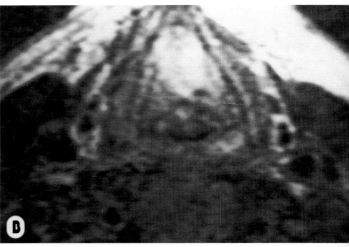

Fig. 3.56 BILATERAL SQUAMOUS CELL CARCINOMA OF THE LARYNX **(A)** T1-weighted axial image. In this case, the abnormal tissue is confined to the vocal cords. **(B)** T2-weighted axial image. The high intensity mass is obvious. The low signal intensity of the thyroid cartilage is preserved bilaterally, indicating that there is no invasion. At biopsy, both vocal cords were found to be positive for squamous cell carcinoma.

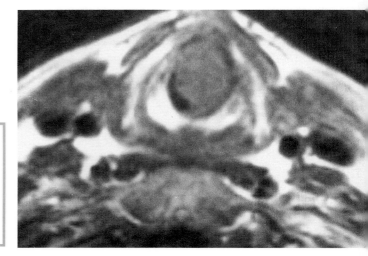

Fig. 3.57 SUBGLOTTIC SQUAMOUS CELL CARCINOMA OF THE LARYNX T1-weighted axial image. This patient presented with stridor and a subglottic mass on endoscopy. The homogeneous, intermediate signal intensity tumor arises from the mucosa on the left side. It almost completely obstructs the airway. The low signal intensity from the calcified edge of the anterior cricoid cartilage indicates that there has not been erosion.

sinuses, anteriorly or posteriorly across the commissures (Fig. 3.56), and inferiorly into the subglottis (Fig. 3.57). Cartilage invasion (see Figs. 3.54 and 3.55), extralaryngeal spread to the base of the tongue, the neck (see Fig. 3.55), and the posterior cricoid region can also be assessed. Evaluation of lymph node involvement completes the examination. Surgical resection, planning, and radiation therapy are determined by the foregoing parameters.

Squamous cell carcinoma occurs much more frequently in the hypopharynx (Fig. 3.58) than in the cervical esophagus. Esophageal carcinoma most often occurs in the middle third of the esophagus. Both are associated with high alcohol and cigarette consumption. Magnetic resonance imaging and CT are used for staging in the neck. To date, neither modality has proven to be superior in the detection of metastatic lymphadenopathy.

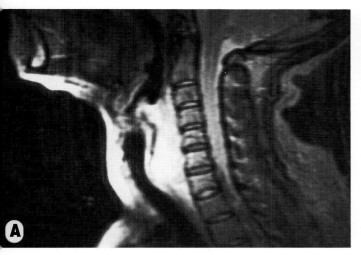
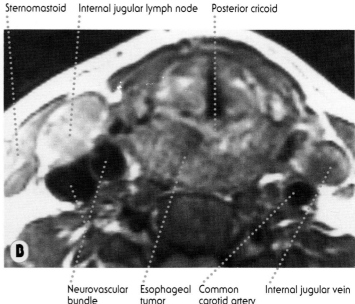

Sternomastoid Internal jugular lymph node Posterior cricoid

Neurovascular bundle Esophageal tumor Common carotid artery Internal jugular vein

Fig. 3.58 CARCINOMA OF THE HYPOPHARYNX AND THE ESOPHAGUS (A) T2-weighted sagittal image. This 60-year-old female presented with dysphagia. There is a high signal intensity mass in the esophagus, displacing the trachea anteriorly. The tumor extends superiorly into the hypopharynx, narrowing the airway at the level of the false and true cords. **(B)** T1-weighted axial image. This section through the supraglottis demonstrates the tumor mass in the hypopharynx, posterior to the airway. It is limited anteriorly by the higher intensity signal of the cricoid and laterally by the fat around the neurovascular bundles. A large metastatic internal jugular lymph node is seen on the right, deep to the sternomastoid. There is a troublesome artifact on the left, involving the internal jugular vein. The high signal within the lumen would suggest thrombosis. However, ultrasound revealed patency of the vessel. Despite the application of presaturation pulses, this artifact could not be eliminated; it is thought to be due to relatively slow blood flow.

THE NECK, THYROID GLAND, AND PARATHYROID GLANDS

NORMAL ANATOMY (Figs. 3.59 to 3.61)

The **neck**, from the floor of the mouth to the lung apex, can be divided into three anatomical compartments: **posterior, visceral**, and **lateral**. The posterior compartment is composed of the bony cervical spine and its neural contents, muscles, fat, blood vessels, and the spinal accessory chain of lymph nodes. The anterior boundary is defined by the prevertebral fascia. The aerodigestive or visceral compartment is the midline compartment incorporating the hypopharynx, larynx, esophagus, thyroid and parathyroid glands, fat, blood vessels, and lymph nodes. The paired lateral compartments contain the sternomastoid muscles, neurovascular bundles, fat, and the internal jugular chain of lymph nodes.

The **thyroid gland** is located just below the level of the cricoid cartilage. The thyroid isthmus, anterior to the trachea, connects the two lobes of the gland that are straddled on either side of the trachea deep to the strap muscles. On MR images, the normal gland is slightly hyperintense to muscle on T1-weighted images (see Fig. 3.61C), and hyperintense to both muscle and fat on T2-weighted images. Internally, it is of uniform signal intensity.

The normal **parathyroid glands** are not routinely demonstrated on MRI studies, although parathyroid tissue is much better visualized by MRI than by CT. Normally there are two pairs of parathyroid glands, superior and inferior; they can be found anywhere from the hyoid bone to the aortic arch. The superior parathyroid glands are more constant in location along the posterior surface of the upper thyroid gland. The inferior glands are less uniformly located just posterior to the lower poles of the thyroid gland. The fat planes located immediately posterior to the thyroid gland help in demonstrating parathyroid masses as structures distinct from the thyroid.

Normal Anatomy of the Head and Neck (Figs. 3.59 to 3.61)

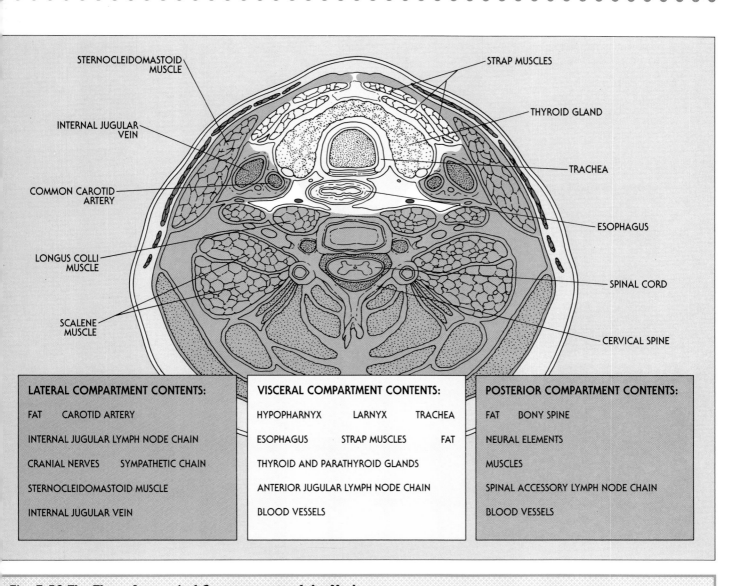

STERNOCLEIDOMASTOID MUSCLE

STRAP MUSCLES

INTERNAL JUGULAR VEIN

THYROID GLAND

COMMON CAROTID ARTERY

TRACHEA

ESOPHAGUS

LONGUS COLLI MUSCLE

SPINAL CORD

SCALENE MUSCLE

CERVICAL SPINE

LATERAL COMPARTMENT CONTENTS:

FAT   CAROTID ARTERY

INTERNAL JUGULAR LYMPH NODE CHAIN

CRANIAL NERVES   SYMPATHETIC CHAIN

STERNOCLEIDOMASTOID MUSCLE

INTERNAL JUGULAR VEIN

VISCERAL COMPARTMENT CONTENTS:

HYPOPHARNYX   LARNYX   TRACHEA

ESOPHAGUS   STRAP MUSCLES   FAT

THYROID AND PARATHYROID GLANDS

ANTERIOR JUGULAR LYMPH NODE CHAIN

BLOOD VESSELS

POSTERIOR COMPARTMENT CONTENTS:

FAT   BONY SPINE

NEURAL ELEMENTS

MUSCLES

SPINAL ACCESSORY LYMPH NODE CHAIN

BLOOD VESSELS

Fig. 3.59 The Three Anatomical Compartments of the Neck

The Neck, Thyroid Gland, and Parathyroid Glands

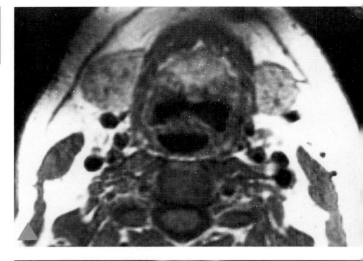

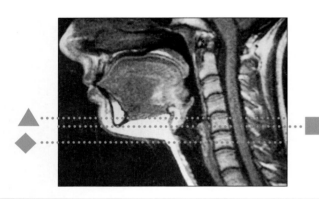

Fig. 3.60 Localizer: Midline T1-Weighted Sagittal Image
The planes of section of three axial sections are indicated: through the epiglottis, through the glottis, and through the subglottic airway.

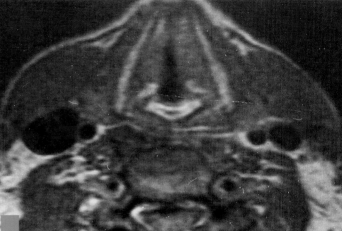

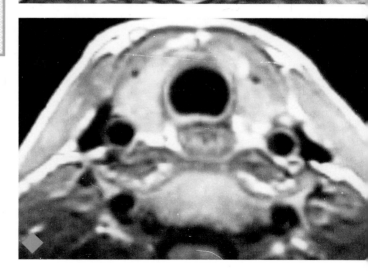

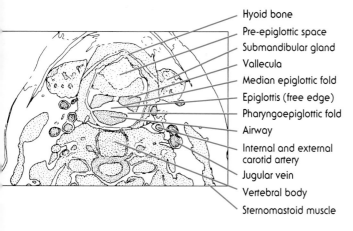

Hyoid bone
Pre-epiglottic space
Submandibular gland
Vallecula
Median epiglottic fold
Epiglottis (free edge)
Pharyngoepiglottic fold
Airway
Internal and external
carotid artery
Jugular vein
Vertebral body
Sternomastoid muscle

Fig. 3.61A T1-Weighted Axial Image Through the Epiglottis The submandibular gland and neurovascular bundle are lateral to the visceral compartment containing the aerodigestive tract. Within the visceral compartment, the epiglottis divides the valleculae from the supraglottic airway.

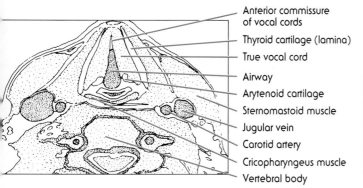

Anterior commissure
of vocal cords
Thyroid cartilage (lamina)
True vocal cord
Airway
Arytenoid cartilage
Sternomastoid muscle
Jugular vein
Carotid artery
Cricopharyngeus muscle
Vertebral body

Fig. 3.61B T1-Weighted Axial Image Through the Glottis At this level the airway is a narrow isosceles triangle, with its base at the cricoid cartilage and its apex at the anterior commissure of the vocal cords. The cords themselves are triangular in the adducted position and are contained within the thyroid cartilage.

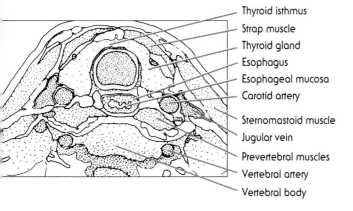

Thyroid isthmus
Strap muscle
Thyroid gland
Esophagus
Esophageal mucosa
Carotid artery
Sternomastoid muscle
Jugular vein
Prevertebral muscles
Vertebral artery
Vertebral body

Fig. 3.61C T1-Weighted Axial Image Through the Subglottic Airway The airway is circular at this level, except posteriorly, where the esophagus indents the soft membranous part of the trachea. The esophageal mucosa is an irregular high intensity ring within the muscular wall. The thyroid gland, higher in intensity than muscle, surrounds the lateral and anterior perimeter of the trachea.

TECHNIQUE

Examination of the neck by MRI is straightforward and, in most cases, limited to a pair of sequences: T2-weighted axial images and T1-weighted axial images. Coronal images may be added for purposes of defining the relationships of lesions high in the neck to the skull base and of lesions low in the neck to the apex of the chest. In a patient with primary hyperparathyroidism, the superior mediastinum must be examined for the possible presence of an ectopic parathyroid adenoma. Axial T2-weighted sections through this area are recommended.

PATHOLOGY

Thyroglossal duct cysts, branchial cleft cysts, and cystic hygromas are the most common benign neck masses occurring in the pediatric population. In that same population, the most common malignancy in the neck is lymphoma, and the second most common, rhabdomyosarcoma. For adults between the ages of 21 and 40, a unilateral neck mass is usually malignant and is most often diagnosed as lymphoma.

Over the age of 40, the most common masses are metastatic lymph nodes (Fig. 3.62).

THE POSTERIOR COMPARTMENT

The most common pathology encountered in the posterior compartment is lymphadenopathy secondary to lymphoma, metastatic disease, or infection. The MRI appearance is nonspecific for all of these pathological processes and does not allow for differentiation. Frequently in children, the spinal accessory chain of lymph nodes is involved with infection, becoming as a result markedly enlarged. Metastatic lymphadenopathy is less often encountered in the spinal accessory chain than in the internal jugular chain; the latter drains most of the head and neck area (see Figs. 3.3B and 3.43).

Infection in the prevertebral space is occasionally seen, usually secondary to an adjacent osteomyelitis of the cervical spine (Fig. 3.63). Bacterial and tuberculous abscesses occur and cannot be distinguished from one another. The small areas of calcification seen within a tuberculous abscess cannot be reliably diagnosed using MRI. The bony spine and its neural elements give rise to tumors presenting in the posterior compartment. (The spine is considered in

Fig. 3.62 PATHOLOGY OF THE NECK (BY COMPARTMENT)

POSTERIOR

SPINE
  Bone Origin Tumor
  Nerve Origin Tumor

LYMPH NODES
  Lymphoma
  Metastases
  Infection

OTHER
  Cystic Hygroma
  Lipoma

VISCERAL

HYPOPHARYNX/ LARYNX
  Infection
  Cysts
    Retention cysts
    Thyroglossal duct cyst
    Laryngocele
  Benign Tumors
    Papilloma
    Chondroma
    Hemangioma
    Neurofibroma
  Malignant Tumors
    Squamous cell carcinoma

THYROID
  Cyst
  Goiter
  Adenoma
  Carcinoma
  Thyroiditis

PARATHYROID
  Adenoma
  Carcinoma
  Hyperplasia

LYMPH NODES
  Metastases
  Lymphoma
  Infection

LATERAL

LYMPH NODES
  Metastases
  Lymphoma
  Infection

NEUROVASCULAR BUNDLE
  Paraganglioma
  Neuroma
  Vascular Thrombosis
  Hematoma

MUSCLE/ FAT/ LYMPHATICS
  Infection
  Lipoma
  Dermoid
  Lymphangioma
  Hemangioma
  Cystic Hygroma
  Branchial Cleft Cyst

greater detail in Chapter 5.) Neurofibromas and schwannomas involve peripheral nerves. These masses present as discrete, well-defined, round or lobulated lesions that can usually be seen to track back along the nerve root into the neural foramen. An oblique coronal plane is often very advantageous in demonstrating the continuity of the mass with the nerve root (Fig. 3.64). On T2-weighted images, a homogeneous high signal intensity is identified, an appearance that is characteristic of a neuroma in any location.

A cystic mass in the posterior compartment is usually a cystic hygroma. In children under two years of age, a cystic hygroma commonly originates in the posterior compartment but often, at the time of presentation, is found to be of massive size and extended into the lateral compartment. As it insinuates through tissue planes, the childhood cystic hygroma is multiloculated but not well-encapsulated. This is in contrast to the more clearly defined and less insinuating cystic hygroma that occurs in adults. A lipoma in the posterior compartment, similar to that in other locations, has a relatively characteristic high signal intensity on T1-weighted images.

THE LATERAL COMPARTMENT

Enlarged lymph nodes account for the most common mass seen in the lateral compartment. Metastatic disease, lymphoma, and infection occur therein frequently and cannot be differentiated from one another—similar in these respects to the related processes of the posterior compartment. Inasmuch as most of the head and neck primary tumors drain to the internal jugular chain, this chain, which lies immediately anterolateral to the neurovascular bundle, is frequently involved with metastatic disease.

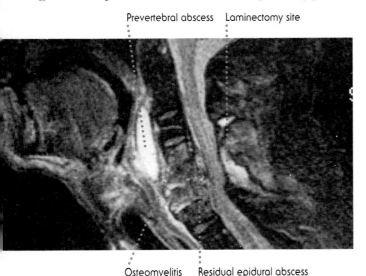

Prevertebral abscess   Laminectomy site

Osteomyelitis   Residual epidural abscess

Fig. 3.63 PREVERTEBRAL STAPHYLOCOCCAL ABSCESS SECONDARY TO OSTEOMYELITIS T2-weighted sagittal image. The homogeneous high signal intensity mass in the prevertebral space immediately overlies several abnormal vertebral bodies. Note, too, the residual epidural abscess at the level of the infected vertebral bodies. This abscess had been surgically drained several days previously by a posterior laminectomy.

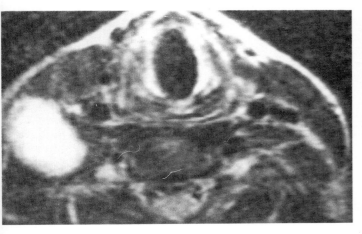

Tumor following nerve root

Fig. 3.64 NEUROFIBROMA **(A)** T2-weighted axial image. There is an extremely hyperintense mass in the right posterior compartment deep to the prevertebral fascia. **(B)** T1-weighted oblique coronal image. This oblique section (approximately 15° from the true coronal) demonstrates the long pedicle on the mass, tracking back along the C6 nerve root.

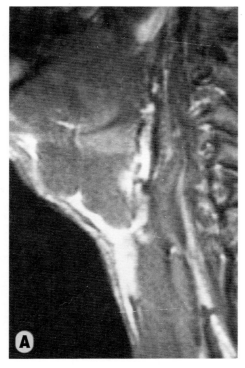

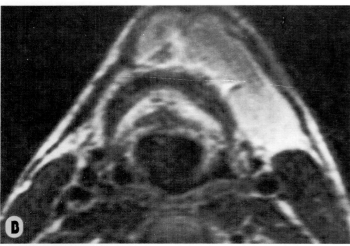

Fig. 3.65 CYSTIC HYGROMA **(A)** T1-weighted sagittal image. There is a multilobulated mass anterior to the sternomastoid muscle. **(D)** T2-weighted axial image. The mass crosses the midline, anterior to the hyoid bone. As compared with the branchial cleft cyst, this mass is less well-defined and not as clearly differentiated from adjacent tissue planes.

Paragangliomas and neuromas are the most common tumors encountered in the neurovascular bundle. These have both been previously described in this chapter's discussion of the nasopharynx. A miscellaneous group of tumors is encountered arising from the muscle, fat, and lymphatics.

Vascular thrombosis, predominantly of the internal jugular vein, and hematomas are also identified in and around the neurovascular bundle. Abscesses are relatively uncommon, although cellulitis is frequently encountered. The most characteristic finding is stranding or obliteration of the fat planes in a diffuse manner throughout the neck.

Cysts are frequent in the neck. These usually are lymphangiomas or lymph-hemangiomas, cystic hygromas, or branchial cleft cysts. Lymphangiomas are very similar to cystic hygromas (Fig. 3.65) but appear much more defined. They tend to insinuate through tissue planes and are frequently lobulated. Lymph-hemangiomas, seen frequently in childhood, also insinuate through tissue planes but over time tend to involute with fatty replacement. They tend to produce bony deformities by virtue of their mass effect. Branchial cleft cysts (Fig. 3.66) are derived from the second branchial cleft and are known to occur anywhere below the angle of the mandible along the anterior border of the sternomastoid muscle. They may be associated with a fistula opening to the skin surface. That these cysts fluctuate in size is the result of their tendency to become infected. Patients between the ages of 10 and 40 years present with encapsulated, well-defined, tubular masses; the normal fascial planes are preserved. These features usually allow for the differentiation of the branchial cleft cyst from a cystic hygroma. On T2-weighted images, the signal intensity is variable, depending on whether the cyst contains simple cyst fluid or infected material.

THE VISCERAL COMPARTMENT

The visceral compartment contains the aerodigestive components, as well as the thyroid and parathyroid glands and the lymph nodes. The hypopharynx and the larynx are considered earlier in this chapter.

THE THYROID GLAND

Diseases of the thyroid gland can be categorized into focal, multifocal, and diffuse lesions. Among the focal lesions are: (a) solitary nodules, usually adenomas, which may be either functional or nonfunctional; (b) cystic masses, which may be simple or hemorrhagic; and (c) malignant tumors (Fig. 3.67). The category of multifocal lesions includes multinodular goiter (Fig. 3.68), multiple adenomas, and multiple cysts. Types of diffuse thyroid disease include Graves' disease and Hashimoto's thyroiditis.

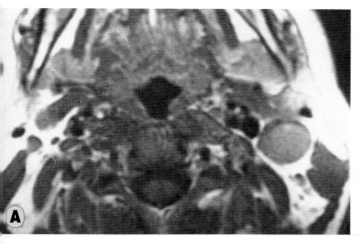

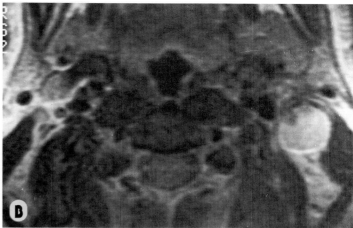

Fig. 3.66 BRANCHIAL CLEFT CYST **(A)** T1-weighted axial image. There is a well-defined, round mass in the left neck posterolateral to the neurovascular bundle and deep to the anterior border of the sternomastoid muscle. The location is classic for this entity. It is slightly hyperintense to muscle, due to the proteinaceous nature of its fluid contents. **(D)** T2-weighted axial image. The lesion is easily visible because of its hyperintensity on this sequence. The intensity pattern is in no way specific for this disease, but the location is highly suggestive of the diagnosis.

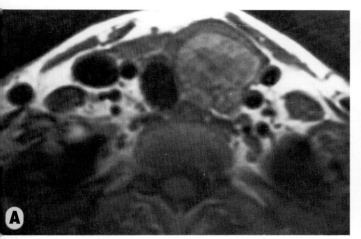

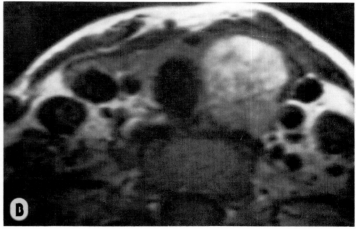

Fig. 3.67 THYROID CARCINOMA **(A)** T1-weighted axial image. There is a large nodule contained within the left lobe of the thyroid gland. It has sharply defined margins and is slightly nonhomogeneous internally. **(D)** T2-weighted axial image. As is typical of most thyroid nodules, this carcinoma is hyperintense on the T2-weighted image. A large adenoma could look identical.

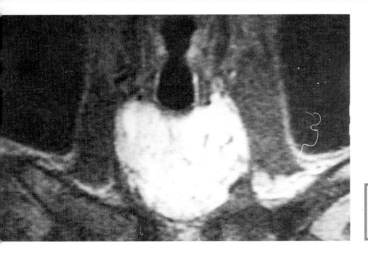

Fig. 3.68 MULTINODULAR GOITER T2-weighted coronal image. The entire thyroid gland is enlarged and hyperintense, as is typical of a goiter.

Because of its capacity for exceptional contrast differentiation, MRI has the potential to detect parenchymal lesions that do not cause enlargement or deformity of the affected lobe. However, adenomas and carcinomas cannot be distinguished by MRI, with the exception of those carcinomas that cause frank cartilage destruction, vascular or esophageal invasion (Fig 3.69), definite lymphadenopathy in the neck, or vocal cord paralysis. In this regard, there is no advantage to MRI over CT. Cystic lesions typically have a uniform high signal intensity on T2-weighted images. Focal lesions that have high signal intensity on both T1-weighted and T2-weighted sequences should raise the suspicion of hemorrhage into a cyst (Fig. 3.70). Multiple thyroid nodules (e.g., multinodular goiter and multiple adenomas) also show high signal intensity on T2-weighted images.

Diffuse thyroid disease, as exemplified by Hashimoto's thyroiditis, demonstrates enlargement of the gland, frequently with a speckled nonhomogeneous increase in signal intensity on T2-weighted images (Fig. 3.71).

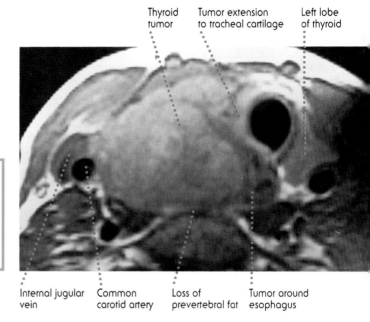

Fig. 3.69 EXTRACAPSULAR EXTENSION IN THYROID CARCINOMA T1-weighted axial image. A large, mixed signal intensity mass extends beyond the capsule of the thyroid gland into the neurovascular bundle. Medially, it erodes the tracheal cartilage and encroaches on the esophagus. Posteriorly, the prevertebral space is invaded. Extracapsular extension indicates malignancy.

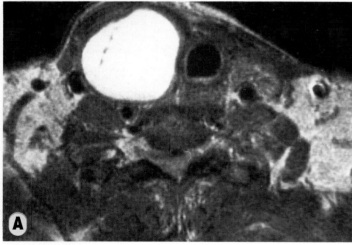
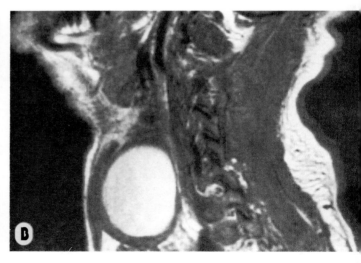

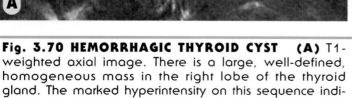

Fig. 3.70 HEMORRHAGIC THYROID CYST **(A)** T1-weighted axial image. There is a large, well-defined, homogeneous mass in the right lobe of the thyroid gland. The marked hyperintensity on this sequence indicates the probability of contained hemorrhagic products. **(B)** T1-weighted sagittal image. The cyst is seen deep to the strap muscles within the thyroid parenchyma.

THE PARATHYROID GLANDS

Diseases of the parathyroid glands are detected on MRI, due to an increase in volume of the gland and/or a demonstration of abnormal signal intensity. A hyperplastic parathyroid gland cannot be reliably distinguished from a parathyroid adenoma or parathyroid carcinoma. In most cases, the enlarged gland shows high signal intensity on T2-weighted images (Fig. 3.72B), regardless of the cause of enlargement. Rarely will an adenoma evidence low signal intensity on T2-weighted sequences. Hyperplasia is suggested when more than one high signal intensity enlarged gland is identified.

The differential diagnosis of a high intensity nodule in the region of the parathyroid glands includes lymphadenopathy and a posterior thyroid nodule. The major purpose of parathyroid imaging is to localize an area for exploration and exclude disease on the contralateral side.

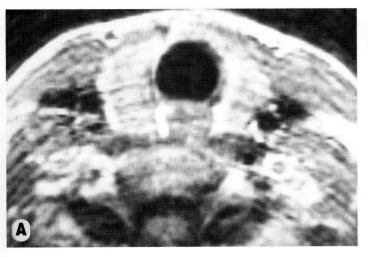
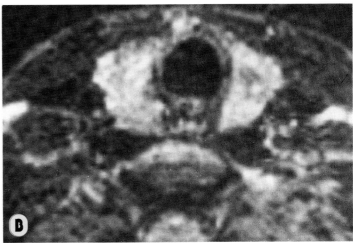

Fig. 3.71 HASHIMOTO'S THYROIDITIS T1-weighted **(A)** and T2-weighted **(B)** axial images. The gland is bilaterally enlarged and nonhomogeneous. It is of considerably greater signal intensity than is normal, particularly on the T2-weighted image. The quality of the scan is degraded by respiratory artifact.

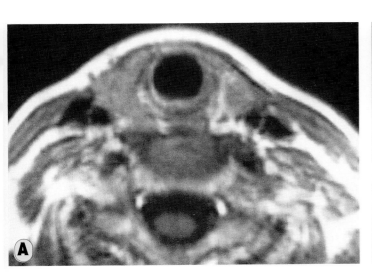
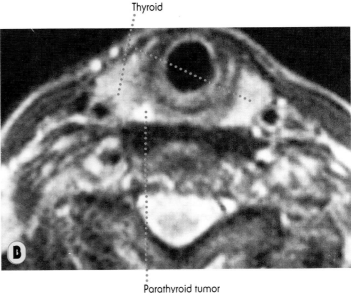

Thyroid

Parathyroid tumor

Fig. 3.72 PARATHYROID ADENOMA T1-weighted **(A)** and T2-weighted **(B)** axial images. There is a distinct, 7- to 8-mm hyperintense focus on the T2-weighted image in the area of the right superior parathyroid gland. An adenoma was surgically confirmed. This appearance is typical.

BIBLIOGRAPHY

BOOKS

Batsakis JG. *Tumors of the head and neck.* Clinical and pathological considerations, 2nd ed. Baltimore: Williams and Wilkins, 1979.

Bergeron RT, Osborn AG, Som PM, eds. *Head and neck imaging.* St. Louis: CV Mosby, 1984.

Mancuso AA, Hanafee WN. *Computed tomography and magnetic resonance imaging of the head and neck,* 2nd ed. Baltimore: Williams and Wilkins, 1985.

JOURNAL ARTICLES AND BOOK CHAPTERS

Casselman JW, Mancuso AA. Major salivary gland masses: comparison of MR imaging and CT. *Radiology* 1987;165:183–189.

Dillon WP, Mills CM, Kjos B, et al. Magnetic resonance imaging of the nasopharynx. *Radiology* 1984;152:731–738.

Glazer HS, Niemeyer JH, Balfe DM, et al. Neck neoplasms: MR imaging part I—initial evaluation. *Radiology* 1986;160:343–348.

Glazer HS, Niemeyer JH, Balfe DM, et al. Neck neoplasms: MR imaging part II—posttreatment evaluation. *Radiology* 1986;160:349–354.

Kier R, Herfkens RJ, Blinder RA, et al. MRI with surface coils for parathyroid tumors: preliminary investigation. *AJR* 1986;147:497–500.

Latack JT, Hutchinson RJ, Heyn RM. Imaging of rhabdomyosarcomas of the head and neck. *AJNR* 1987;8:353–359.

Lufkin R, Hanafee WN. Imaging the laryngopharynx. *Semin US CT MR* 1986;7:166–180.

Lufkin R, Hanafee WN, Wortham D, Hoover L. Larynx and hypopharynx: MR imaging with surface coils. *Radiology* 1986;158:747–754.

Lufkin RB, Wortham DG, Dietrich RB, et al. Tongue and oropharynx, findings on MR imaging. *Radiology* 1986;161:69–75.

Mandelblatt SM, Braun IF, Davis PC, et al. Parotid masses: MR imaging. *Radiology* 1987;163:411–414.

Som PM. Lymph nodes of the neck. *Radiology* 1987;165:593–600.

Som PM, Biller HF, Lawson W, et al. Parapharyngeal space masses: an updated protocol based upon 104 cases. *Radiology* 1984;153:149–156.

Som PM, Braun IF, Shapiro MD, et al. Tumors of the parapharyngeal space and upper neck: MR imaging characteristics. *Radiology* 1987; 164:823–829.

Som PM, Sacher M, Lanzieri CF, et al. Parenchymal cysts of the lower neck. *Radiology* 1985;157:399–406.

Spritzer CE, Gefter WB, Hamilton R, et al. Abnormal parathyroid glands: high resolution MR imaging. *Radiology* 1987;162:487–491.

Teresi LM, Lufkin RB, Vinuela F, et al. MR imaging of the nasopharynx and floor of the middle cranial fossa: part I—normal anatomy. *Radiology* 1987; 164:811–816.

Teresi LM, Lufkin RB, Vinuela F, et al. MR imaging of the nasopharynx and floor of the middle cranial fossa: part II—malignant tumors. *Radiology* 1987; 164:817–821.

Teresi LM, Lufkin RB, Wortham DG, et al. Parotid masses: MR imaging. *Radiology* 1987;163:405–409.

chapter four

the orbit

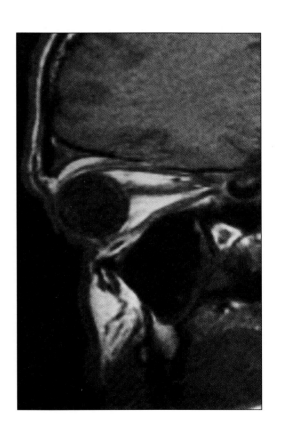

M. ANNE KELLER   ROGER M.L. SMITH

INTRODUCTION

Examination of the superficial tissues of the orbit is easily accomplished by direct visual inspection, and the globe and its contents are accessible to ophthalmoscopic techniques. Diagnostic imaging tests are therefore most useful for lesions in areas that are inaccessible to these simpler techniques—i.e., the retroglobar region, the extraocular muscles, the lacrimal gland—and as supplementary examinations in the evaluation of the globe itself. Computed tomography (CT) and magnetic resonance imaging (MRI) are the most important of these diagnostic imaging modalities. Computed tomography is ideal for evaluation of the orbital osseous anatomy and also displays the orbital soft tissues very well. Fine osseous detail is much poorer on MRI but soft tissue detail is superb. Magnetic resonance imaging is particularly useful for lesions at the orbital apex and in the optic canal or orbital fissures, and for evaluation of the optic nerve. This visualization is facilitated by the multiplanar display and the freedom from bone artifact. The absence of ionizing radiation to the lens is, of course, a distinct additional advantage of MRI. The major drawbacks of MRI are principally due to artifacts induced by eye movement during the examination, and to the inability to delineate fine bone details.

NORMAL ANATOMY (Figs. 4.1 to 4.7)

The orbit can be divided anatomically into three compartments: intraocular, intraconal, and extraconal. Each of these compartments is a well-defined space separated by distinct, easily recognizable boundaries.

The **intraocular compartment** consists of the globe and its contents: the cornea, the aqueous, the lens, the iris, the vitreous, the retina, the choroid, and the sclera. The anterior aspect of the globe is bounded by the conjunctiva. The posterior surface is surrounded by a separate fibrous sheath known as Tenon's capsule, which is pierced by the optic nerve and the extraocular muscles. Tenon's capsule has a limiting effect on the spread of both inflammatory and malignant processes.

The **intraconal compartment** contains the muscle cone, the connective tissue space within the muscle

Normal Anatomy of the Orbit (Figs. 4.1 to 4.7)

●●

The Intraocular Compartment

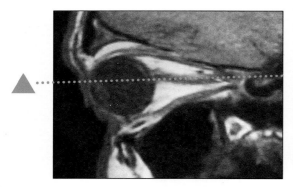

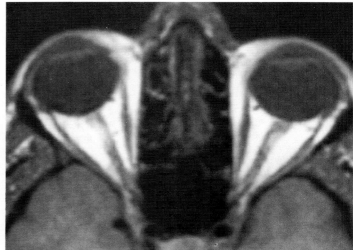

Fig. 4.1 Localizer: T1-Weighted Sagittal Image Through the Optic Nerve Axis The plane of section of the axial image is indicated.

cone, and the optic nerve. The optic nerve is, in fact, an extension of the brain. The axons of cell bodies lying in the retina extend via the optic nerve, cross in the chiasm, and follow the optic tracts to synapse in the lateral geniculate body. Subarachnoid space lies between the optic nerve and its dural sheath and is intracranially continuous with the suprasellar cistern. The extraocular muscles, which form the peripheral margin of the intraconal space, are surrounded by a continuous musculofascial sheath that begins at the orbital apex and continues to the point at which the extraocular muscles are attached to the globe. Within the intraconal compartment is a variable amount of fat that is traversed by nerves and vascular structures, including the ophthalmic artery.

The **extraconal compartment** is circumscribed on its inner margin by the musculofascial sheath that surrounds the extraocular muscles. The periorbita (periosteum), an extension of the dura from the middle cranial fossa, lines the bony orbit, thus forming the outer margin of the extraconal space. A variable amount of fat extends between the two fascial planes. The most important structure in this compartment is the lacrimal gland, which is situated in the superolateral aspect of the orbit.

Cranial nerve III innervates all of the extraocular muscles, with the exception of the superior oblique and lateral rectus muscles, which are innervated by cranial nerves IV and VI, respectively. Cranial nerve V_1 (with the exception of its nasociliary branch), cranial nerve IV, and the superior ophthalmic vein are extraconal structures as they enter the orbit through the superior orbital fissure; they become intraconal in mid-orbit. The nasociliary branch of V_1, and cranial nerves III and VI enter the orbit through the superior orbital fissure and immediately become intraconal; they lie within the tendinous ring surrounding the optic nerve. Cranial nerve V_2, the infraorbital artery and vein, and the inferior ophthalmic vein enter the orbit through the inferior orbital fissure and remain extraconal until mid-orbit.

The optic nerve becomes intraconal immediately upon entering the orbit through the optic foramen. Along with the optic nerve and its meninges, the optic foramen provides orbital access for the ophthalmic artery and sympathetic nerves.

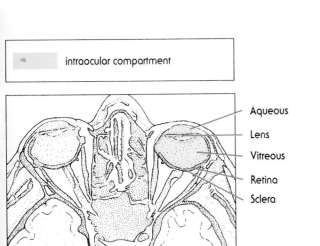

intraocular compartment

Aqueous

Lens

Vitreous

Retina

Sclera

Fig. 4.2 T1-Weighted Axial Image Demonstrating the Intraocular Compartment at the Level the Optic Nerves The lens is clearly defined anteriorly as separating the aqueous and the vitreous. The retina and the sclera appear as a band of low signal surrounding the globe.

The Intraconal Compartment

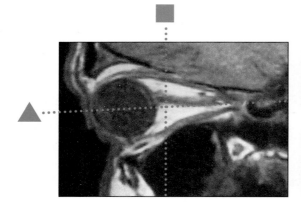

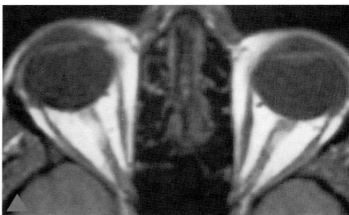

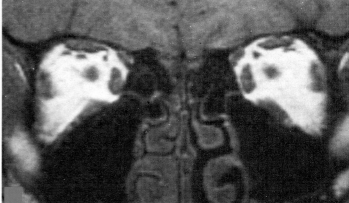

Fig. 4.3 Localizer: T1-Weighted Sagittal Image Through the Optic Nerve Axis   The planes of section of the axial and coronal images are indicated.

The Extraconal Compartment

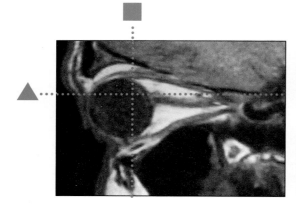

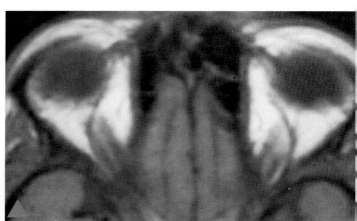

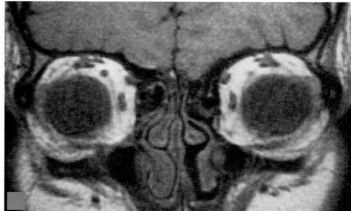

Fig. 4.5 Localizer: T1-Weighted Sagittal Image Through the Optic Nerve Axis   The planes of section of the axial and coronal images are indicated.

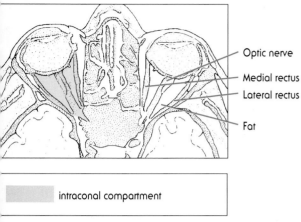

Optic nerve

Medial rectus

Lateral rectus

Fat

intraconal compartment

Fig. 4.4A T1-Weighted Axial Image Demonstrating the Intraconal Compartment at the Level of the Optic Nerves The medial and lateral rectus muscles and the optic nerves are sharply defined by the large amount of fat surrounding them. The blood vessels within the intraconal fat are visible, but the nerves to the extraocular muscles cannot be identified.

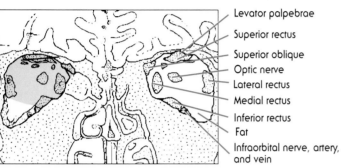

Levator palpebrae

Superior rectus

Superior oblique

Optic nerve

Lateral rectus

Medial rectus

Inferior rectus

Fat

Infraorbital nerve, artery, and vein

Fig. 4.4D T1-Weighted Coronal Image Demonstrating the Intraconal Compartment, Posterior to the Globe The extraocular muscles are best evaluated on the coronal view, as the superior rectus and superior oblique can be readily distinguished from one another. The inferior muscle group is less easily separated.

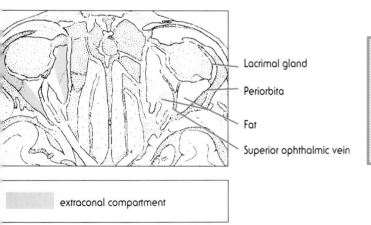

Lacrimal gland

Periorbita

Fat

Superior ophthalmic vein

extraconal compartment

Fig. 4.6A T1-Weighted Axial Image Demonstrating the Extraconal Compartment at the Level of the Superior Extraocular Muscle Group The lacrimal gland is in the superolateral aspect of the orbit, external to the muscle cone. The periorbita forms the peripheral margin of the extraconal space and is identified, together with the cortical bone of the orbital walls, as a band devoid of signal.

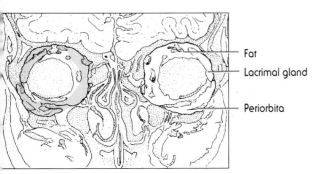

Fat

Lacrimal gland

Periorbita

Fig. 4.6D T1-Weighted Coronal Image Demonstrating the Extraconal Compartment at the Level of the Midglobe The lacrimal gland is interposed between the globe and the periorbita and is closely related to both.

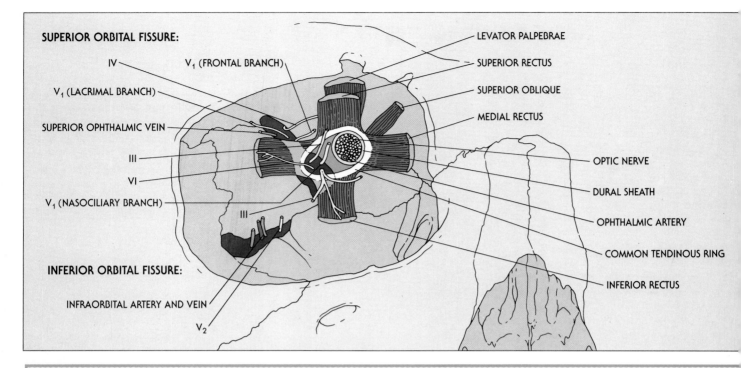

SUPERIOR ORBITAL FISSURE:

IV
V₁ (FRONTAL BRANCH)
V₁ (LACRIMAL BRANCH)
SUPERIOR OPHTHALMIC VEIN
III
VI
V₁ (NASOCILIARY BRANCH)
III

INFERIOR ORBITAL FISSURE:

INFRAORBITAL ARTERY AND VEIN
V₂

LEVATOR PALPEBRAE
SUPERIOR RECTUS
SUPERIOR OBLIQUE
MEDIAL RECTUS
OPTIC NERVE
DURAL SHEATH
OPHTHALMIC ARTERY
COMMON TENDINOUS RING
INFERIOR RECTUS

Fig. 4.7 The Orbital Fissures and Their Contents All of the cranial nerves enter the orbit through the superior orbital fissure except V₂ and the optic nerve. The optic nerve traverses the optic foramen, and V₂ enters via the inferior orbital fissure.

TECHNIQUE

The patient should be supine with the head in the neutral position (canthomeatal line perpendicular to the table top). To minimize the artifacts from eye movement, the patient's gaze should be fixed in one direction—preferably straight ahead—for the entire scan period. Either a surface coil or a circumferential head coil may be used for the examination. A surface coil has signal-to-noise advantages in the near-field, but there is significant signal dropoff at the orbital apex and within the cranium. For this reason, the orbital apex, optic canal, and intracranial optic pathways are better demonstrated on head coil images which are very uniform in intensity regardless of depth. The head coil is also preferable if the entire optic pathway is to be evaluated and has the added flexibility of permitting examination of the entire brain, if necessary. If the lesion is superficial, surface coil examination is preferred.

A multislice spin echo technique is used in the majority of cases. T1-weighted images [spin echo (SE), short repetition time (TR), short echo time (TE)] provide excellent image contrast in the orbit and are the mainstays of the examination protocol. Multiple image planes—in particular, axials, coronals and oblique sagittals along the long axis of the optic nerve—facilitate the accurate localization of pathological processes.

Usually, one set of T2-weighted images is also obtained, generally in the plane that best demonstrates the pathology as determined on the basis of the T1-weighted images. T2-weighted images are particularly useful in two settings: the requisite additional characterization of any lesion seen or suspected on the T1-weighted images, and the evaluation of the brain for any associated diseases.

STIR sequences (short inversion time, inversion recovery) are a means of achieving cumulative T1 and T2 contrast and also of nulling the extremely high signal of intraorbital fat. Experience with this sequence is limited, and its use has not been widespread, due in part to the lack of availability on all commercial scanners.

Excellent spatial resolution on MR images of the orbit is essential; it is achieved by using thin slices, small fields of view, and fine matrix sizes. Two or four excitations are generally necessary to obtain images of adequate quality (Fig. 4.8).

Paramagnetic contrast agents will one day have an important role in MRI of the orbit, particularly in regards to the detection and staging of neoplasms and inflammatory lesions. To date, the application of these agents in the clinical area has yet to be defined.

PATHOLOGY

The types of lesions found in the intraocular, intraconal, and extraconal compartments of the orbit are presented in Fig. 4.9 and are discussed below.

FIG. 4.8 MRI TECHNIQUE FOR EXAMINATION OF THE ORBIT[a]

Parameter	No. 1 T1-Weighted	No. 2 T1-Weighted	No. 3 T1-Weighted[b]	No. 4 T2-Weighted
Plane	Axial	Coronal	Oblique[c]	Variable[d]
TR (msec)	500–800	500–800	500	2000–3000
TE (msec)	20	20	20	70–100[e]
Slice thickness (mm)	3-5	3-5	3-5	5
Matrix	256	256	256	128
Field of view (cm)	16	16	16	16
No. of excitations	2-4	2-4	2-4	2
Examination time (min)	5-10	5-10	5-10	10

[a]All sequences: spin echo, multislice.
[b]Optional sequence, performed if optic nerve lesion suspected.
[c]Parallel to axis of optic nerve.

[d]Plane that best displays lesion.
[e]Second echo of two-echo study.

FIG. 4.9 ORBITAL LESIONS (BY COMPARTMENT)

INTRAOCULAR

NEOPLASMS
  Primary Tumors
    Retinoblastoma
    Melanoma
  Metastases
    Breast carcinoma
    Lung carcinoma
    Lymphoma
    Leukemia
    Melanoma

INFECTION
  Secondary to Trauma
  Hematogenous

TRAUMA/ HEMATOMA

OTHER
  Primary Hyperplastic Vitreous
  Coats' Disease

INTRACONAL

OPTIC NERVE LESIONS
  Neoplasms
    Glioma
    Meningioma
    Leukemia
    Retinoblastoma
  Pseudotumor
  Optic Neuritis

MUSCLE LESIONS
  Graves' Ophthalmopathy
  Myositis
  Pseudotumor
  Metastases

INTRACONAL CONNECTIVE TISSUE
  Neoplasms
    Lymphoma
    Metastases
    Neuroma
  Vascular
    Hemangioma
    Varix
    Arteriovenous malformations
  Pseudotumor

EXTRACONAL

NEOPLASMS
  Lacrimal Gland Origin
    Salivary gland type
    Lymphoma
    Dermoid
  Meningioma
  Metastases
    Hematogenous spread
      Melanoma
      Breast carcinoma
      Lung carcinoma
    Contiguous spread
      Nasopharyngeal
      Sinus carcinoma

INFLAMMATION
  Noninfectious
    Pseudotumor
    Wegener's
  Infectious
    Cellulitis
    Abscess

MUCOCELE

TRAUMA/HEMATOMA

Retinal detachment
with hemorrhage   Tumor

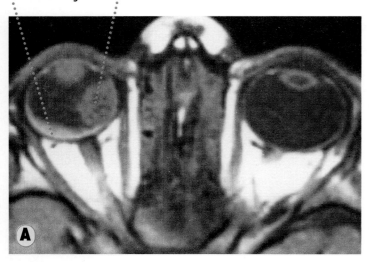

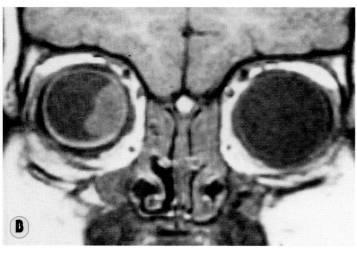

Fig. 4.10 RETINOBLASTOMA Axial **(A)** and coronal **(B)** T1-weighted images. The right globe contains a homogeneous mass that does not appear to infiltrate the sclera. Note the retinal detachment with subretinal hemorrhage.

INTRAOCULAR LESIONS

The most common intraocular mass found in children is the retinoblastoma (Fig. 4.10), which is primarily seen in patients under the age of three. The tumor is derived from primitive neuroblastic cells in the retina. Typically, the child presents with a white pupillary reflex (leukocoria), strabismus, or poor vision. Retinoblastoma is multicentric and/or bilateral in 30% of the cases. It originates in the globe but tends to spread beyond that region by tracking along the optic nerve and the surrounding meninges and ultimately gaining intracranial access. The tumor can also extend directly through the sclera and into the intraconal compartment. Associated vitreous hemorrhage may be demonstrated by MRI, although the calcification seen on CT may not be appreciated. Because subtle calcification may be the only evidence of the tumor, and MRI is known to be insensitive to such calcification, CT remains the primary means of diagnosis. Magnetic resonance imaging may be useful in determining extraocular extent. On T1-weighted images, the tumor is hyperintense to vitreous, slightly hyperintense to muscle, and hypointense to fat. On T2-weighted images, the retinoblastoma may be dark compared with vitreous and approximately isointense to muscle. Dense calcification in a tumor may further reduce the apparent signal.

The appearance of retinoblastoma on T2-weighted images is distinct from that of Coats' disease and primary hyperplastic vitreous (PHPV), two rare causes of leukocoria in childhood. In contrast to retinoblastoma, the lipoproteinaceous, subretinal exudate in Coats' disease and the intravitreal hemorrhage in PHPV cause the globe to be hyperintense on both T1- and T2-weighted images. These two diseases can be distinguished from one another by the fact that the eye is small in PHPV, but not in Coats' disease.

Malignant melanoma (Fig. 4.11) is the most common primary intraocular neoplasm in adults, occurring most frequently in the fifth decade of life. Thickening of the sclera and the presence of a contiguous mass in the intraconal compartment indicate tumor extension or spread beyond the retina. The tumor may also originate in the ciliary body. Extraconal melanomas do occur but are more often metastatic than primary. Melanotic melanoma usually displays both T1 and T2 shortening because of the melanin pigment. It is, therefore, one of the few tumors that is markedly hyperintense to muscle on T1-weighted images.

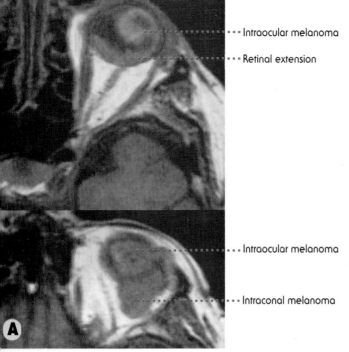

··· Intraocular melanoma

··· Retinal extension

··· Intraocular melanoma

··· Intraconal melanoma

A

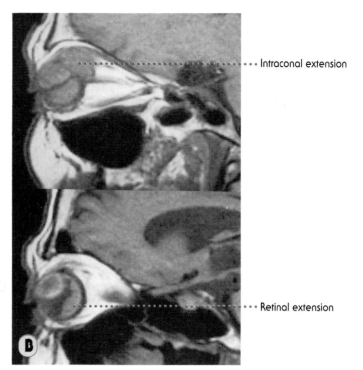

··· Intraconal extension

··· Retinal extension

B

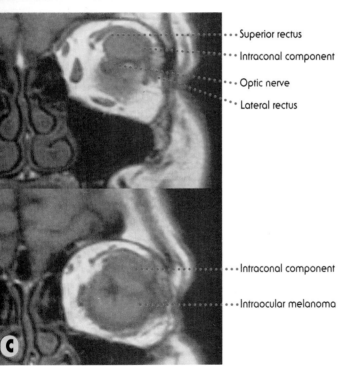

··· Superior rectus

··· Intraconal component

··· Optic nerve

··· Lateral rectus

··· Intraconal component

··· Intraocular melanoma

C

Fig. 4.11 MALIGNANT MELANOMA T1-weighted axial **(A)**, sagittal **(B)**, and coronal **(C)** images. A nonhomogeneous lobulated mass in the left globe extends to the retina and fungates through the superolateral aspect of the sclera into the intraconal compartment. There is no significant T1 or T2 shortening, as seen in some melanomas.

Metastases within the globe (Fig. 4.12) are relatively common. They most often spread from breast or lung carcinoma, lymphoma, leukemia, or melanoma. They rarely extend into the intraconal space. These metastases do not have characteristic MRI features; like most other tumors, they usually appear bright on T2-weighted images. Leukemia tends to differ from other metastases by diffusely infiltrating along the arachnoid sheath of the optic nerve and extending intracranially. The MR images are nonspecific, showing only a thickening of the meningeal sheath.

Intraocular hematoma, with or without retinal detachment, has a characteristic appearance of marked hyperintensity on T1-weighted images. The retina can be identified as a low signal band relative to the signal of the normal vitreous (Fig. 4.13)

INTRACONAL LESIONS

It is useful to consider the intraconal space as three subcompartments: the optic nerve and meninges, the muscle cone, and the connective tissue space within the muscle cone.

The optic nerve and meninges give rise to optic nerve gliomas and meningiomas. Optic nerve glioma

Retinal metastasis   Optic nerve   Retinal metastasis

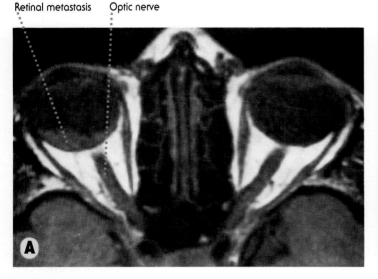

Fig. 4.12 RETINAL METASTASES T1-weighted axial **(A)** and sagittal **(B)** images. This soft tissue mass involves the retina and is confined to the globe. There are no features to distinguish this metastatic lesion from a localized primary melanoma. This patient had a primary breast carcinoma.

Hemorrhage   Retina   Vitreous   Sclera band

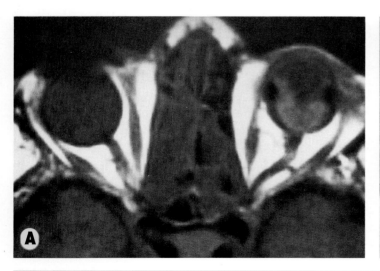
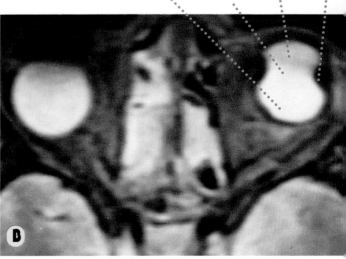

Fig. 4.13 SCLERAL BAND WITH SUBRETINAL HEMORRHAGE T1-weighted **(A)** and T2-weighted **(B)** axial images. Scleral banding is noted in the left globe. A large hemorrhage, hyperintense on both T1 and T2-weighted images, is present behind the retina. The retina is seen on the T2-weighted image as a thin band of low signal intensity relative to both the hemorrhage and the vitreous.

Fig. 4.14) is the most common intraconal lesion in children; it occurs between the ages of two and six. The tumor may be bilateral and is frequently associated with neurofibromatosis. Histologically, the tumor in children is a benign pilocytic astrocytoma, whereas the tumor in adults is more often a malignant astrocytoma. The glioma typically remains intradural, growing to the optic chiasm along the length of the optic nerve, which becomes thickened or tortuous; occasionally, the tumor grows along the optic radiation. Gliomas that remain entirely intraorbital tend to be spindle-shaped. The tumor is relatively bright on T2-weighted MR images; the characteristic extension along the visual pathway leads to a confident diagnosis.

Primary meningioma within the orbit generally originates eccentrically from the dura along the course of the optic nerve (Fig. 4.15). On MR images, the optic nerve can usually be clearly defined on the basis of its dural investment and the tumor mass. Infrequently, a meningioma arising from ectopic arachnoidal cells lies within the muscle cone but does not attach to the dura. It may also take its origin extraconally from the periorbita. Most commonly, however, an orbital meningioma arises by secondary extension from a primary intracranial tumor located on the greater wing of the sphenoid. Magnetic resonance imaging is especially helpful in detecting meningiomas that occur at the orbital apex, because it best demonstrates the tumor's relationship to the optic nerve at this difficult level. The tumor may be bright on T2-weighted images, but, unlike the high signal of an optic nerve glioma, is more often isointense.

Optic nerve glioma

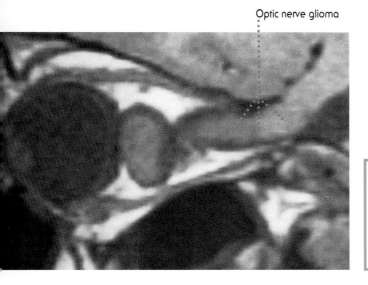

Fig. 4.14 OPTIC NERVE GLIOMA T1-weighted oblique sagittal image. This child has a lobulated mass that involves the entire length of the optic nerve and extends intracranially to the optic chiasm. This appearance is characteristic of an optic nerve glioma. The image plane is oriented along the long axis of the optic nerve.

Meningioma   Optic nerve

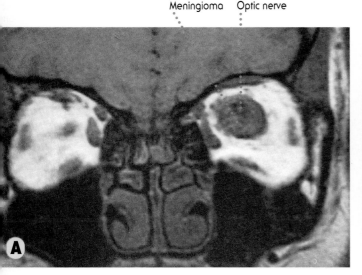

Fig. 4.15 OPTIC NERVE MENINGIOMA T1-weighted (**A**) and T2-weighted (**B**) coronal images. An eccentric mass surrounds the optic nerve. Yet, characteristically, the nerve is clearly defined within it, allowing for differentiation from optic nerve glioma. This meningioma is slightly hyperintense on T2-weighted images. Most optic nerve meningiomas, like those intracranially situated, are isointense or mildly hyperintense on T2-weighted images.

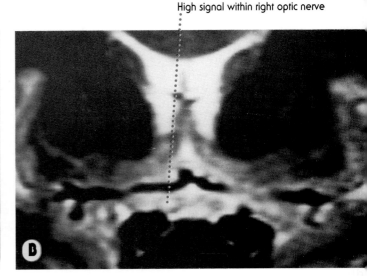

Carotid arteries   Optic nerves   Pituitary stalk

High signal within right optic nerve

Fig. 4.16 OPTIC NEURITIS   T1-weighted **(A)** and T2-weighted **(B)** coronal images. Both optic nerves appear slightly enlarged — the right more than the left. The T2-weighted image reveals a focal area of high signal in the right nerve. Over time, the size of both nerves returned to normal, confirming the diagnosis.

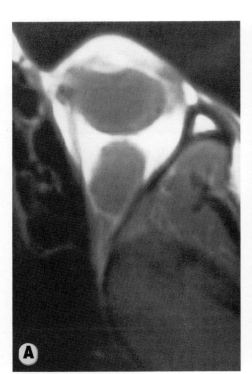
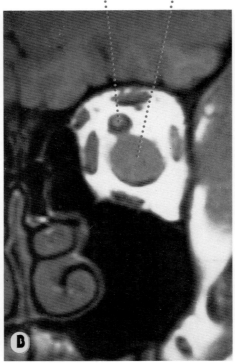
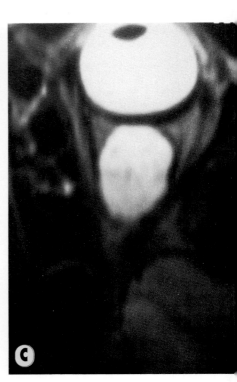

Optic nerve   Hemangioma

Fig. 4.17 CAVERNOUS HEMANGIOMA   T1-weighted axial **(A)**, T1-weighted coronal **(B)**, and T2-weighted axial **(C)** images. Hemangiomas have a relatively characteristic appearance—well-defined and homogeneous; more often than not, they are intraconal rather than extraconal. On T2-weighted images, hemangiomas classically have a very bright, homogeneous signal.

Optic neuritis (Fig. 4.16) is a common entity, as either an isolated event or in association with multiple sclerosis. If the inflammatory process incites sufficient edema within the nerve, optic nerve enlargement may be appreciated. In the appropriate clinical setting, an increased signal on T2-weighted images suggests the diagnosis of neuritis, although resolution with time is necessary for confirmation. The finding of multiple white matter lesions in the brain further confirms the diagnosis, given that one third of patients with optic neuritis have multiple sclerosis.

The intraconal connective tissue subcompartment is a relatively loosely organized grouping of fat, small nerves, and blood vessels. It gives rise to masses of vascular origin and frequently becomes involved in inflammatory processes. Varices, arteriovenous (AV) fistulas, and AV malformations occasionally occur intraconally. A signal void is seen in varices and in a dilated superior ophthalmic vein due to high flow AV fistulae or AV malformations. The absence of signal is a helpful indicator of these vascular lesions within the orbit. Varices may involve either the superior or the inferior ophthalmic vein.

In adults, the cavernous hemangioma (Fig. 4.17) is the most common tumor within the orbit. It appears as a well-defined, encapsulated mass that may contain phleboliths. The tumor may be intraconal or extraconal and may involve the lacrimal gland. Pathologically, large, dilated vascular lakes are seen, but the flow is too slow to produce a signal void. These lakes are characteristically very hyperintense on T2-weighted images. Phleboliths are not observed on MR images. The capillary hemangioma that typically occurs in the childhood years is nonencapsulated, infiltrative, and highly vascular. It may spontaneously involute. Magnetic resonance imaging can clearly differentiate encapsulated from diffuse varieties. As with cavernous hemangiomas, internal venous lakes produce a bright signal on T2-weighted images.

Idiopathic inflammatory pseudotumor of the orbit usually produces hazy distortion in the normally well-defined orbital fat, although it can appear as a discrete intraconal mass. Occasionally, the process is bilateral. The lymphocytic infiltration can involve any tissue in the orbit, including the extraocular muscles, the musculofascial sheath, the extraconal fat, the choroid, and the retina. Involvement of the extraconal fat is probably more clearly visualized by MRI than it is by CT. In most cases, the lesion is a poorly defined process, approximately isointense to muscle on T1-weighted images and usually slightly hypointense to muscle on T2-weighted images; in contrast, many tumors display hyperintensity as a prominent feature on T2-weighted images. However, the appearance of pseudotumor is not pathognomonic and can be confused with arteritis (Fig. 4.18), lymphoma (Fig. 4.19), metastases (Fig. 4.20), and various granulomatous processes (e.g., sarcoid and Wegener's granulomatosis).

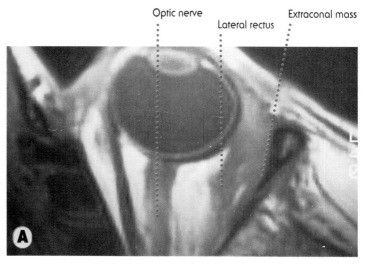

Optic nerve   Lateral rectus   Extraconal mass

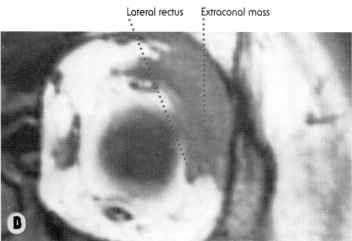

Lateral rectus   Extraconal mass

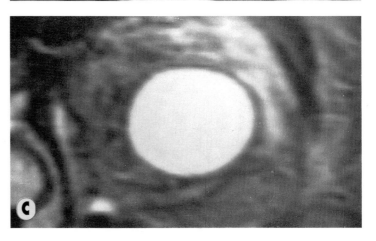

Fig. 4.18 POLYARTERITIS T1-weighted axial **(A)**, T1-weighted coronal **(B)**, and T2-weighted coronal **(C)** images. This irregular, infiltrative extraconal mass involves the extraconal fat, the lateral rectus muscle, and the lacrimal gland. It illustrates a nonspecific appearance. The differential diagnosis includes polyarteritis, granulomatous disease, lymphoma and metastases. The bright signal on T2-weighted images does not aid in the diagnosis.

Optic nerve   Medial rectus   Intraconal mass

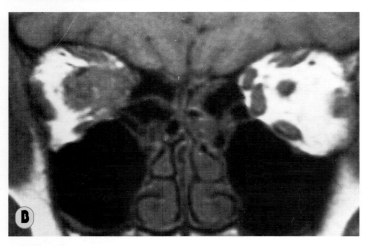

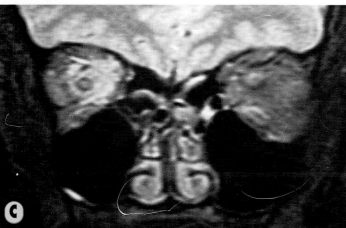

Rhabdomyosarcoma is the most common primary malignant orbital tumor found in children, presenting most frequently in males younger than 10 years old. Most are of the embryonal type and are thought to arise from undifferentiated pluripotential mesenchymal cells. Rhabdomyosarcoma occurs within the intraconal soft tissues and is not associated with the extraocular muscles. Rare cases derived from an extraocular muscle have been described in adults.

The muscle cone itself is less often affected by tumor than it is by endocrine abnormality, the most common being Graves' disease (thyroid ophthalmopathy). Graves' disease (Fig. 4.21), may occur in the hyperthyroid, euthyroid, or hypothyroid patient. The extraocular muscle belly is most markedly infiltrated with fibroblasts that produce mucopolysaccharides; the tendinous insertions remain least affected. Despite considerable muscle enlargement in many cases, no consistent change in muscle signal intensity has been observed. The inferior and medial rectus muscles are most often involved; lesser degrees of involvement have been noted with respect to the lateral rectus and the superior muscles, or any combination thereof. The coronal plane is ideal for assessing comparative muscle size. Initially, the volume of orbital fat may increase, but as fibrosis develops in chronic disease, the fat volume will decrease. Other diseases that can cause extraocular muscle enlargement are metastases and myositis. Occasionally, orbital apex masses that obstruct venous orbital drainage also enlarge the muscles.

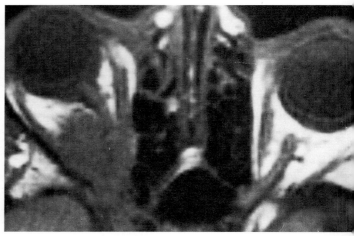

Fig. 4.19 LYMPHOMA T1-weighted axial **(A)**, T1-weighted coronal **(B)**, and T2-weighted coronal **(C)** images. An infiltrative, intraconal mass surrounds the optic nerve and involves the proximal portion of the medial rectus muscle. This pattern is nonspecific and occurs in many pathologies. A similar appearance is seen with metastases. The medium intensity signal on the T2 sequence is, again, nonspecific.

Fig. 4.20 INTRACONAL METASTASES T1-weighted axial image. An aggressive mass at the orbital apex infiltrates the muscle cone and extends through the optic foramen and into the cavernous sinus. This behavior indicates an aggressive malignant lesion, rather than a granulomatous reaction.

Lacrimal gland masses, either neoplastic or inflammatory, occur in the superolateral aspect of the extraconal compartment. Approximately one half of lacrimal gland tumors are benign, mixed tumors (Fig. 4.22), which are seen as encapsulated, septated masses. They appear bright on T2-weighted images. The malignant counterpart, adenocystic carcinoma, has no capsule and is infiltrative along the nerves. Extension along the periosteum—with or without attendant bone involvement—differentiates a malig-

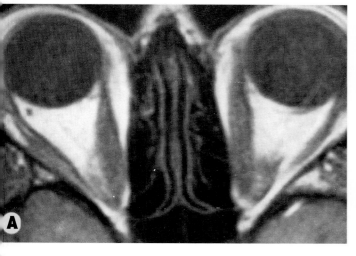

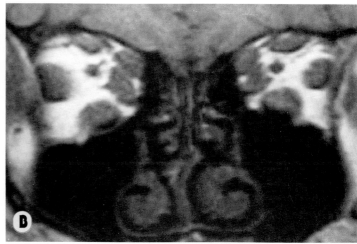

Fig. 4.21 GRAVES' OPHTHALMOPATHY T1-weighted axial **(A)** and coronal **(B)** images. All of the extraocular muscles are enlarged bilaterally and affected to varying degrees. The characteristic muscle belly involvement with tendinous insertion sparing is demonstrated particularly well in the right medial and lateral rectus muscles, best seen in the axial plane.

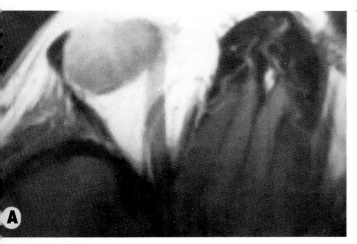

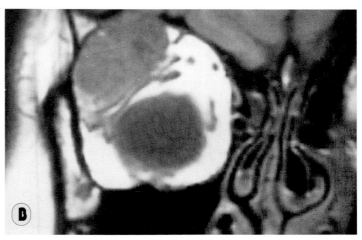

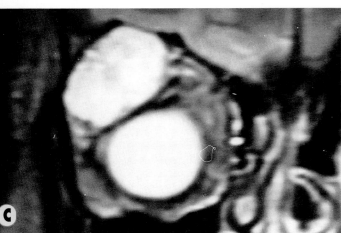

Fig. 4.22 BENIGN MIXED LACRIMAL GLAND TUMOR T1-weighted axial **(A)**, T1-weighted coronal **(B)**, and T2-weighted coronal **(C)** images. A flat surface coil was used in the axial examination, thus accounting for the poor depth resolution. A large mass involving the lacrimal gland has a slightly septated internal architecture. This suggests the diagnosis of benign mixed tumor. It is well-defined and appears confined to the gland, becoming bright on the T2-weighted sequence. The coronal plane accurately localizes the tumor to an extraconal area within the lacrimal gland.

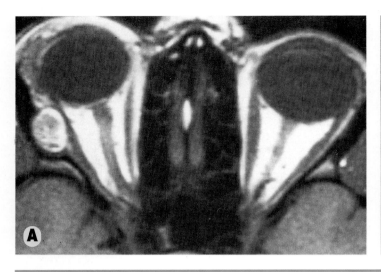

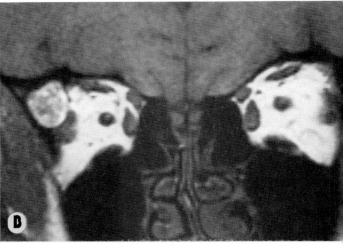

Fig. 4.23 DERMOID T1-weighted axial **(A)** and coronal **(D)** images. The superolateral, extraconal location and hyperintense signal of this lesion are characteristic of a dermoid tumor. The hyperintensity on the T1-weighted images indicates the presence of fat.

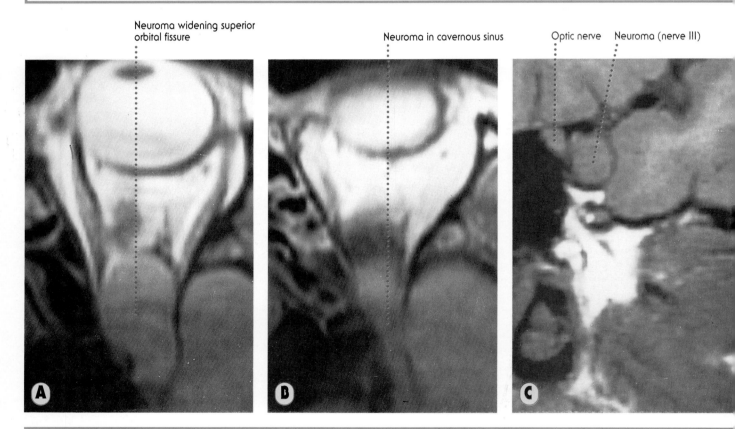

Neuroma widening superior orbital fissure

Neuroma in cavernous sinus

Optic nerve   Neuroma (nerve III)

Fig. 4.24 NEUROMA T1-weighted proton density axial **(A** and **B)** and coronal **(C)** images. A well-defined mass is seen at the orbital apex, extending posteriorly into the cavernous sinus. On the coronal image, the mass lies inferolateral to the optic nerve and is clearly separate from it. This appearance most suggests a neuroma that involves one of the nerves traversing the superior orbital fissure. Clinically, cranial nerve III was involved.

nancy from an inflammatory process within the gland. Magnetic resonance imaging is not helpful in distinguishing an inflamed, enlarged gland from a neoplasm in the absence of direct tumor extension beyond the capsule of the gland.

Lymphoma quite frequently involves the orbit. In all but the rarest of cases this is a manifestation of widespread, systemic disease. Extraconally situated lymphoma tends to occur in the anterior aspect of the orbit under the lid. It also commonly infiltrates the lacrimal gland. Metastases, particularly those derived from breast carcinoma, also occur somewhat frequently in an extraconal location, accompanied at times by destruction of the surrounding bone.

Epidermoids and dermoids tend to occur in a younger population. Although an epidermoid cyst is extremely common on the skin surrounding the orbit, it is very uncommon within the orbit. Conversely, dermoids (Fig. 4.23) characteristically occur within the orbit or the orbital wall. In the osseous form, the bony orbit is expanded by a benign, slow-growing dermoid, usually along the superolateral margin in the region of the lacrimal gland. It may be attached to the underlying bone and extended intracranially through foramina. Orbital dermoids may also occur in the lacrimal gland or the orbital soft tissues. The mixed composition of these tumors is well-demonstrated on MR images. Confirming the presence of calcification may necessitate the use of CT. The tumor typically is bright on T1-weighted images, depending on the amount of fat present. A fat-fluid level is present in some cases. Epidermoids are distinctly different in appearance on T1-weighted images; they are hypointense to muscle, similar to the dark gray of the vitreous.

Neuromas (Fig. 4.24) are derived from the nerve sheaths, usually from those nerves passing through the superior orbital fissure. They may be plexiform and infiltrate along the nerve. Many are associated with neurofibromatosis. Magnetic resonance imaging is excellent for assessing the extent of the well-defined lesion, which is homogeneously bright on T2-weighted images.

Orbital hematomas occur with direct, physical trauma to the orbit or with barotrauma (usually scuba diving). Where direct or penetrating trauma is involved, the resultant hematoma may be in either the globe or the orbit proper; the tumor is usually subperiosteal when associated with diving (Fig. 4.25). High signal intensity on T1-weighted images generally indicates the presence of hematoma. In the very acute phase of the hematoma, hyperintensity may be minimal or nonapparent. Marked hypointensity on the T2-weighted image, then, is the clue to the diagnosis.

Orbital abscess is an uncommon entity. However, it is extremely important to establish this diagnosis early in the course of the disease because of the rapidity with which it can progress. Orbital abscess occurs either by direct extension of infection from the paranasal sinuses (in which case it is usually subpe-

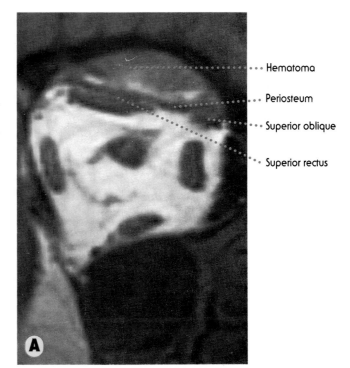

··· Hematoma

··· Periosteum

··· Superior oblique

··· Superior rectus

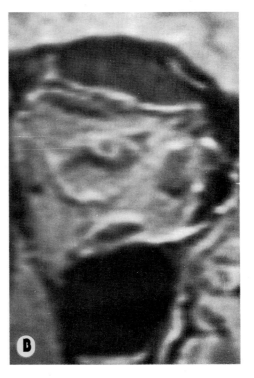

Fig. 4.25 SUBPERIOSTEAL HEMATOMA T1-weighted **(A)** and T2-weighted **(B)** coronal images. The thin, low signal margin of the periosteum is clearly defined, indicating the presence of an extraorbital mass between the periosteum and the intact cortical bone of the orbital roof. Scattered, bright signal within this mass indicates that there is very little methemoglobin, suggesting an acute hemorrhage. The marked hypointensity on the T2-weighted image (due to deoxyhemoglobin) confirms the diagnosis.

riosteal), or from penetrating trauma (Fig. 4.26). It may appear identical to any other intraorbital mass, but the detection of air in any lesion should be considered indicative of abscess until proven otherwise.

EXTRAORBITAL LESIONS

Inflammatory and malignant lesions of the paranasal sinuses frequently extend into the extraconal compartment of the orbit, following destruction of the bony sinus walls. Mucoceles and mucopyoceles commonly encroach on the extraconal fat but do not extend intraconally due to the musculofascial sheath. The very bright signal on T2-weighted images is helpful in differentiating mucoceles from carcinomas of the sinuses (see Chapter 3). Carcinoma of the ethmoid sinus invariably erodes early into the medial aspect of the orbit. Similarly, malignancies of the maxillary sinus, nasopharynx, infratemporal fossa, and the parapharyngeal space gain orbital access via the orbital fissures or by frank bone erosion. These have been previously illustrated in Chapter 3.

Tumors originating within bone, either primary or metastatic, often extend into the orbit. The fine bone detail of these tumors is better visualized by CT, but the extent of the tumor spread along dural planes is much better evaluated by MRI.

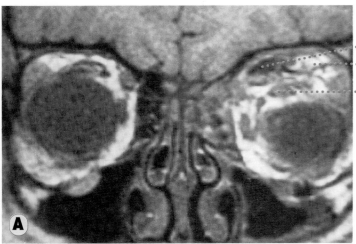

··· Air in abscess

··· Stranding in fat

··· Superior rectus

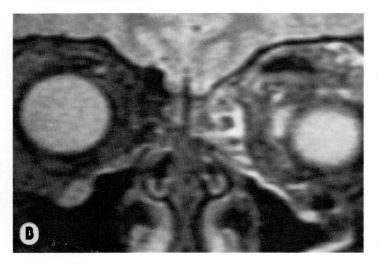

Fig. 4.26 EXTRACONAL ABSCESS T1-weighted coronal **(A)** and proton density coronal **(B)** images. There is a mixed density mass in the superior aspect of the orbit that is external to the muscle cone. The signal void within the lesion is due to air. This abscess developed secondary to a penetrating injury.

BIBLIOGRAPHY

BOOKS

Duane TD, Jaegar EA, eds. *Diseases of the orbit, clinical ophthalmology,* 2nd ed. Philadelphia: JB Lippincott, 1988.

Jones JS, Jakobiec FA. *Diseases of the orbit.* New York: Harper and Row, 1979.

Mafee MF, ed. *Imaging in ophthalmology. Part I— Radiologic Clinics of North America.* Philadelphia: WB Saunders, 1987.

Mafee MF, ed. *Imaging in ophthalmology. Part II— Radiologic Clinics of North America.* Philadelphia: WB Saunders, 1987.

JOURNAL ARTICLES AND BOOK CHAPTERS

Atlas SW, Bilaniuk LT, Zimmerman RA. Orbit. In: Stark DD, Bradley WG, eds. *Magnetic resonance imaging.* St Louis: CV Mosby, 1988.

Raden DT, Savino PJ, Zimmerman, RA. Magnetic resonance imaging in orbital diagnosis. *Radiol Clin North Am* 1988;26:535.

Sobel DF, Mills C, Char D, et al. NMR of the normal and pathologic eye and orbit. *AJNR* 1983;5:345–350.

Sullivan JA, Harms SE. Surface-coil MR imaging of orbital neoplasms. *AJNR* 1986;7:29.

Sullivan JA, Harms SE. Characterization of orbital lesions by surface coil MR imaging. *Radiographics* 1987;7:9–28.

Zimmerman RA, Bilaniuk LT. Ocular MR imaging. *Radiology* 1988;168:875.

chapter five

the spine

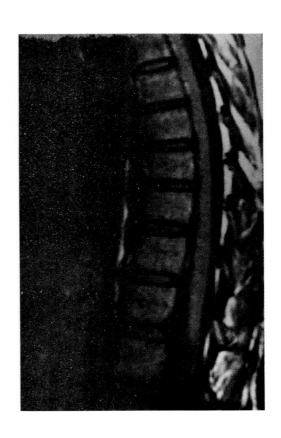

BLAKE McCLARTY   SCOTT SUTHERLAND   E.G. BERTRAM

INTRODUCTION

Spinal disorders are the most common indication for magnetic resonance imaging (MRI) in North America, accounting for approximately one half of all MRI examinations performed. Among the many reasons for the widespread use of MRI in spinal diagnosis is the frequency of spinal disease (in particular, degenerative disc disease) and the lack of a noninvasive diagnostic alternative. Computed tomography (CT) and myelography both involve ionizing radiation, and myelography also requires a lumbar puncture with injection of intrathecal contrast. Other advantages of MRI include its capacity for direct multiplanar imaging and the absence of bone artifact. Yet, perhaps MRI's prime virtue is that it was the first, and remains the only, method available for direct visualization of the spinal cord and its internal structure. In a very short time, MRI has emerged as the diagnostic imaging modality of choice for most diseases of the spine.

NORMAL ANATOMY (Figs. 5.1 to 5.10)

THE CERVICAL SPINE (Figs. 5.1 to 5.4)

THE VERTEBRAE, INTERVERTEBRAL JOINTS, AND LIGAMENTS

There are seven cervical vertebrae. The first two, the atlas and the axis, are unique. The atlas (C1) does not have a body and is composed of the anterior arch, the right and left lateral masses, and a posterior arch. A small transverse process projects from each lateral mass. The lateral masses have large, upper weight-bearing facets that support the skull. A tubercle for the transverse ligament projects medially from each lateral mass. This retains the odontoid process in position. The axis (C2) has an odontoid process (the displaced body of C1) that projects from the upper surface of the body. The odontoid process, which is easily identified on MRI, serves as an important landmark for determining the segmental level. A dark horizontal band, a remnant of the subdental synchondrosis, is often visible at the base of the odontoid process. The transverse processes of C2 are short, and its spinous process is large and bifid.

The lower five (C3-C7) are typical and are each composed of a body, a vertebral arch (pedicle and lamina), and the spinous, transverse, and articular processes. These vertebrae are of equal depth (anteroposterior direction) but become broader and increase in height from C3 to C7. The paired pedicles arise from the posterior surface of the body and pro-

ject dorsolaterally. They form the superior and inferior margins of the neural foramen and the lateral margins of the spinal canal. The paired laminae (part of each vertebral arch) join at an obtuse angle in the midline to form the base of the spinous process, which is short, bifid, directed inferiorly, and V-shaped in cross-section. The spinous process of the seventh cervical vertebra is longer, thicker, and tilted more inferiorly than the more rostral cervical spinous process.

The articular processes are located at the junction of the pedicles and laminae. These processes form an oblique, long column. The superior processes arise from the pedicles and face posteriorly and superiorly; the inferior processes arise from the laminae and face in contrary directions. The concave surface of the superior process and the convex surface of the inferior process form the diarthrodial facet joints. The transverse processes arise between the superior and inferior articular processes at the junctions of pedicles with laminae, and they course laterally. The transverse processes have two roots (anterior and posterior), a perforation (foramen transversarium), and two tubercles. The circular, transverse foramina transmit the vertebral artery and small veins.

On T1-weighted images, the cancellus bone of the adult spine is of intermediate-to-high signal intensity, reflecting the primarily fatty nature of mature bone marrow. In children, the axial skeleton is less intense because of more active hematopoiesis in the marrow. The cortex of each bone is a thin, dark outline, framing the bright marrow space.

The intervertebral disc is composed of the cartilaginous end-plate, the anulus fibrosus, and the nucleus pulposus. The cartilaginous end-plate is composed of hyaline cartilage covering the superior and inferior body surfaces of adjacent vertebrae. The anulus fibrosus, a collagenous capsular ligament of the nucleus pulposus, is circular. It is composed of short, thick fibers attached to the adjacent vertebral bodies at the site of the fused epiphyseal ring. The nucleus pulposus, the remnant of the embryonic notochord, is composed of loose, fine fibrous strands in a gelatinous matrix. Peripherally, it blends imperceptibly with the anulus fibrosus. The nucleus consists of approximately 90% water and the anulus 80% water. On T1-weighted images, the peripheral portion is of higher signal intensity than the central portion. On T2-weighted images, the relative signal intensities are reversed.

The intervertebral joints are opposed bony surfaces firmly bound together by the anterior and posterior longitudinal ligaments that extend from the base of the skull to the sacrum. These ligaments are attached to the intervertebral discs and adjacent margins of the vertebral bodies. In the cervical area the anterior ligament becomes a cord that attaches to the anterior tubercle of the atlas, and then to the pharyngeal tubercle of the basioccipital. The posterior ligament widens at its disc attachments and is known as the membrana tectoria at the base of the skull. On MR images, the anterior and posterior longitudinal ligaments are hypointense; they blend with the peripheral anulus and the compact bone of cervical vertebral bodies. The ligamentum flavum unites adjacent laminae. Weak, interspinous ligaments unite the adjacent spinous processes, and the strong supraspinous ligament (ligamentum nuchae) unites the tips of the spinous processes. In the neck, the ligamentum nuchae is triangular with a free posterior border. The most rostral part of this ligament, also called the atlanto-occipital membrane, attaches to the inion and external occipital crest.

THE SPINAL CANAL AND ITS CONTENTS

The cervical spinal canal is triangular in transverse section with its apex directed posteriorly. It is of uniform size from C7 to C3 (anteroposterior diameter of approximately 12 mm) but enlarges from C3 to C1 (anteroposterior dimension, 15 mm at C2 and 16 mm at C1). The spinal canal is composed of a set of concentric compartments with the epidural space outermost and the spinal cord at its center.

The epidural space is located between the bone confines of the spinal canal and the dura mater. It is filled with epidural fat, nerves, and the external venous plexus. Its most visible component is epidural fat, seen as high signal intensity on T1-weighted sequences. The dura mater—a tough, fibrous, tubular sheath—extends from the foramen magnum to the level of the second sacral vertebra where it ends as a blind sac. The subdural space is a potential space between the dura and the underlying arachnoid. The arachnoid is a thin, transparent sheath separated from the pia mater by the subarachnoid space, which is filled with cerebrospinal fluid (CSF). The CSF is hypointense and hyperintense on T1- and T2-weighted images, respectively. The arachnoid and the pia are not visible on MRI. The microscopic layer of pia lies immediately adjacent to the spinal cord. An elongated fold of pia mater, the dentate ligament, originates from the lateral margins of the spinal cord, and courses laterally in the subarachnoid space between the dorsal and the ventral rootlets to pierce the arachnoid and attach to the inside of the dura mater at regular intervals (21 on each side). It is an important landmark in neurosurgery but is not visible on MR images.

The cervical spinal cord is larger in cross-sectional area between C4 and T1 (the first thoracic vertebra) than between C1 and C3. This is referred to as the brachial enlargement and should not be confused with a tumor. The shape and size of the cord are well-shown on T1-weighted images, the cord having a higher signal intensity than the dark CSF. The relative signal intensities of spinal cord and CSF are reversed on T2-weighted images. Gray-white differentiation is visible on many axial images, particularly through the higher cervical levels. The gray matter is central and is H-shaped. The anterior, lateral, and posterior columns of white matter are arranged around this "H."

Eight pairs of spinal nerves arise from the cervical cord and are attached to the cord by dorsal (sensory) and ventral (motor) roots. The respective dorsal roots (composed of many root fibers) course through the subarachnoid space, piercing the dura at intervals of approximately 2 mm; then, they continue laterally to the intervertebral foramen, where each dorsal root is enlarged to contain the spinal root ganglion cells. Just distal to the ganglion, the ventral root unites with it to form a typical spinal nerve. The roots of each spinal nerve (C1-C7) leave the vertebral canal through the intervertebral foramina, above the corresponding vertebrae. The first cervical nerve emerges between the atlas and the occipital bone, and the eighth leaves through the foramina between C7 and T1. The dorsal and ventral roots can be identified as coursing through the subarachnoid space toward the intervertebral foramina, particularly on transverse images. High signal intensity often surrounds the nerve roots. This represents fat and the extensive venous network in both the ventral epidural space and the intervertebral foramina.

THE THORACIC SPINE (Figs. 5.5 and 5.6)

THE VERTEBRAE, INTERVERTEBRAL JOINTS, AND LIGAMENTS

There are 12 thoracic vertebrae each composed of a body, a vertebral arch, and the spinous, transverse, and articular processes. There is a progressive decrease in size from T1 to T12 of the vertebral bodies. On the lateral sides of each vertebra is an upper and lower demifacet for the articulation of a rib. The short and thick laminae overlap and are directed posteriorly and medially. The spinous processes pass posteriorly and inferiorly and are longer than those of the cervical or lumbar vertebrae. The pedicles, also directed posterolaterally, are attached to the superior half of each vertebral body. Each adjacent pedicle contributes to the boundaries of the intervertebral foramen. The transverse processes extend laterally from the articular pillars (junction of pedicles and laminae) in a posterosuperior direction. Their tips have articular facets for the ribs. The four articular processes (two superior and two inferior) are similar to those of the cervical vertebrae.

Although the structure of the discs is similar to that of cervical discs, they are thinner than their cervical counterparts. Each disc is thicker posteriorly than ventrally, contributing to the normal thoracic kyphosis. The anterior longitudinal ligament is thicker in the thoracic region than elsewhere. It also has posterolateral attachments to the crests of the ribs. The posterior longitudinal ligament, the ligamentum flava and nuchae, and the other articular joints do not differ significantly from their counterparts in the cervical spine.

THE SPINAL CANAL AND ITS CONTENTS
In the thoracic region, the spinal canal is round and uniform in size throughout its length. It is surrounded anteriorly by vertebral bodies and discs, posteriorly by laminae and spinous processes, and laterally by pedicles.

The contents of the thoracic canal are similar to the contents of the cervical canal, except that posteriorly there is more epidural fat between the dura and the neural arch. The dural sheath is larger than in the cervical area and extends along the nerves for a longer distance in the thoracic area than the cervical region. The intra-arachnoid compartment contains the thoracic cord, the dorsal and ventral roots, the dentate ligament, and the spinal and radicular arteries and veins, all of which are surrounded by CSF.

The thoracic cord is rounded, with a prominent, indented, anterior median sulcus and very shallow posterior median and posterolateral sulci. The spinal cord normally terminates at the vertebral level of L1 (first lumbar vertebra) or the T12-L1 disc space. Its terminal portion is expanded at the T11-T12 vertebral level to form the conus medullaris (lumbosacral enlargement). The anteroposterior diameter of the conus may normally be as much as 80% of the spinal canal. The cord at this level may be round or oval; the anterior median sulcus is shallow. On axial sections at the conus level, the roots have a spider-like appearance at their points of connection to the cord.

In the upper thoracic spine, there is a difference of two levels—and in the lower thoracic spine, three levels—between cord and vertebra (i.e., cord segment T10 lies at the T7 vertebral level). Dorsal and ventral roots must descend two or three vertebral body segments to exit in the proper intervertebral foramen.

THE LUMBOSACRAL SPINE (Figs. 5.7 to 5.10)

THE VERTEBRAE, INTERVERTEBRAL JOINTS, AND LIGAMENTS
There are five lumbar and five sacral vertebrae. The sacral segments unite to form the sacrum. The lumbar vertebrae are composed of a body, a vertebral arch, and the same processes as in the cervical and

thoracic spine (spinous, transverse, and articular).

The bodies of the lumbar vertebrae are kidney-shaped (long diameter transverse) with a flat upper and lower surface. Their bodies are convex ventrally and are thicker anteriorly. The bodies of the sacral vertebrae are thicker posteriorly than they are anteriorly, conforming to the lumbar lordosis and the sacral kyphosis, respectively. Basivertebral venous channels are seen in the middle of the lumbar vertebral bodies as high signal intensity horizontal bands on T1-weighted sagittal images. The transverse processes of the lumbar vertebrae are low and flat. The spinous processes are thick, oblong plates.

The lumbar discs are thickest (vertical height greatest) in the lower lumbar region. The lumbar discs are the largest in the spine, but their structure is otherwise identical to those in the cervical and thoracic regions. Likewise, the anterior and posterior longitudinal ligaments, the ligamentum flava, and the articular joints are similar in structure and function.

THE SPINAL CANAL AND ITS CONTENTS

The lumbar spinal canal is larger than the thoracic and is triangular in cross-section. As is the case with the other parts of the spine, it is surrounded by bone (body, pedicles, laminae, and spinous processes).

The lumbar epidural space has a very rich venous plexus, and there is more epidural fat in the anterior half of the lumbar epidural space than in the thoracic region. The dense fibrous dura extends caudally, terminating as a sac at the S2 vertebral segment. Laterally, on each side of the cord, the dura (along with the arachnoid) surrounds the lumbar nerve roots (dorsal and ventral) to form a tubular sheath that courses inferiorly and laterally into the respective intervertebral foramen.

The filum terminale (fibrous filament) extends caudally from the caudal tip of the cord to the fundus of the dural sac (S2 segment of sacrum). It has a signal intensity similar to the other neural elements. The cauda equina, composed of long dorsal and ventral lumbosacral nerve roots, originates from the cord at the conus. The lumbar and sacral roots descend in the subarachnoid space toward their point of exit from their respective intervertebral foramina that lie at a distant caudal level. On midline sagittal images, the collection of nerve roots appears as a single linear area of intermediate signal intensity, which gradually tapers from the conus to the sacrum. Parasagittal images show the roots dispersing in a radiating manner, as they extend inferiorly to exit from their respective intervertebral foramina. On axial images at L2 and L3, these roots are grouped together posteriorly in the canal. More inferiorly, pairs of roots separate from this posterior collection to traverse the thecal sac and exit from their respective foramina.

Normal Anatomy of the Spine (Figs. 5.1 to 5.4)

The Cervical Spine

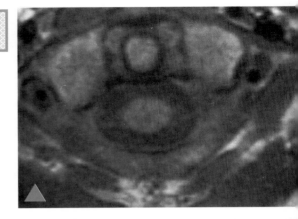

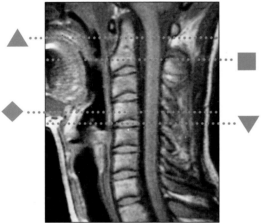

Fig. 5.1 Localizer: Midline T1-Weighted Sagittal Image
The planes of section of four axial images are indicated: through the dens, the C2 body, the C4-C5 neural foramen, and the C4-C5 disc space. The dens is the best landmark for determining segmental level.

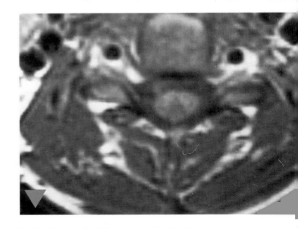

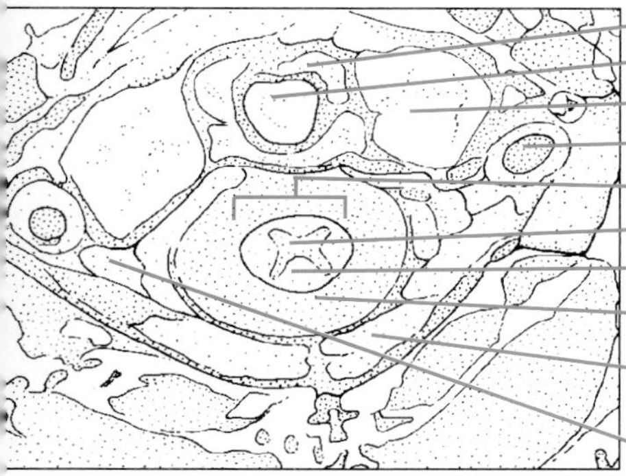

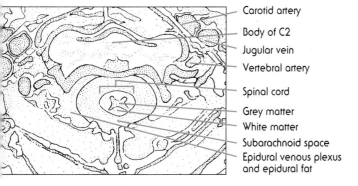

Atlantoaxial joint
Odontoid process
C1 (lateral mass)
Vertebral artery
Spinal cord
Spinal cord grey matter
Spinal cord white matter
Subarachnoid space
Posterior arch (neural arch)
Epidural venous plexus

Fig. 5.2A T1-Weighted Axial Image Through the Dens
The dens is situated directly between the lateral masses of C1. The posterior arch encloses the vertebral canal. The subarachnoid space around the cord at this level is larger than at any other point in the spine. The gray matter is a faint central "H"-shaped area within the spinal cord.

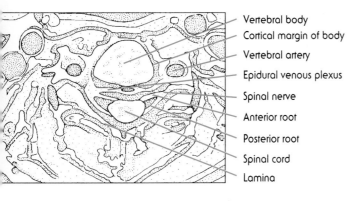

Carotid artery
Body of C2
Jugular vein
Vertebral artery
Spinal cord
Grey matter
White matter
Subarachnoid space
Epidural venous plexus and epidural fat

Fig. 5.2B T1-Weighted Axial Image Through the C2 Body   The body of C2 has a distinctive, easily recognized shape. The epidural space contains fat and a rich venous plexus.

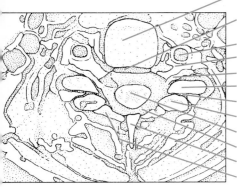

Vertebral body
Cortical margin of body
Vertebral artery
Epidural venous plexus
Spinal nerve
Anterior root
Posterior root
Spinal cord
Lamina

Fig. 5.2C T1-Weighted Axial Image Through the Neural Foramen   The vertebral arteries occupy the foramina of the transverse processes on either side. The exiting nerve roots are directly anterior to the superior facet and course anterolaterally. The facet joint, on the lateral aspect of the spinal canal, may be difficult to see on axial sections because it is almost horizontally oriented.

Vertebral body and Intervertebral disc
Posterior longitudinal ligament
Vertebral artery
Neural foramen (with fat)
Exiting nerve roots
Superior facet
Facet joint
Inferior facet
Spinal cord
Subarachnoid space
Lamina
Spinous process

Fig. 5.2D T1-Weighted Axial Image Through the Disc Space   The cervical discs are considerably thinner than their lumbar counterparts, and, therefore, axial sections through them are subject to partial averaging from the end-plates. The outer anulus is inseparable from the posterior longitudinal ligament (both dark). In turn, both are difficult to distinguish from the CSF on which they border. Sequences that produce white CSF are suggested to overcome this problem (see Fig. 5.20).

The Cervical Spine

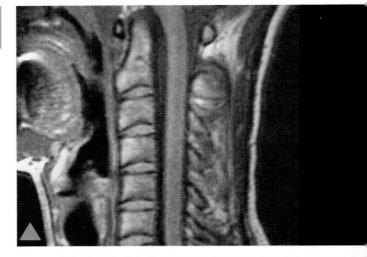

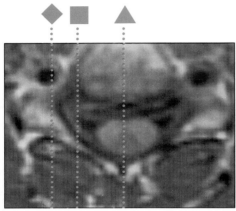

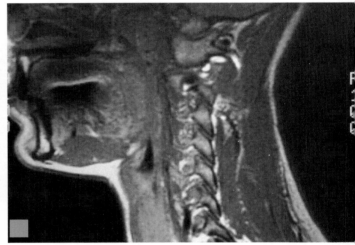

Fig. 5.3 Localizer: T1-Weighted Sagittal Image Through C4 The planes of section of three sagittal images are indicated: through the midline, the neural foramen, and the foramen transversarium.

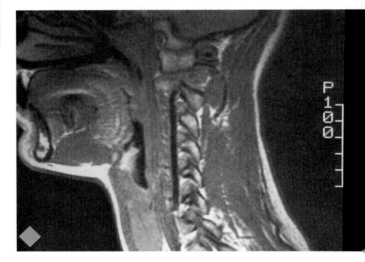

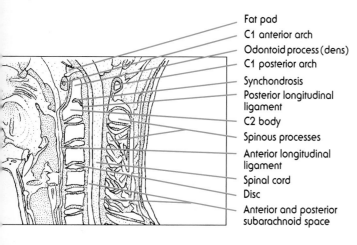

Fat pad
C1 anterior arch
Odontoid process (dens)
C1 posterior arch
Synchondrosis
Posterior longitudinal ligament
C2 body
Spinous processes
Anterior longitudinal ligament
Spinal cord
Disc
Anterior and posterior subarachnoid space

Fig. 5.4A Midline T1-Weighted Sagittal Image The anterior and posterior arches of the atlas (C1) lie immediately inferior to the occipital condyles. The dens (odontoid process) is fused to C2 at the synchondrosis. The homogeneous cancellous bone of the bodies of C3-C7 is separated from the intervening discs by bony end-plates. The bodies are joined by strong anterior and posterior longitudinal ligaments. The spinal cord enlarges slightly from C5 to T1 and is surrounded by CSF.

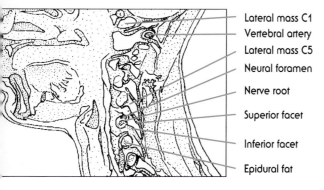

Lateral mass C1
Vertebral artery
Lateral mass C5
Neural foramen
Nerve root
Superior facet
Inferior facet
Epidural fat

Fig. 5.4B T1-Weighted Sagittal Image Through the Neural Foramen The pedicles in the cervical spine are oriented posterolaterally and therefore the neural foramen is not in good profile on sagittal sections. Several foramina are visible, each with exiting nerve roots and two or more epidural veins embedded in fat. The articular processes (facet joints) form a bony column with the inferior and superior facets articulating with one another at an angle of approximately 30° from the horizontal.

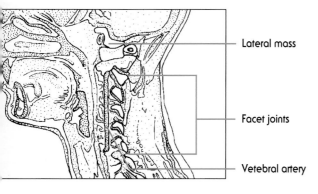

Lateral mass

Facet joints

Vetebral artery

Fig. 5.4C T1-Weighted Sagittal Image Through the Foramen Transversarium The vertebral artery on each side enters the spinal column at C6, ascends through the foramen transversarium to C2, exits, and loops around the lateral mass of C1 to enter the cisterna magna. It is distinctly visible because of the flow void from the high velocity blood flow in the vessel.

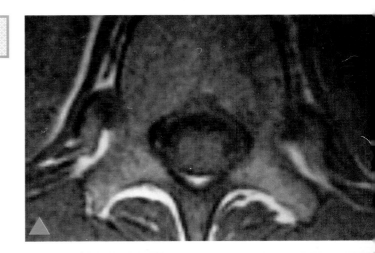

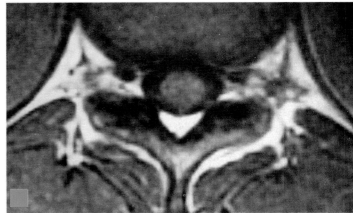

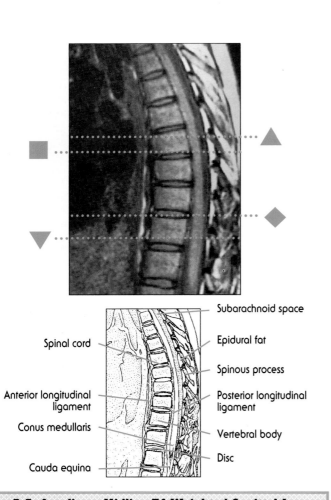

Subarachnoid space

Spinal cord

Epidural fat

Spinous process

Anterior longitudinal ligament

Posterior longitudinal ligament

Conus medullaris

Vertebral body

Cauda equina

Disc

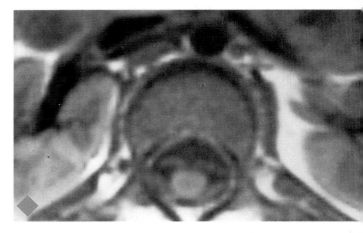

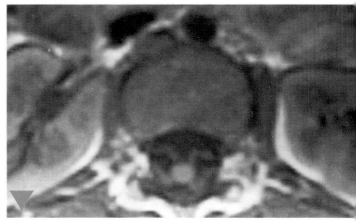

Fig. 5.5 Localizer: Midline T1-Weighted Sagittal Image
The planes of section of four axial images are indicated: through the pedicle, the neural foramen, the superior portion of the conus, and the inferior tip of the conus. On the sagittal image, the conus is a bulbous enlargement of the distal cord, usually at the T12 level. At the midthoracic level, the cord is anterior; it follows the shortest path around the thoracic kyphus.

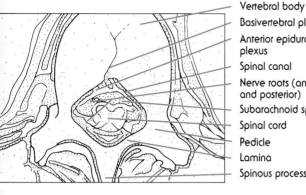

Vertebral body
Basivertebral plexus
Anterior epidural venous plexus
Spinal canal
Nerve roots (anterior and posterior)
Subarachnoid space
Spinal cord
Pedicle
Lamina
Spinous process

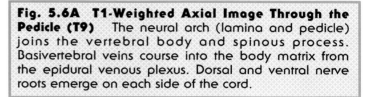

Fig. 5.6A T1-Weighted Axial Image Through the Pedicle (T9) The neural arch (lamina and pedicle) joins the vertebral body and spinous process. Basivertebral veins course into the body matrix from the epidural venous plexus. Dorsal and ventral nerve roots emerge on each side of the cord.

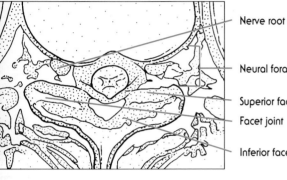

Nerve root

Neural foramen

Superior facet
Facet joint

Inferior facet

Fig 5.6B T1-Weighted Axial Image Through the Neural Foramen (T9-T10) The vertebral body and the facet joint form the anterior and posterior boundaries of the neural foramen, which contains fat, a venous plexus, and a nerve root.

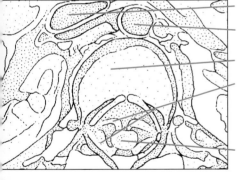

Inferior vena cava

Aorta

T12

Nerve roots (anterior and posterior)

Superior part of conus medullaris

Fig 5.6C T1-Weighted Axial Image Through the Superior Conus Medullaris The thickest portion of the spinal cord is the conus medullaris, which occupies about 80% of the spinal canal. The spider-like origin of the nerve roots is a landmark of the conus.

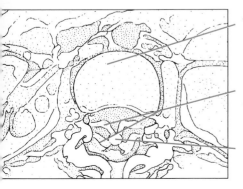

T12

"Spider-like" nerve root origins of cauda equina

Inferior conus medullaris

Fig. 5.6D T1-Weighted Axial Image Through the Inferior Conus Medullaris The conus tapers to a fine tip at its inferior end, running into the filum terminale. Axial images are the most definitive method of establishing the level of the cord's termination.

The Lumbosacral Spine

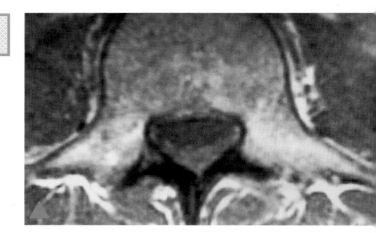

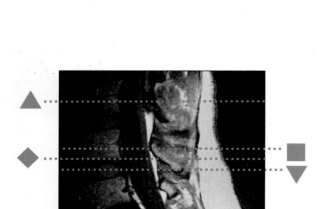

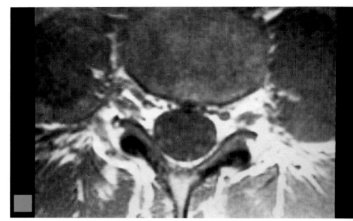

Fig. 5.7 Localizer: Midline T1-Weighted Sagittal Image
The planes of section of four axial images are indicated: through the L3 pedicle, the superior portion of the L4-L5 neural foramen, the inferior portion of the L4-L5 neural foramen, and the L4-L5 disc space.

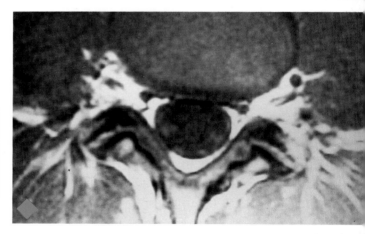

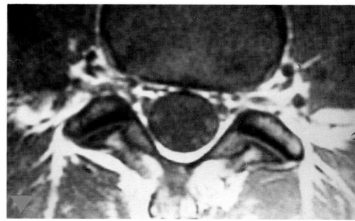

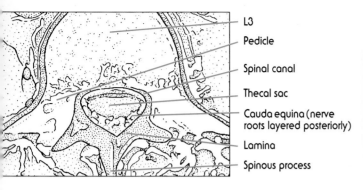

L3
Pedicle
Spinal canal
Thecal sac
Cauda equina (nerve roots layered posteriorly)
Lamina
Spinous process

Fig. 5.8A T1-Weighted Sagittal Image Through the Pedicle The large lumbar pedicles form the lateral boundaries of the spinal canal. The laminae are continuous with the midline spinous process. The anterior two thirds of the subarachnoid space is occupied by CSF; the posterior one third is filled by the nerve roots of the cauda equina, which, layered together as a group, simulate a soft tissue mass.

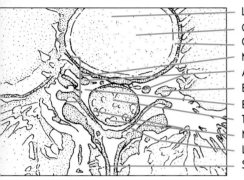

L4
Cancellous bone
Cortical bone
Neural foramen
Anterior epidural veins
Exiting L4 nerve root
Epidural fat
Thecal sac
Nerve roots
Lamina
Spinous process

Fig. 5.8B T1-Weighted Sagittal Image Through the Superior Neural Foramen The superior half of the foramen is relatively large. The L4 spinal nerve exits through the foramen immediately below the pedicle, surrounded by abundant epidural fat. Multiple epidural veins are found throughout the anterior epidural space.

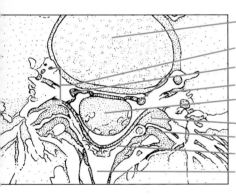

Inferior portion of L4 vertebral body
Neural foramen
Epidural veins
"Exited" L4 nerve
Thecal sac with nerve roots
Tip of superior facet
Facet joint
Lamina
Spinous process

Fig. 5.8C T1-Weighted Sagittal Image Through the Inferior Neural Foramen The exiting L4 spinal nerve continues to course laterally and inferiorly. The nerve roots remaining in the thecal sac have separated and are more individually distinct, as compared with those in the upper lumbar canal. The facet joints are visible on each side. Prominent epidural veins are located posterior to the posterior longitudinal ligament.

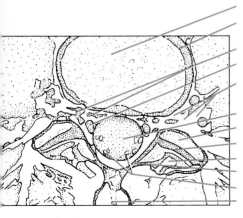

L4-L5 disc space
Cortical bone of end-plate
Epidural veins
"Traversing" nerve of L5
Epidural fat (bright areas)
Thecal sac
Superior facet
Facet joint
Inferior facet
Lamina
Nerve roots
Spinous process

Fig. 5.8D T1-Weighted Sagittal Image Through the Disc Space The intervertebral disc space is identified by its lesser signal intensity relative to the cancellous bone of the vertebral body. The anulus forms a hypointense ring around the nucleus. The next pair of roots (L5) is beginning to arise from the anterolateral aspects of the thecal sac; the L5 spinal nerve will "traverse" the spinal canal until the roots "exit" through the (L5-S1) neural foramen.

The Lumbosacral Spine

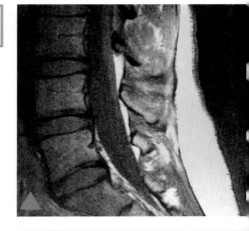

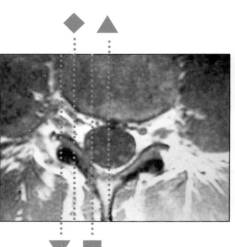

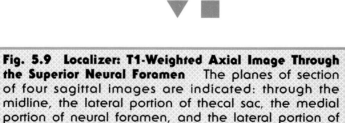

Fig. 5.9 Localizer: T1-Weighted Axial Image Through the Superior Neural Foramen The planes of section of four sagittal images are indicated: through the midline, the lateral portion of thecal sac, the medial portion of neural foramen, and the lateral portion of neural foramen.

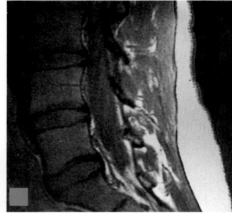

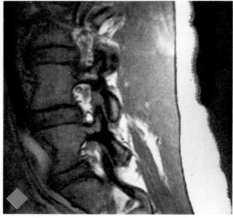

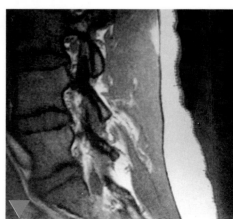

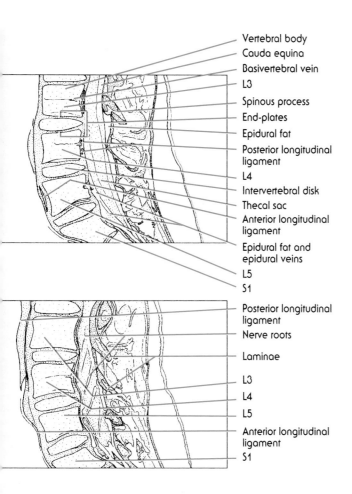

Vertebral body
Cauda equina
Basivertebral vein
L3
Spinous process
End-plates
Epidural fat
Posterior longitudinal ligament
L4
Intervertebral disk
Thecal sac
Anterior longitudinal ligament
Epidural fat and epidural veins
L5
S1

Fig. 5.10A Midline T1-Weighted Axial Image The L5-S1 disc is the thinnest of the lumbar discs and is typically oriented at the steepest angle from the horizontal. Epidural fat is most prominent anteriorly, particularly at L4 and L5. Multiple small veins are interspersed through the fat. In the spinal canal, the cauda equina is posteriorly positioned and thins out inferiorly.

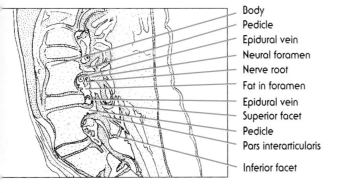

Posterior longitudinal ligament
Nerve roots
Laminae
L3
L4
L5
Anterior longitudinal ligament
S1

Fig. 5.10B T1-Weighted Axial Image Through the Lateral Thecal Sac The nerve roots of the cauda equina course at a steep angle through the subarachnoid space to their points of exit through the neural foramina. The anterior and posterior surfaces of the vertebral bodies and discs are covered by the anterior and posterior longitudinal ligaments. The laminae and their ligaments complete the bony spinal canal.

Body
Pedicle
Epidural vein
Neural foramen
Nerve root
Fat in foramen
Epidural vein
Superior facet
Pedicle
Pars interarticularis
Inferior facet

Fig. 5.10C T1-Weighted Image Through the Medial Neural Foramen The neural foramen is a keyhole-shaped opening, which leads out of the spinal canal. It contains fat, nerve roots, and multiple small veins. The synovial facet joint is formed by the superior and inferior articular processes.

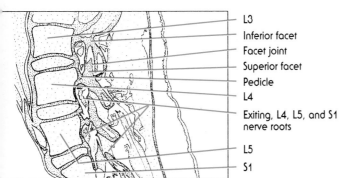

L3
Inferior facet
Facet joint
Superior facet
Pedicle
L4
Exiting, L4, L5, and S1 nerve roots
L5
S1

Fig. 5.10D T1-Weighted Axial Image Through the Lateral Neural Foramen The borders of the neural foramen are formed by the vertebral body and disc (anterior), pedicles (above and below), and facet joint (posterior). Note the exiting L4, L5, and S1 nerves.

TECHNIQUE

Proper MRI examination of the spine is very much technique-dependent, more so than any other body part (the reason being that there is a large selection of surface coils and pulse sequences from which to choose). The appropriate technique used depends on the segment to be examined, the length of spine to be included in the examination, and the specific clinical concerns. A good clinical history is thus of paramount importance, especially if it localizes the suspected pathology to a specific segment of spine.

In most circumstances, an initial sagittal localizer, or scout view, is obtained, using a body coil and a large field of view. These localizer images should encompass either C2 or the L5-S1 interspace. Inclusion of one of these easily recognized landmarks facilitates identification of other spinal levels for the remainder of the examination. The diagnostic portion of the study is then performed exclusively with surface coils.

The choice of surface coil is important because they vary markedly in size and shape. In general terms, the depth and length of tissue covered by a circular surface coil is equal to its diameter, but the signal-to-noise ratio (SNR) decreases with increasing coil size. Therefore, for the optimum SNR, the diameter of the coil should be kept to the least that would still enable one to examine the region of interest.

A rectangular surface coil provides depth of coverage approximately equal to the short axis of the coil, and length of coverage approximately equal to the long axis of the coil. Rectangular coils are therefore useful when longer segments of the spine must be examined; these coils maintain the signal advantages of a smaller circular surface coil while covering a greater length of spine.

If the entire spine is to be examined, multiple surface coils can be laid end to end and connected to the coil port by an adapter. This maneuver maintains the SNR advantages of surface coil examinations without necessitating undesirable repeated changes in coil positions.

Molding the contour of the surface coil to the shape of the body part being examined is another modification of coil geometry that can improve image quality. Molding brings the edges of the coil closer to the region of interest, thereby improving signal strength and image uniformity. The cervical spine is well-suited to examinations performed with such molded coils.

The choice of pulse sequence depends on whether the examination is to be of the cervical, thoracic, or lumbosacral areas, or of the entire spine. It depends as well on the type of pathology suspected.

Most examinations of the lumbosacral spine are performed for degenerative disc disease, spondylosis, and spinal stenosis. Postoperative assessment, congenital deformities, and vertebral and epidural neoplasms are also relatively common indications, whereas intrinsic disease of the spinal cord is not a major concern (given that the spinal cord ends at the thoracolumbar junction). The images should be designed, therefore, for good contrast between the vertebral column, the intervertebral discs, the neural foramen, and the nerve roots. The best technique for achieving this contrast is one that is relatively T1-weighted [spin echo, repetition time (TR) = 500-1000 msec, echo time

Fig. 5.11 MRI TECHNIQUE FOR EXAMINATION OF THE LUMBOSACRAL SPINE

Parameter	Sequence[a]			
	No. 1 Scout view	No. 2 T1-Weighted	No. 3 T1-Weighted	No. 4[b] T2-Weighted
Plane	Sagittal	Sagittal	Axial	Sagittal or axial
TR (msec)	400	600-1000	600-1000	2000
TE (msec)	20	20[c]	20	70-100
Slice thickness (mm)	5	3-5	5	5
Matrix[d]	128	256	256	128
Field of view	48	24-28	16-20	16-24
No. of excitations	1	2-4	2-4	2
Examination time (min)	1	5-17	5-17	8-12

[a] All sequences: spin echo, multislice.
[b] Useful for tumors and arachnoiditis.
[c] Double echo study with echo time of 20 msec (80 msec is optional).
[d] Matrix of 192 may be used (if available).

TE) = 20 msec]. A second echo (e.g., TE = 100 msec) may be added during the same acquisition to get a second set of images that are slightly T2-weighted, but this usually adds little diagnostic information. Sagittal images should have a field of view large enough to include the thoracolumbar junction so as not to overlook possible lesions at the level of the conus medullaris that are not clinically evident. T2-weighted images may be substituted or added if tumor is the primary consideration. Axial images are recommended, as the radiologic axiom that two perpendicular views should always be obtained is most appropriate in MRI of the spine. Axial sections should at least go through the lower three disc spaces. If the symptoms indicate a higher level, or if a lesion is seen on the sagittal sections above the suspected levels, the axial sections should, of course, be shifted accordingly (Fig. 5.11).

Pulse sequence strategies for the cervical and thoracic spine are different than those for the lumbosacral spine. At these levels, the spinal cord, as well as the vertebral column and intervertebral discs, must be examined. Furthermore, CSF motion is of greater magnitude here than lower in the spinal axis and, therefore, must be compensated for by either cardiac gating or flow compensating gradients (gradient moment nulling). The examination is similar to that in the lumbosacral region with respect to initial T1-weighted sagittal images. If a congenital lesion or a syrinx is demonstrated, the examination may stop at this point (although T1-weighted axial sections are often a useful supplement). However, if the patient has a myelopathy, or if there is any other reason to suspect intrinsic spinal cord disease or spinal cord compression, T2-weighted images are essential.

T2-weighted images are obtained in one of three ways: a long TR, long TE spin echo sequence or either of the two gradient recalled echo sequences listed (Fig. 5.12). All of these methods produce good contrast between the vertebral column, the subarachnoid space, and the spinal cord (the "MR myelogram"). The spin echo method produces the best contrast within the spinal cord and is recommended when an intrinsic spinal cord lesion is suspected. The second of the two gradient recalled echo methods listed is also adequate for this purpose. If an intrinsic spinal cord lesion is not suspected, the very short TR gradient recalled echo sequence produces a satisfactory "MR myelogram" and has the added benefit of being very fast. It adequately delineates the margin between the vertebral column and the thecal sac.

Regardless of which sagittal technique is used, axial sections are performed to better define identified or suspected lesions. Of particular interest in this regard is a given lesion's precise location relative to the spinal canal and spinal cord. Coronal sections are valuable in such select circumstances as nerve sheath tumors, in that they define the precise relationship of this tumor to the spinal cord, the neural foramen, and the paravertebral soft tissues.

The recent introduction of paramagnetic contrast agents will change many imaging strategies. At this early stage, it appears that they will be particularly useful in the improved detection of neoplasms and in the assessment of the postoperative back. The optimal modifications of current imaging techniques remain to be defined, as experience is gained with contrast agents.

Fig. 5.12 MRI TECHNIQUE FOR EXAMINATION OF THE CERVICAL AND THORACIC SPINE

Parameter	No. 1 Spin Echo Scout view	No. 2 Spin Echo T1-Weighted	No. 3 Spin Echo T1-Weighted	No. 4 Spin Echo[a] T2-Weighted	No. 5 Gradient Echo T2-Weighted	No. 6 Gradient Echo T2-Weighted
Plane	Sagittal	Sagittal	Axial	Sagittal or axial	Axial or sagittal	Axial or sagittal
TR (msec)	400	600	500-1000	2000-3000	25-50	400-600
TE (msec)	20	20	20	80-100	10-12	20-25
Flip angle (degrees)	90	90	90	90	6-10	30-40
Slice thickness (mm)	5	3	5	5	5	5
Matrix[b]	128	256	256	256	256	256
Field of view	48	20-28	20	20-28	20-24	20-24
No. of excitations	1	2-4	2-4	1	6	4
Examination time (min)	1	5-10	10-15	8-12	Depends on no. of slices[c]	4-6

[a]T2-weighted sequences require cardiac gating or flow compensating gradients (or both).
[b]Matrix of 192 may be substituted (if available).
[c]Acquired as sequential single slices.

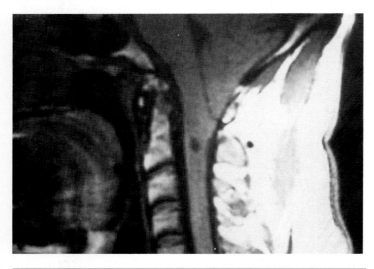

Spinal cord and
nerve roots ···

Dural sac ···

Sacrum ···

Fig. 5.13 REPAIRED MENINGOMYELOCELE T1-weighted sagittal image. The posterior elements are absent from L5 to S3. The fluid-filled dural sac prolapsed through the defect into the subcutaneous tissue of the lower back, together with the distal spinal cord and nerve roots. Repair consisted simply of closure of the exposed sac by a skin flap.

Fig. 5.14 TYPE I CHIARI MALFORMATION T1-weighted sagittal image. The cerebellar tonsils are pointed and extended inferiorly to the level of the C1 posterior arch. A very small hydromyelia cavity is present.

CONGENITAL MALFORMATIONS

MENINGOCELE AND MENINGOMYELOCELE

Failure of neural tube closure, especially in the lumbosacral region, results in a morphological continuum of spinal dysraphism from spina bifida occulta (midline bony defect) through meningocele (dural sac outside canal), and from meningomyelocele (spinal cord and/or roots within sac), to myeloschisis (exposed spinal cord). In addition, the exposed sac frequently contains fat, or rarely cartilage, and other hamartomatous elements. Meningomyelocele is frequently associated with multiple anomalies of the brain, particularly the Chiari II malformation. Associated clinical and neurological defects vary with the severity of the defect—from no defect to small patches of pigmentation or hair, to lower limb spastic paraparesis, to profound paralysis and lack of both bowel and bladder control. The exposure of the neural tube to the environment also leads to central nervous system (CNS) infections.

The reported incidence of these clinically significant defects is between one and two per thousand live births. Reconstructive surgery prevents ulceration and CNS infections, and surgical release of the spinal cord (if possible) prevents tethering and progressive neurological impairment.

Coronal and sagittal T1-weighted images best demonstrate the distal spinal cord and the nerve root relationship to the dural defect and any associated lipomas. In meningomyelocele, the cord ends in a malformed mass of tissue at the level of the defect. This placode is posteriorly positioned in the spinal canal or is given to prolapse through the defect [together with the roots of the cauda equina (Fig. 5.13)]. In a simple meningocele, all the neural elements remain in the spinal canal.

CHIARI MALFORMATION

In 1891, Chiari described three congenital malformations of the hindbrain. Although they share many similar morphological features, they are felt by many authors to be unrelated developmentally. There is, however, a continuum of severity in the Chiari malformations.

Patients with Chiari I malformation have low-lying tonsils adjacent to the foramen magnum. They usually present in the third decade with symptoms of ataxia or central cord symptoms related to coexisting hydromyelia. Occipital pain and headache are frequent symptoms. The craniocervical junction and cervical vertebra may be anomalous, e.g., assimilation of C1, basilar impression, and fusion deformities of the cervical vertebra (Klippel-Feil syndrome).

Normally, the inferior aspect of the cerebellar tonsils lies immediately at or above the foramen magnum and has a rounded shape (see *Normal Anatomy*). In the Chiari I malformation, the inferior aspect of the tonsils is pointed and deformed, often closely applied to the posterior aspect of the spinal cord. The tonsils extend inferiorly, often to the level of the C1 posterior arch or lower. The cervicomedullary junction is compressed by both the low-lying tonsils and a thickened dural-arachnoid band posteriorly at the foramen magnum. T1-weighted sagittal series best demonstrate the anatomical relationship between the brainstem, cerebellum, and spinal cord, on the one hand, and the foramen magnum, on the other. These images offer good contrast between neural tissue and the low signal intensity of the adjacent CSF (Fig. 5.14).

The most significant associated lesion is coexisting hydromyelia which occurs in half of the patients with Chiari I malformation. Hydrocephalus is rare.

In Chiari II malformation (frequently referred to as the Arnold-Chiari malformation), there is elongation and downward displacement of the brainstem and spinal cord, resulting in marked kinking at the low cervicomedullary junction. The low position of the spinal cord causes an upward course of the cervical nerve roots. The vermis, the fourth ventricle, and the tonsils are all displaced inferiorly. There are many associated brain anomalies. Patients present at birth with a meningomyelocele and concomitant neurological deficits.

T1-weighted sagittal images best demonstrate the anatomy of the Chiari II malformation: caudal displacement of cerebellar tissue, with the inferior tip of the vermis located near the C2-C3 level in a majority of cases; cervicomedullary kinking; and lengthening of the mesencephalon, with an increase in the mamilopontine distance (Fig. 5.15). The coronal plane allows for visualization of the relationship of the incisura to the cerebellum and the medial aspect of the temporal lobes.

In the Chiari III malformation, there is an occipitocervical encephalocele (Fig. 5.16). The condition is rare and almost always associated with other severe neurologic abnormalities.

HYDROMYELIA AND SYRINGOMYELIA

Hydromyelia implies enlargement of the central canal. True hydromyelia has an ependymal lining. It is frequently associated with anomalies of the craniocervical junction, notably Chiari I and II malformations. Hydromyelia has been variably reported to be associated with as many as one half and three quarters of Chiari I and Chiari II malformations, respectively. Whereas hydromyelia represents enlargement of the central canal, it does not ascend beyond the inferior aspect of the fourth ventricle. It is often segmented into compartments by axial bands. Syringomyelia signifies cavity formation in the spinal cord outside the central canal. Syringomyelia may develop spontaneously, following trauma, or in association with spinal cord tumors. Syringomyelia may occur in any segment of the cord and may ascend into the brainstem. The classical presentation is that of a dissociative sensory loss in the upper extremities due to interruption of the crossing pain and temperature fibers in the anterior commissure.

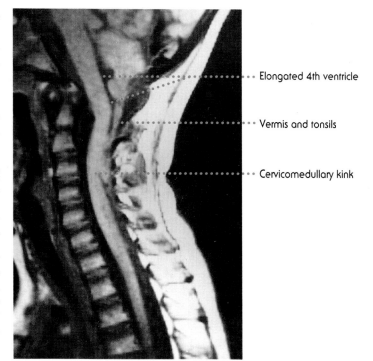

···· Elongated 4th ventricle

···· Vermis and tonsils

···· Cervicomedullary kink

Fig. 5.15 TYPE II CHIARI MALFORMATION T1-weighted sagittal image. The vermis and tonsils are flattened and inferiorly positioned well below the foramen magnum. The fourth ventricle and brainstem are elongated and inferiorly situated. There is a prominent cervicomedullary kink.

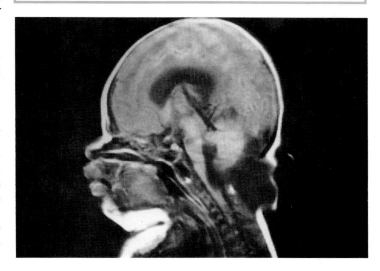

Fig. 5.16 TYPE III CHIARI MALFORMATION T1-weighted sagittal image. There is a large occipital meningocele and many other congenital abnormalities, including agenesis of the corpus callosum.

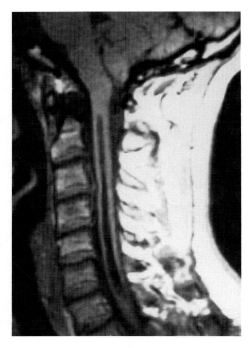

Fig. 5.17 HYDROMYELIA T1-weighted sagittal image. The tonsils are pointed and somewhat inferiorly displaced at the foramen magnum. A clearly defined hydromyelia cavity is present.

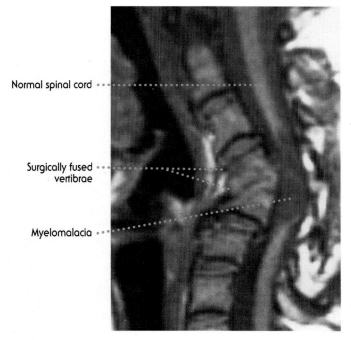

Normal spinal cord ·········

Surgically fused ·······
vertibrae

Myelomalacia ········

Fig. 5.18 MYELOMALACIA T1-weighted sagittal image. This patient became quadriplegic as a result of a motor vehicle accident 6 months prior to this scan. The C4 and C5 vertebrae have been surgically fused. There is a focal area of myelomalacia in the spinal cord at the C4 and C5 levels. It is not as dark as the signal from a syrinx cavity nor does it have well-defined margins.

Syringomyelia and hydromyelia are morphologically indistinguishable on MR images. In either case the cavity is well-defined and distinctly hypointense relative to neural tissue on T1-weighted images (usually matching CSF intensity). Sagittal and axial T1-weighted images best demonstrate the intramedullary cavities (Fig. 5.17). Initial reports from work on early scanners suggested that in thick (10 mm) sections, where partial volume effects were a factor, MRI did not consistently reveal small cavities within atrophic spinal cords. The improved spatial capabilities brought about by the use of surface coils and higher field MR imagers have minimized these problems. Magnetic resonance imaging is now clearly the best method for the diagnosis of these lesions.

The occasional inability to distinguish between noncystic myelomalacia and syringomyelia remains a problem. As surgical therapy for the latter is direct cyst drainage, this distinction is important. Both conditions are very hypointense on T1-weighted images, usually the syrinx more so than myelomalacia. A useful differential feature is that the margins of a syrinx are sharp, whereas in myelomalacia they are indistinct (Fig. 5.18). Intraoperative ultrasound examination may be required to distinguish between these two entities.

Syrinx-like artifacts are common on sagittal MR images. These truncation artifacts are related to the high contrast spinal cord–CSF interface that leads to artifactual signal patterns in the central portion of the spinal cord. Truncation or edge-ringing artifacts (Gibb's phenomena) occur where there is a large change in signal intensity over a small distance. Artifactual striations occur parallel to the interface. The effect is maximum when two interfaces are in proximity to one another, with superimposition of the striations from either interface. The artifact is most frequently seen in the sagittal T1-weighted images (Fig. 5.19). It also occurs frequently with the gradient recalled echo technique. The CSF is intense on these images relative to the spinal cord, and the artifact is a high intensity line parallel to the surface of the cord (Fig. 5.20). Truncation artifacts can be minimized through pixel size reduction, which is achieved by using a smaller field of view or a finer matrix size. The syrinx-like artifact can be recognized by its typical central position, by the maximum signal intensity change—which is usually small compared with that seen with true cavitary lesions—and by the failure to confirm a cavity on axial sections.

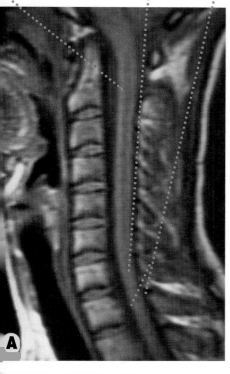

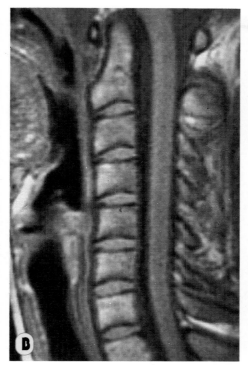

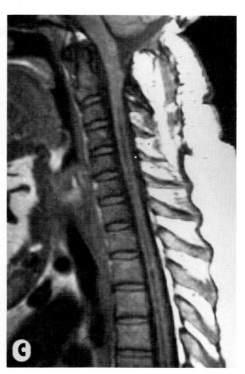

Truncation artifact central stripe   Spinal cord   CSF

Fig. 5.19 COMPARISON OF TRUNCATION ARTIFACT AND COLLAPSED SYRINX **(A)** T1-weighted sagittal image (256 x 128): normal volunteer. The phase-encoding direction is front to back (128 steps). Truncation errors occur at both the anterior and posterior cord-CSF interfaces and reinforce one another exactly in the center of the cord, resulting in a very prominent hypointense central stripe. It is not as dark as a true syrinx and it disappears when the diameter of the cord changes. **(B)** T1-weighted sagittal image (256 x 256):

same volunteer. The pixel size has been halved by increasing the number of phase-encoding steps to 256. The truncation errors no longer reinforce and consequently either disappear or become much less apparent. **(C)** T1-weighted sagittal image (256 x 256): syrinx. A true syrinx cavity has sharper margins and is more hypointense than a truncation artifact, even though it may be thinner than the artifactual central stripe. Furthermore, it will be visible independent of matrix size and image plane.

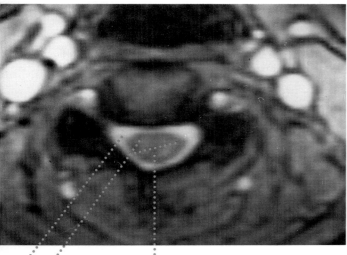

CSF   Truncation artifacts   Spinal cord

Fig. 5.20 TRUNCATION ARTIFACT Axial gradient recalled echo image. Truncation artifacts will occur on any image reconstructed by Fourier transform methods, where there is a marked change in signal intensity over a short distance. This image demonstrates artifactual areas of high intensity superimposed on the spinal cord. It does not represent the normal internal architecture of the cord or any abnormality.

Intradural dermoid · · · · ·

Dermal sinus · · · · ·

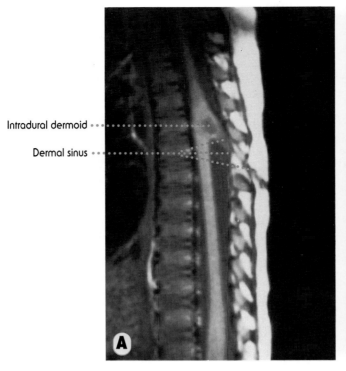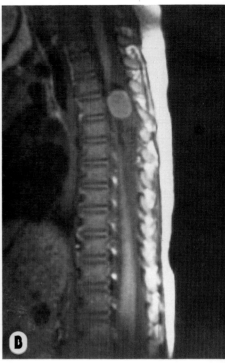

Fig. 5.21 DERMAL SINUS AND INTRADURAL DERMOID TUMOR **(A)** T1-weighted sagittal image. A dermal sinus extends from the skin into the spinal canal. A dermoid tumor is closely applied to the spinal cord. **(B)** T1-weighted sagittal image. The tumor is to the right of the midline. It is cystic with a well-defined wall. It does not contain fat.

Enterogenous cyst · · · · ·

Spinal cord · · · · ·

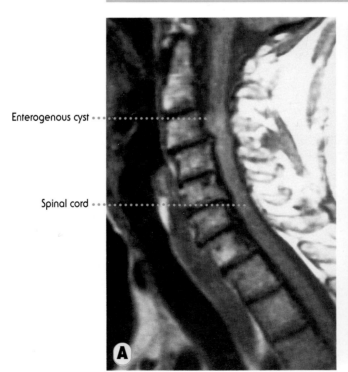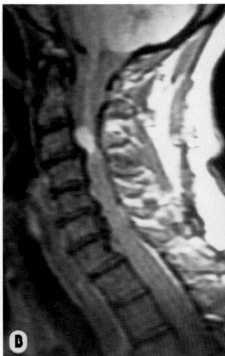

Fig. 5.22 ENTEROGENOUS CYST **(A)** T1-weighted sagittal image. A small nodule isointense to the spinal cord is seen at C3. **(B)** Proton density sagittal image. The cyst is hyperintense on this sequence, a feature which distinguishes it from a simple arachnoid cyst.

DERMAL SINUS

Other anomalies related to failure of midline closure are the dermal sinus and midline dermoid tumors. These are most frequently seen in the occipital and lumbosacral regions. They are thought to be caused by failure of the caudal neural pore to close during the fourth fetal week. In most cases, a fibrous band joins a skin dimple to the dura. If a true sinus or tract is present, it may leak CSF, and recurrent meningitis may ensue. Ectodermal remnants in the spinal canal may give rise to an intradural dermoid tumor.

Sagittal T1-weighted images best demonstrate the dermal sinus tract (Fig. 5.21). Associated dermoid tumors frequently, but not invariably, have a lipomatous element. These are hyperintense on T1-weighted images, but the tumor may contain other ectodermal elements, such as keratin or hair that cause reduction of signal intensity.

CONGENITAL CYSTS

Arachnoid cysts occur most often in the midthoracic spine. They are posteriorly placed, CSF-containing cysts, which may compress the spinal cord. Their origin has been variously described as congenital, traumatic, and postinflammatory. Ependymal cysts are true cysts with a ciliated, cuboidal lining. They appear most frequently in the anterior cervical canal in children. Enterogenous cysts, also common in the cervical or upper thoracic spine, arise from the primitive endoderm (Fig. 5.22) and may be associated with duplication of the gastrointestinal tract. Communication to the gastrointestinal tract via an anterior, bony spinal dysraphic abnormality is always present but may not be visible. Teratomatous cysts occur anywhere in the spinal canal and have cells of all three primitive layers. Magnetic resonance imaging characteristics depend chiefly on the predominance of material present within the congenital cysts. Associated bony defects may also be seen, but are better defined by axial computed tomographic (CT) images.

DIASTEMATOMYELIA

The term diastematomyelia implies sagittal division of the spinal cord, the conus medullaris, and/or the filum terminale. The arachnoid and the dura may or may not be divided. In the former, there is frequently a bony or fibrous spur extending from the vertebral body to the posterior arch. Diastematomyelia most often involves the lower thoracic or upper lumbar spine. Progressive spastic paraparesis of the lower limbs due to tethering of the spinal cord is the presenting symptom. Scoliosis is frequent. There has been recent emphasis placed on the uncommon association of syringohydromyelia with diastematomyelia. As their clinical presentations are similar, but the prescribed surgical treatments for them are distinctly different, it is important to recognize their possible coexistence.

Given that the clefting is in the sagittal plane, thin coronal or axial sections are best for displaying the abnormal anatomy (Fig. 5.23). If there is an associated scoliosis, the coronal and sagittal images are difficult both to obtain and to interpret; axial images are then required for best delineation.

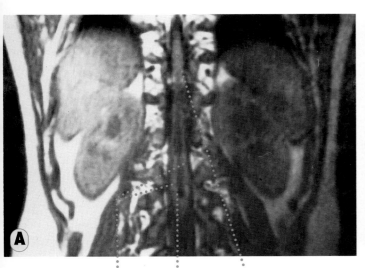

Hemicords   Bone spur   Spinal cord

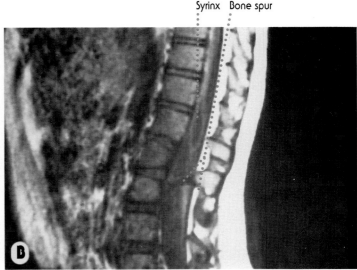

Syrinx   Bone spur

Fig. 5.23 DIASTEMATOMYELIA **(A)** T1-weighted coronal image. The spinal cord splits sagittally into two hemicords. A hypointense bone spur is present at the caudal end of the diastematomyelia. **(B)** T1-weighted sagittal image. The bone spur extends from the posterior lamina to the vertebral body. A syrinx cavity is present in the spinal cord above the diastematomyelia.

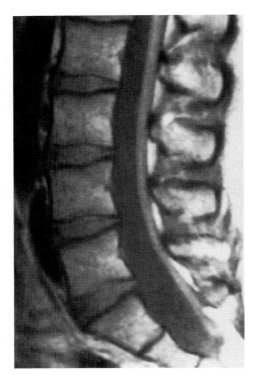

Fig. 5.24 TETHERED CORD T1-weighted sagittal image. The spinal cord ends low and merges into a thickened filum terminale, which, in turn, runs posteriorly to the spinal canal to attach to a collection of extradural fat at S2.

TETHERED CORD SYNDROME

Patients with tethering of the spinal cord by a thickened filum terminale usually present in adolescence or early adulthood with spastic paresis of the lower limbs. A thickened filum terminale extends from the low-lying, but otherwise normal, spinal cord to the posterior sacrum. There may or may not be an associated lipoma within—or at the end of—the filum. There is no meningocele but always some form of dysraphism. Lumbosacral spine examination is designed to show the conus medullaris and nerve roots. Sagittal T1-weighted images demonstrate the approximate position of the conus within the lumbar CSF (Fig. 5.24), but axial images define its precise location. The relationship of the cord to the thickened filum and the orientation of the nerve roots are best demonstrated on the axial images.

ANTERIOR SACRAL MENINGOCELE AND PERINEURAL CYST

Anterior sacral meningoceles present as a CSF-filled mass posterior to the rectum (Fig. 5.25). They cause neurological deficit only when they are of sufficient size to deviate from the sacral nerve roots.

Tarlov's cysts are expansions of the nerve sheath that may cause local erosion of the sacral foramina. Typically, they demonstrate symmetric, uniform enlargement of the sacral foramina (Fig. 5.26).

NEOPLASMS

EPIDURAL AND VERTEBRAL BODY TUMORS

Due to the abundant fat in normal bone marrow, vertebral bodies appear of high signal intensity on T1-weighted images. Bone cortex has few free protons and is of very low signal intensity. The vertebral body is, therefore, white and framed in a thin black outline of cortical bone. Most pathological processes in bone replace marrow and, therefore, appear as areas of decreased signal intensity against the background of bright marrow. With increased T2-weighting, the fatty marrow decreases in signal intensity, becoming isointense or hypointense relative to the surrounding soft tissue. Metastases or other marrow-replacing processes are, then, isointense or hyperintense relative to marrow.

VERTEBRAL HEMANGIOMA   Thin-walled blood vessels replace medullary bone and marrow in benign vertebral hemangiomas. Histologically, the dilated, vascular channels surround thickened bony trabeculae in a matrix of adipose tissue. They are a frequent autopsy finding (15% incidence). Most are asymptomatic. Plain radiographic and CT features are well-known and characteristic. The thickened trabeculae cause vertical striations in the vertebral body. Hemangiomas are most frequent in the lower thoracic and upper lumbar spine. They rarely become symptomatic unless associated with compression fractures or extravertebral extension.

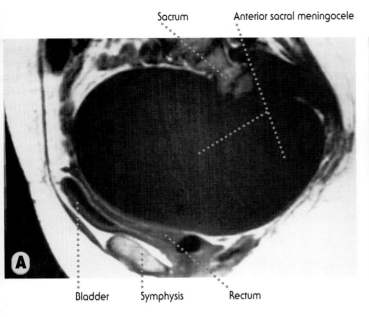

Sacrum   Anterior sacral meningocele

Bladder   Symphysis   Rectum

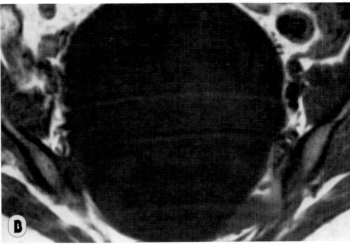

Fig. 5.25 ANTERIOR SACRAL MENINGOCELE   (A) T1-weighted sagittal image. A very large CSF-filled sac extends into the pelvis, compressing the rectum and bladder against the symphysis pubis. **(B)** T1-weighted axial image. The anterior sacral meningocele fills the pelvis.

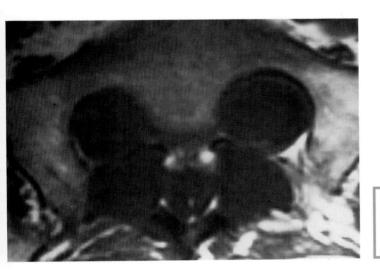

Fig. 5.26 PERINEURAL (TARLOV'S) CYSTS T1-weighted axial image. The dark, round, CSF-filled cysts expand the nerve root foramina of the sacrum bilaterally.

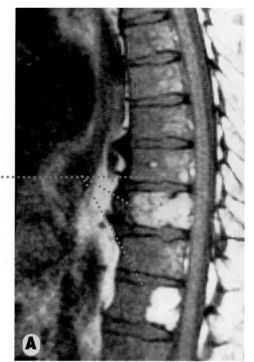

Multiple hemangiomas · · · ⋯⋯

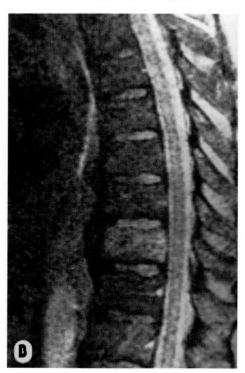

The MRI appearance of vertebral hemangiomas is variable. Virtually all hemangiomas are hyperintense on T1-weighted images but of variable intensity on T2-weighted images (Fig. 5.27). Histological study supports the theory that the presence of abundant adipose tissue causes the increased signal intensity on T1-weighted images. This has been further supported by chemical shift images, as well as by the demonstration that the extraosseous component of the hemangiomas tends not to be hyperintense on T1-weighted images, as fat is not present on histological examination of the extraosseous portion of the tumor. Hemangiomas have variable signal intensity on T2-weighted images, but generally tend to be hyperintense. The reason for this appearance is uncertain.

FOCAL FAT DEPOSITION   Focal areas of high signal intensity on T1-weighted images of the spine are seen in over one half of patients examined. These areas are due to localized fat deposition in hematopoietic bone marrow. Their signal intensity decreases with increasing T2-weighting. The focal fat depositions are typically 0.5 to 1.5 cm in diameter and may involve any region of the spine (Fig. 5.28). Their frequency increases with advancing age (from being comparatively rare in the pediatric age group to an over 90% representation in patients older than 60 years of age).

LIPOMA   Lipomas may occur as localized tumor masses in the epidural space. They occur most frequently in the upper thoracic and cervical regions. They are well-defined and uniformly hyperintense on T1-weighted images. Extradural lipomas are less common than those in the intradural space.

LIPOMATOSIS   Epidural lipomatosis is a condition of fatty proliferation in the epidural space, usually in the thoracic spine. It can cause spinal cord compression. It occurs almost exclusively with exogenous steroid use, although it has been described in hypothyroidism and obesity. The lipomatous tissue has typical MRI characteristics of being hyperintense on T1-weighted images and has decreasing signal intensity on T2-weighted sequences (Fig. 5.29).

Fig. 5.27 VERTEBRAL HEMANGIOMAS **(A)** T1-weighted sagittal image. Multiple vertebral bodies are affected. The hemangiomas are hyperintense, and the cortical bone of the vertebral bodies is preserved. **(B)** T2-weighted sagittal image. The hemangiomas remain hyperintense. This pattern is typical of most vertebral hemangiomas.

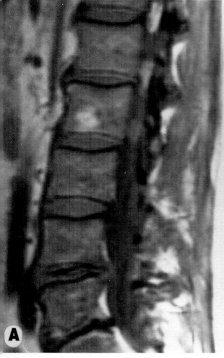

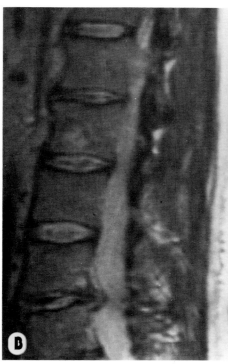

Fig. 5.28 FOCAL FAT DEPOSITION **(A)** T1-weighted sagittal image. A well-defined, high-intensity nodule of fat is present in the L2 vertebra. **(B)** T2-weighted sagittal image. The nodule of focal fat deposition is relatively hypointense with increased T2-weighting. In this T2-weighted image, it is only faintly visible.

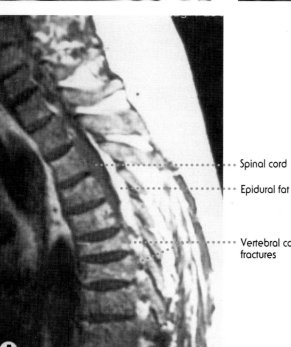

Spinal cord

Epidural fat

Vertebral compression fractures

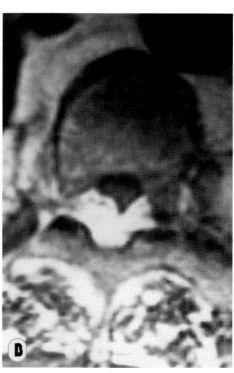

Fig. 5.29 EPIDURAL LIPOMATOSIS **(A)** T1-weighted sagittal image. High signal intensity fat in the posterior epidural space displaces the spinal cord. Note the vertebral compres-sion fractures secondary to steroid-induced osteoporosis. **(B)** T1-weighted axial image. Fat fills the posterior epidural space, displacing and compressing the spinal cord.

LYMPHOMA   Lymphomas have a predilection for the midthoracic spine. An epidural mass related to direct extension from the paraspinal space without bone destruction favors the diagnosis. The prognosis of the patient with paraplegia secondary to a lymphomatous epidural mass, either of the Hodgkin's or non-Hodgkin's type, is far brighter than for the prognosis of one with a metastatic carcinoma. T1-weighted images typically demonstrate a paravertebral lesion isointense to muscle with direct epidural extension. The lack of vertebral body destruction is a characteristic, but not a constant, feature. In fact, due to the high sensitivity of MRI to marrow disease, intraosseous extension is seen more often with MRI than with other modalities (Fig. 5.30). T2-weighted images can be used to confirm the epidural extension, the lymphoma being hyperintense.

METASTATIC CARCINOMA   Most metastases are marrow-replacing and appear on T1-weighted images as hypointense regions within the normal hyperintense marrow (Fig. 5.31). Diffuse metastases cause uniform decrease in signal intensity on T1-weighted images. Metastases from prostatic carcinoma cause reduction in vertebral signal intensity on both T1- and T2-weighted images due to their sclerotic nature (Fig. 5.32).

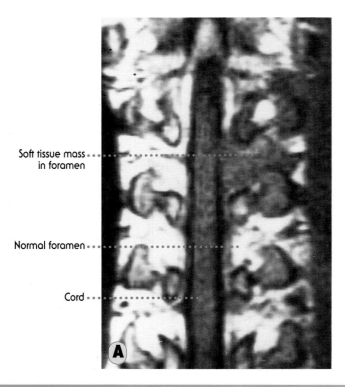

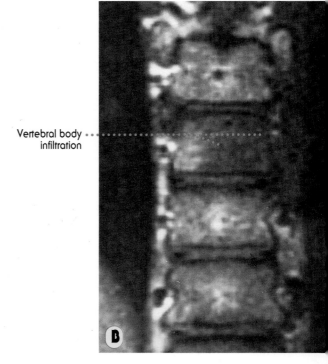

Fig. 5.30 LYMPHOMA   (A) and **(B)** T1-weighted coronal images. This young man's thoracic radiculopathy had been attributed to herpetic neuralgia for several months. X-ray films and bone scan were normal. MRI shows a distinct soft tissue mass in one neural foramen on the left with infiltration of the vertebral body.

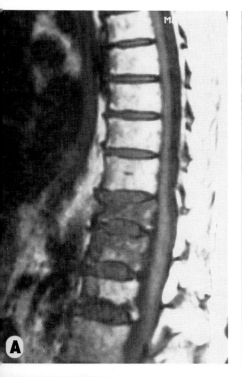

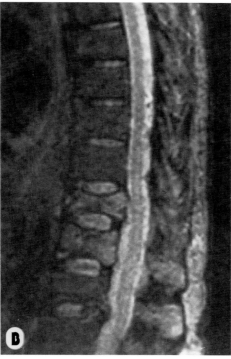

Fig. 5.31 METASTATIC BREAST CARCINOMA **(A)** T1-weighted sagittal image. There are compression fractures of T11, T12, and L1. Low signal intensity metastases replace the entire normal marrow space at T11 and T12, and the anterior one third of L1. **(B)** T2-weighted sagittal image. The metastases are now relatively hyperintense to the normal vertebrae. This pattern of hypointensity and hyperintensity on T1- and T2-weighted images is the most common observed for both metastases and myeloma.

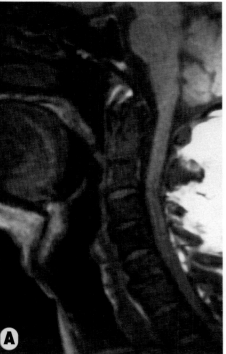

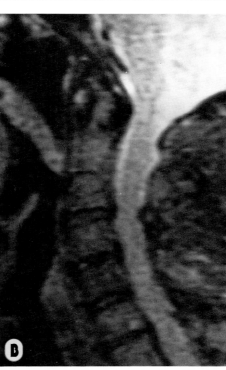

Fig. 5.32 PROSTATIC METASTASES **(A)** T1-weighted sagittal image. Diffuse, sclerotic, prostatic metastases cause a uniform decrease in the vertebra's signal intensity on the T1-weighted image. **(B)** T2-weighted sagittal image. The sclerotic bone metastases are hypointense on the T2-weighted images as well. Hypointensity on T2-weighted images is usually found only in those metastatic tumors that are sclerotic.

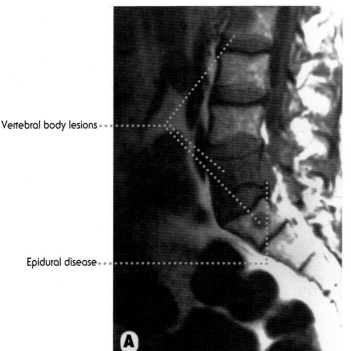

Vertebral body lesions

Epidural disease

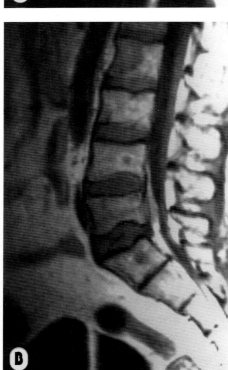

Epidural extension from vertebral metastases causes spinal cord compression and paralysis. In the majority of patients, local bone pain precedes the onset of neurological symptoms. Lung and breast carcinoma are the most common primary sites. Myelographic examination followed by CT has been the gold standard for the diagnosis of epidural metastases with spinal cord compression. Magnetic resonance imaging has been shown to be equally as effective in diagnosing the level of obstruction and more beneficial in demonstrating additional lesions, particularly those above the level of the myelographic block.

Paramagnetic contrast agents are useful in detecting or highlighting otherwise radiologically occult or subtle epidural tumors. However the enhancement of osseous metastases is an undesirable effect, as an otherwise obvious hypointense lesion may become isointense to normal bone marrow. Therefore, in metastatic work-ups both noncontrast and contrast-enhanced MRI should be performed (Fig. 5.33).

MULTIPLE MYELOMA   Due to the relative abundance of marrow in the vertebra, involvement of the spine with myeloma is common. Myelomatous deposits are marrow-replacing and, therefore, of decreased signal intensity relative to adjacent marrow on T1-weighted images. Magnetic resonance imaging has proven to be superior to plain radiography, bone scanning, and CT in the diagnosis of myeloma. Bone scans frequently produce false negatives, due to the lack of osteoblastic reaction to the myelomatous deposits. The lesions are well-demonstrated, if focal (Fig. 5.34). In elderly patients, it is difficult to distinguish diffuse myeloma in a background of normal fatty marrow from normal marrow undergoing focal fatty replacement. Solitary myelomatous lesions are indistinguishable from a metastasis.

CHORDOMA   A chordoma is a neoplasm of notochordal remnants and is, therefore, restricted to the cranial-spinal axis. Forty percent of all chordomas occur in the clivus and the majority of the remainder in the sacrum. They are locally invasive and may metastasize. Peak age incidence is in the fourth to sixth decade. On CT images, they are lytic masses, half of which contain some calcification.

Chordomas are usually either mildly hypointense or isointense on T1-weighted MR images. Essentially, all chordomas demonstrate moderately to extremely high signal intensity on T2-weighted images. The tumors are often lobulated, with septa of decreased intensity between nodules of high signal intensity on the T2-weighted images (Fig. 5.35). Histologically, chordomas have been divided into typical and chondroid types due to predominance of cartilaginous matrix in the latter. The cartilaginous component is less intense on T2-weighted images than the gelatinous tissue of the typical chordoma. In terms of prognosis, those with chondroid chordomas have a life expectancy exceeding 15 years, as opposed to 4 years for those with typical chordomas.

Fig. 5.33 METASTATIC COLON CARCINOMA   (A) T1-weighted sagittal image. Multiple lesions involve the bodies of L2 and L5 and the epidural space adjacent to L5. **(B)** Post-gadolinium-DTPA. All the metastases enhance. The epidural tumor becomes more evident but the bone lesions become isointense to normal marrow and, thus, less evident. The masking of bone metastases is a known pitfall in the use of gadolinium-DTPA. (Courtesy of Dr. G. Sze, Department of Radiology, Yale University, New Haven, CT)

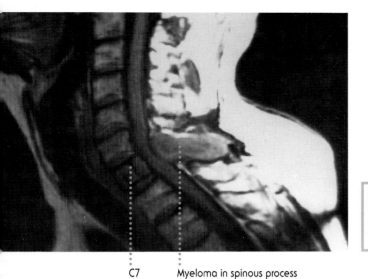

C7   Myeloma in spinous process

Fig. 5.34 MULTIPLE MYELOMA   T1-weighted sagittal image. The C7 vertebral body and spinous process are diffusely involved. The spinal cord is compressed. These features are identical to those of metastases.

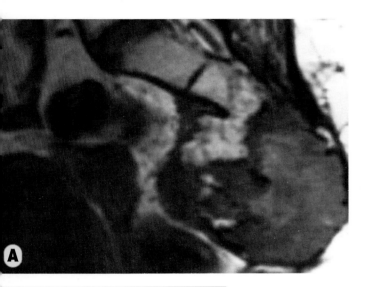

A

→ arrows point to tumor

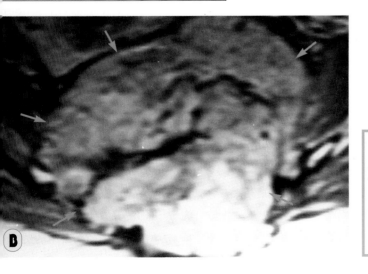

B

Fig. 5.35 CHORDOMA   **(A)** T1-weighted sagittal image. There is a large lobulated tumor, originating from the lower sacrum and extending into the pelvis. This is a common location and the typical appearance of a chordoma. **(B)** T2-weighted axial image. This tumor displays several features of chordomas: lobulation, heteregeneous signal, and areas of marked hyperintensity.

INTRADURAL TUMORS

MENINGIOMA Twenty to 35% of all primary spinal canal tumors are meningiomas. Most occur in the sixth decade, with a female predominance of ten to one. The thoracic spine is the most common site. Most are nodular (Fig. 5.36) but the "en-plaque" configuration is not infrequent. Psammomatous calcification is common but difficult to appreciate on MR images. Meningiomas can be difficult tumors to detect with noncontrast MRI, particularly if they are small and/or the en-plaque type (Fig. 5.37). As in the brain, they enhance intensely with paramagnetic contrast agents.

NERVE SHEATH TUMOR Nerve sheath tumors have an incidence approximately equal to that of meningiomas. There are basically two histologic varieties—schwannomas and neurofibromas. Unlike meningiomas, there is no female predominance and no predilection to the thoracic region. The peak age of incidence is the fourth or fifth decade. These tumors develop on the sensory nerve roots.

Neurofibromas are far less common than schwannomas and usually are associated with neurofibromatosis. Axons penetrate the body of a neurofibroma, in contrast to the eccentric relationship of tumor to axons in a schwannoma.

Nerve sheath tumors are isointense or mildly hyperintense on T1-weighted images and markedly hyperintense on T2-weighted images (relative to neural tissue). Many have central areas of decreased signal intensity on T2-weighted images. Extension through the neural foramen is a characteristic finding (Fig. 5.38). The relationship to the spinal cord, the nerve root, the neural foramen, and the extradural space is best defined on the T1-weighted coronal or axial images.

LIPOMA Isolated intradural lipomas are most frequent in the cervical spine (Fig. 5.39) and filum terminale (Fig. 5.40); however, the most frequent lipomas are those associated with meningoceles occurring at the lumbosacral level. The tumor is characterized by hyperintense signal on T1-weighted images.

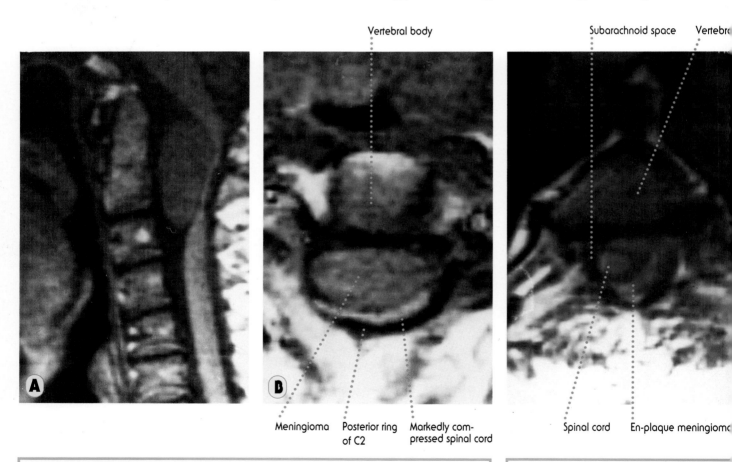

Vertebral body

Subarachnoid space   Vertebra

Meningioma   Posterior ring   Markedly com-
of C2   pressed spinal cord

Spinal cord   En-plaque meningioma

Fig. 5.36 MENINGIOMA **(A)** T1-weighted sagittal image. A large extra-axial tumor is present in the spinal canal at C2. The spinal cord is compressed posteriorly and deviates over the large tumor. **(B)** T1-weighted axial image. The cord is compressed into a ribbon of tissue behind the large tumor.

Fig. 5.37 EN-PLAQUE MENINGIOMA T1-weighted axial image. The en-plaque meningioma coats the left lateral aspect of the thecal sac. It is isointense with the spinal cord, which is displaced to the right.

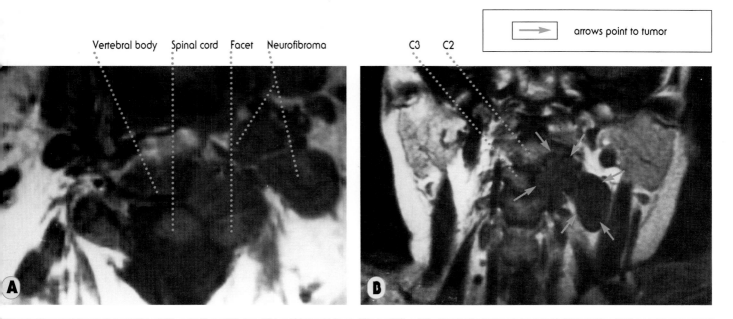

Vertebral body   Spinal cord   Facet   Neurofibroma

C3   C2

arrows point to tumor

A

B

Fig. 5.38 NEUROFIBROMA   (A) T1-weighted axial image. A large lobulated neurofibroma enlarges the left C3 foramen. It has both intradural and paravertebral extension. **(B)** T1-weighted coronal image. This tumor has the typical "dumbbell" configuration. There is erosion of the adjacent C2 and C3 vertebrae.

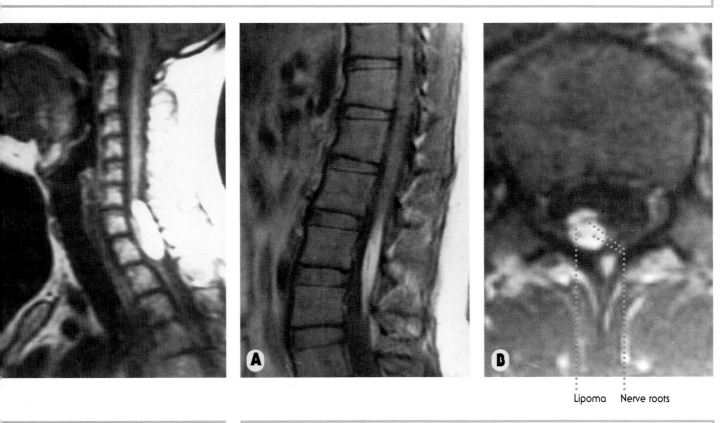

A

B

Lipoma   Nerve roots

Fig. 5.39 INTRADURAL LIPOMA
T1-weighted sagittal image. The high signal intensity on T1-weighted images of the mass at C7-T1 is characteristic of a lipoma.

Fig. 5.40 FILUM LIPOMA   (A) T1-weighted sagittal image. A hyperintense oblong lesion envelops the filum terminale and cauda equina. The signal is typical of fat. **(B)** T1-weighted axial image. The lesion is predominantly right-sided. It is inseparable from the nerve roots of the cauda.

Iodinated organic compounds previously used for myelography may simulate a lipoma. They are slowly absorbed from the subarachnoid space and are frequently seen, in the years following myelography, as a collection in the caudal sac or as small droplets in the spinal canal. These compounds are oil-based and appear similar to fat on MR images. They are hyperintense on T1-weighted images and of decreased signal intensity on T2-weighted images. If present in the caudal sac, they may appear as a lipomatous mass and simulate a fibrolipoma of the filum terminale (Fig. 5.41). Plain radiography readily confirms the presence of the high density contrast agent in the spinal canal.

METASTASES   Intradural metastases are uncommon, compared with bony and epidural metastases. Carcinoma of the lung, breast, and melanoma are the most common primaries. "Drop" metastases from intracranial primaries, particularly medulloblastoma, ependymoma, and pineal germinomas, are a result of dissemination of tumor cells through the subarach-

noid space (Fig. 5.42). Multiple nodules of varying sizes are found on the nerve roots or surface of the cord. These nodules are an intermediate gray on T1-weighted images or are seen as dark nodules within white surrounding CSF on T2-weighted images (Fig. 5.43). As with other spinal tumors, contrast agents markedly improve visualization of the nodules (Fig. 5.44). Diagnosis can be confirmed by CSF cytology.

INTRAMEDULLARY TUMORS

ASTROCYTOMA   The incidence of spinal astrocytomas is about 3% of that of brain gliomas, which is a close approximation of the ratio of spinal cord weight to brain weight. Peak incidence is in the third to fifth decade. Any segment of the spinal cord may be affected. These tumors rarely occur in the filum terminale. They tend to be infiltrating, low-grade astrocytomas, diffusely enlarging the spinal cord without a localized mass (Fig. 5.45). Central necrosis may occur, accompanied possibly by an adjacent cyst. These cysts are secondary phenomena and do not contain tumor.   Cystic and solid portions of a

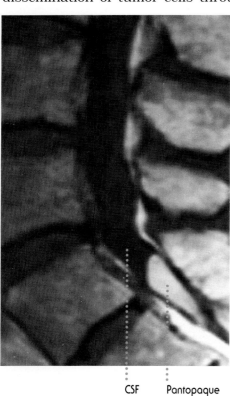

CSF   Pantopaque

Fig. 5.41 PANTOPAQUE T1-weighted sagittal image. The oil-based contrast is hyperintense on this T1-weighted image. As the patient was scanned in the supine position, a fluid-fluid level is present.

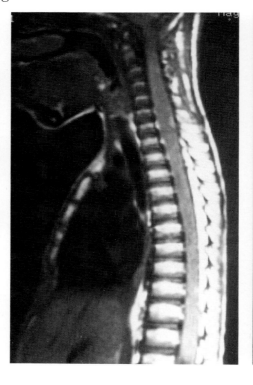

Fig. 5.42 MEDULLOBLASTOMA METASTASES T1-weighted sagittal image. Subarachnoid metastases from a cerebellar medulloblastoma coat the entire spinal cord and diffusely enlarge it.

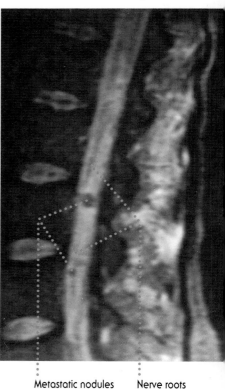

Metastatic nodules   Nerve roots

Fig. 5.43 SUBARACHNOID METASTASES FROM LUNG CARCINOMA T2-weighted sagittal image. Low intensity metastatic nodules are attached to the caudal nerve roots.

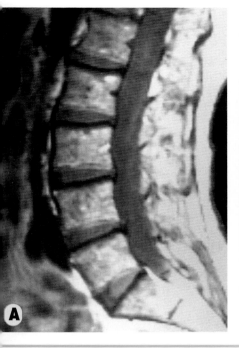

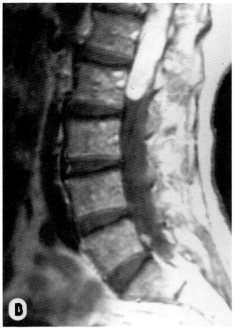

Fig. 5.44 CONUS EPENDYMOMA WITH DROP METASTASES (A) T1-weighted sagittal image. No definite abnormality is seen. **(B)** Post-gadolinium-DTPA. Two lesions enhance intensely: a large oblong ependymoma in the upper lumbar spinal canal and a small lesion behind L5. (Courtesy of Dr. G. Sze, Department of Radiology, Yale University, New Haven, CT)

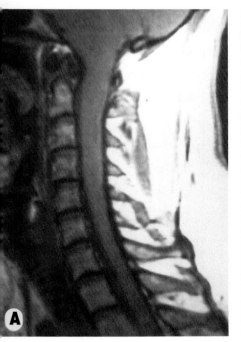

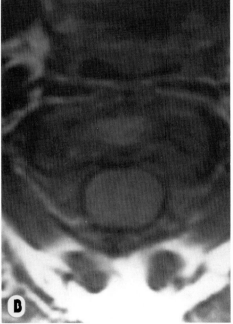

Fig. 5.45 CERVICAL ASTROCYTOMA (A) T1-weighted sagittal image. The entire medulla and the upper cervical cord from the foramen magnum to C4 are diffusely enlarged, with obliteration of the inferior fourth ventricle and subarachnoid space. **(B)** T1-weighted axial image. The spinal canal is filled with the enlarged spinal cord. The tumor is inseparable from the normal spinal cord.

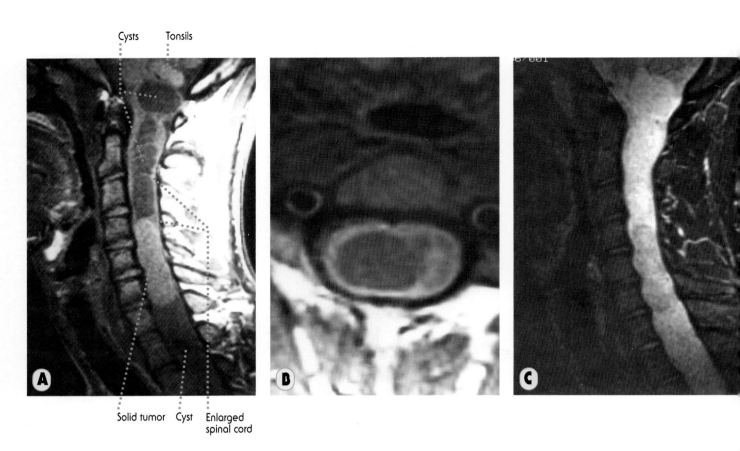

Cysts   Tonsils

Solid tumor   Cyst   Enlarged spinal cord

Fig. 5.46 CERVICAL ASTROCYTOMA **(A)** T1-weighted sagittal image. A mixed solid and cystic tumor enlarges the spinal cord. The tonsils are elevated and posteriorly displaced. **(B)** T1-weighted axial image. The solid and cystic components of the astrocytoma expand the cervi-cal cord, filling the spinal canal. **(C)** T2-weighted sagittal image. With this technique, the cystic components are isointense relative to CSF. The solid component is clearly defined as an ovoid hypointense nodule (compare with the T1-weighted image).

Cyst   Astrocytoma   Cyst

Fig. 5.47 GRADE II SPINAL CORD ASTROCYTOMA **(A)** T1-weighted sagittal image. The cervical spinal cord is enlarged without distinct evidence of a tumor mass. **(B)** Post-gadolinium-DTPA. The astrocytoma enhances intensely, facilitating accurate surgical planning. Small cysts are present in the cord below and above the tumor. (Courtesy of Dr. G. Sze, Department of Radiology, Yale University, New Haven, CT)

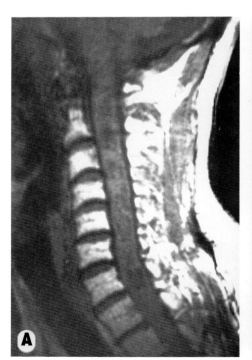

neoplastic lesion are best separated on T1-weighted images, the cyst being darker (Fig. 5.46). Contrast administration may enhance the solid portion as an additional diagnostic feature (Fig. 5.47).

EPENDYMOMA   Ependymomas develop from the ependymal lining cells of the central canal and filum terminale. They represent over one half of all primary spinal cord tumors. The majority occur in the region of the filum terminale. Peak incidence is in the fourth to fifth decade. The tumors themselves are rarely cystic but are frequently associated with an adjacent syrinx. Their imaging characteristics are identical to astrocytomas (Fig. 5.48).

HEMANGIOBLASTOMA   Spinal hemangioblastomas are benign tumors, closely associated with the cerebellar hemangioblastoma, in terms of when peak incidence occurs (third to fifth decade), multiplicity, and the connection with von Hippel–Lindau syndrome. These highly vascular tumors often show arterial-venous shunting and enlarged veins on angiography. Associated cysts are common. Their appearance can be very characteristic: a vascular nodule in the cord, an adjacent syrinx, and large vessels alongside the cord leading to the tumor (Fig. 5.49). Not all three findings are always present. The nodule enhances intensely with contrast administration (Fig. 5.50).

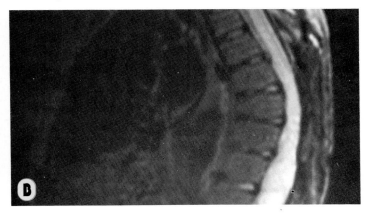

Fig. 5.48 EPENDYMOMA   (A) T1-weighted sagittal image. A partially cystic ependymoma expands the lower thoracic spinal cord from the apex of the thoracic kyphus to the conus. **(B)** T2-weighted sagittal image. The upper border of the hyperintense tumor at the apex of the kyphus is relatively well-delineated from the normal spinal cord above.

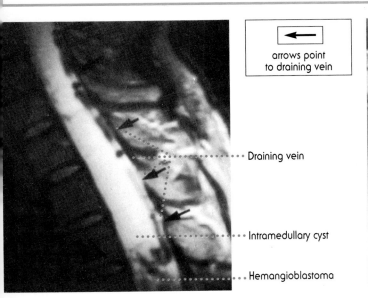

arrows point to draining vein

- Draining vein
- Intramedullary cyst
- Hemangioblastoma

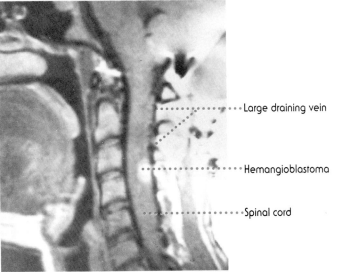

- Large draining vein
- Hemangioblastoma
- Spinal cord

Fig. 5.49 HEMANGIOBLASTOMA   T2-weighted sagittal image. This highly vascular tumor is visible as an irregular low-intensity nodule in the cord. The irregular structures are the large vessels. The draining vein, also enlarged, is on the dorsal aspect of the spinal canal. The high intensity in the cord cephalad to the tumor nodule is a cyst, a common associated finding.

Fig. 5.50 HEMANGIOBLASTOMA   T1-weighted sagittal image (contrast enhanced). This woman had von Hippel–Lindau disease. The noncontrast scan showed only subtle cord widening (not shown). This contrast-enhanced scan demonstrates intense enhancement of a focal nodule—a prominent feature of hemangioblastomas—and a draining vein dorsal to the spinal cord.

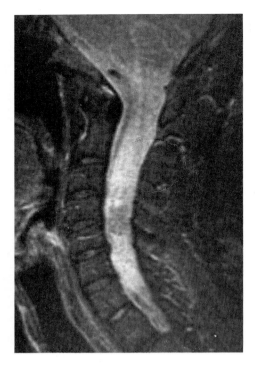

Fig. 5.51 INTRAMEDULLARY METASTASIS T2-weighted sagittal image. A round, hypointense metastatic nodule is present in the cervical spinal cord at the C4-C5 disc space level. The surrounding edema in the spinal cord is hyperintense and extends above and below the metastasis.

INTRAMEDULLARY METASTASES Intramedullary metastases occur rarely. Lung and breast carcinoma are the most common primary sources outside the CNS. An area of spinal cord enlargement due to mass effect and adjacent edema is visible (Fig. 5.51). Enhancement with paramagnetic contrast agents best demonstrates metastatic nodules.

VASCULAR MALFORMATION

There are basically two types of spinal vascular malformations seen in clinical practice—cavernous hemangiomas and arteriovenous malformations. Two other types found in the brain, the capillary telangiectasia and the venous angioma, are not clinically encountered in the spine.

CAVERNOUS HEMANGIOMA

Cavernous hemangiomas are discrete lesions of thin walled vessels. The intervening cells are gliotic and stained with hemosiderin. They are frequently calcified and may be ossified. They lack arterial-venous shunting and enlarged arteries or veins. The hemosiderin staining results from diffusion of hemoglobin breakdown products from the intermittently thrombosed vascular spaces into the adjacent parenchyma. The MRI characteristic of cavernous hemangiomas is typically that of a high intensity center, with a markedly hypointense periphery, the latter being particularly prominent on the T2-weighted images. This is related to the presence of methe-

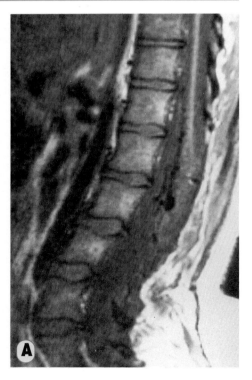

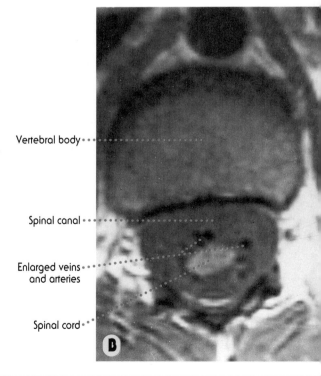

Vertebral body

Spinal canal

Enlarged veins and arteries

Spinal cord

Fig. 5.52 RECURRENT ARTERIOVENOUS MALFORMATION **(A)** T1-weighted sagittal image. There has been a previous laminectomy. The conus medullaris is surrounded by enlarged veins and arteries that display the typical signal void of high flow vesses. **(B)** T1-weighted axial image. The enlarged veins and arteries encircle the spinal cord.

moglobin in the center, and hemosiderin along the peripheral aspects of the lesion. Hemosiderin is hypointense on T1-weighted images and markedly hypointense on T2-weighted images. Reports of cavernous hemangiomas of the spinal cord, though distinctly uncommon, demonstrate an appearance identical to those described in the brain.

ARTERIOVENOUS MALFORMATION

True arteriovenous malformations represent a focal absence of a capillary bed, resulting in arterial-venous shunting and arterialization of draining veins. They may occur either in the spinal cord (intramedullary) or the dura (radiculomeningeal). The classic appearance is of a cluster of blood vessels on the dorsal aspect of the thoracic cord. The clinical presentation is that of sudden paresis following hemorrhage into the spinal cord, or slowly progressive symptoms related to venous hypertension or focal ischemia induced by the lesion.

The elongated, serpentine blood vessels on the dorsal surface of the spinal cord are equally well-seen on T1- or T2-weighted sagittal images (Fig. 5.52). Gradient recalled echo images demonstrate the blood vessels extremely well, due to their depiction of flow-related signal enhancement.

The abnormal circulatory dynamics generated by arteriovenous malformations cause secondary effects in the spinal cord. Myelomalacia is considered to be related to the increased venous pressure of the arterialized veins and appears as intramedullary edema on MR images. The edematous central portion of the cord is of low signal intensity on T1-weighted images and hyperintense on T2-weighted images.

INFLAMMATORY CONDITIONS

RHEUMATOID ARTHRITIS

Involvement of the craniocervical junction with rheumatoid arthritis results in a variety of neurological impairments. Instability of the atlantoaxial joint, which is due to transverse ligament disruption and odontoid erosion, leads to narrowing of the spinal canal and results in cord compression. These changes are most marked with respect to neck flexion. Associated erosive changes in the atlantooccipital and lateral atlantoaxial facet joints result in extension of the odontoid process above the foramen magnum, which may, in turn, compress the cervicomedullary junction.

T1-weighted sagittal images best show the relationship of the spinal cord to the adjacent bone (Fig. 5.53). Instability can be demonstrated on flexion and extension views. Morphological distortion of the spinal cord and medulla is well-seen.

Pannus, abnormal synovial proliferation, and inflammation are the pathognomonic features of rheumatoid arthritis. Pannus destroys the adjacent articulating cartilage and fills the joint space. Although the bony cortex is not optimally evaluated by MRI, the soft tissue abnormality of pannus forma-

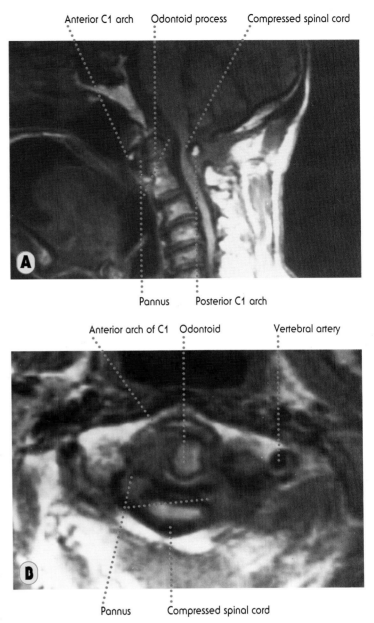

Fig. 5.53 RHEUMATOID ARTHRITIS WITH ATLANTOAXIAL SUBLUXATION **(A)** T1-weighted sagittal image. The spinal cord is compressed by the odontoid and adjacent pannus. The distance between the anterior arch of C1 and the odontoid is increased, indicating atlantoaxial subluxation. **(B)** T1-weighted axial image. The spinal cord is flattened posteriorly by the odontoid and pannus.

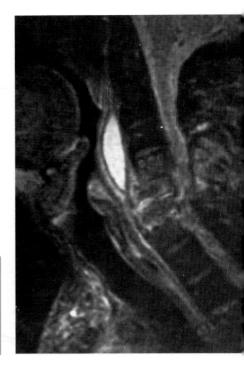

Fig. 5.54 RETROPHARYNGEAL ABSCESS, DISCITIS, AND OSTEOMYELITIS T2-weighted sagittal image. A hyperintense abscess cavity is present in the prevertebral space. The C5-C7 vertebrae are of increased signal intensity due to osteomyelitis. The C5-C6 and C6-C7 discs are irregular and hyperintense.

Roots of cauda equina   Clumped nerve roots

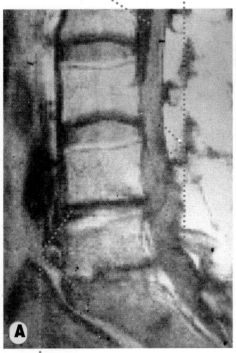
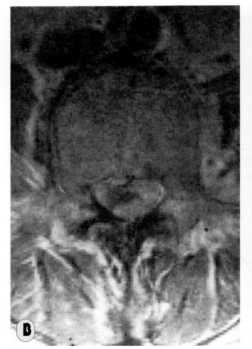
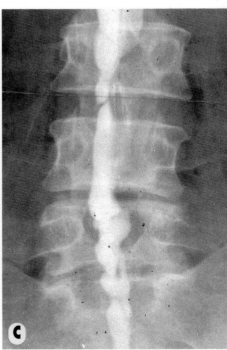

Previous L4-L5 L5-S1 discectomies

Fig. 5.55 ARACHNOIDITIS **(A)** T1-weighted sagittal image. The discs at L4-L5 and L5-S1 are reduced in height and intensity due to previous discectomies. The spinal canal between L3 and S1 is filled with an amorphous mass of clumped nerve roots rather than the distinct linear structures that nerve roots should be. **(B)** T2-weighted axial image. The roots are inseparable from one another and are adherent to the dural sac. **(C)** Myelogram. This study confirms the MRI findings of severe nerve root matting; in addition, it demonstrates obliteration of normal nerve root sleeves and a featureless outline to the thecal sac. This is a severe case of arachnoiditis. (Courtesy of Dr. S. Rosenbloom, Cleveland Clinic, Cleveland, OH)

tion in the relationship of the spinal cord to the bony structures is well-demonstrated. Pannus is demonstrated as a soft tissue mass of intermediate intensity frequently filling the preodontoid space (Fig. 5.53). A fibrofatty proliferation above the level of the preodontoid pannus has been described in a high percentage of patients.

OSTEOMYELITIS AND DISCITIS
Hematogenous spread to the intervertebral disc results in infective discitis and adjacent osteomyelitis. The intervertebral disc represents the largest area of essentially avascular tissue in the body. This predisposes the disc and end-plate to infection. The most frequent organism is *Staphylococcus*. Destruction of the end-plates and the adjacent vertebral body is best demonstrated on plain radiographs. Sagittal and axial MR images best show changes in the disc. There is increased signal on T2-weighted images due to the inflammation and edema in the disc and adjacent marrow. The disc is irregular and diffusely hyperintense (Fig. 5.54).

ARACHNOIDITIS
Spinal arachnoiditis is an inflammatory condition of the spinal subarachnoid space. A fibrin exudate coats the nerve roots and thecal sac. Fibrocyte proliferation and collagenous matrix adhere the nerve root and arachnoid to one another. It is most frequently seen following lumbar spine surgery. Patients present with continuing or recurrent back pain.

Three patterns of arachnoid adhesions occur in the lumbar spine: (a) the nerve roots may stick to form a thickened, cord-like structure; (b) they may adhere to the arachnoid posteriorly; or (c) if the proliferation is extensive, a solid mass of nerve roots and fibrous tissue may be formed, thereby filling the thecal sac.

Magnetic resonance imaging demonstrates the change of severe arachnoiditis well, but it may be difficult to assess small, localized nerve root changes. Axial T1- or T2-weighted images can demonstrate the spatial relationship of the lumbar nerve roots. The normal nerve roots are seen evenly distributed in a butterfly pattern posteriorly in the subarachnoid space. In arachnoiditis, the roots are irregularly clumped together posteriorly in a cord-like shadow or in a solid, intermediate intensity, fibrous mass at the base of the thecal sac (Fig. 5.55).

RADIATION

Diffuse increased signal intensity of the vertebrae on T1-weighted images occurs following radiotherapy related to replacement of normal hematopoietic marrow with fatty or yellow marrow (Fig. 5.56). The etiology is presumably associated with radiation-induced vasculopathy and reduced blood supply to the marrow. Similar changes occur in aplastic anemia and prolonged inactivity or bed rest. Aplastic anemia in remission may demonstrate islands of normal hematopoietic marrow in a background of high intensity fatty marrow.

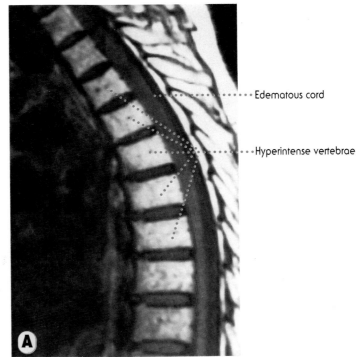

Edematous cord

Hyperintense vertebrae

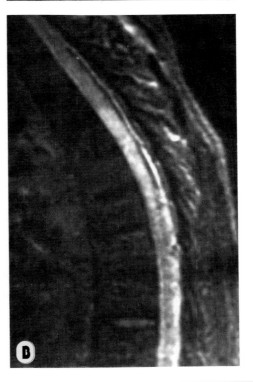

Fig. 5.56 RADIATION-INDUCED VERTEBRAL BODY CHANGES AND MYELITIS (A) T1-weighted sagittal image. The midthoracic vertebrae demonstrate increased signal intensity due to fatty replacement of marrow secondary to radiation. The spinal cord is enlarged in its upper and midthoracic portions. **(B)** T2-weighted sagittal image. Radiation myelitis causes increased intensity in the midthoracic spinal cord.

The abnormalities seen in the spinal cord following radiotherapy are also secondary to a vasculopathy. Radiation causes thickening and hyalinization of the arterial wall. Secondary demyelination occurs in areas adjacent to the vascular changes. Diffuse interstitial edema and subsequent necrosis occurs. As with other forms of myelitis, the cord swells acutely and is hyperintense on T2-weighted images (Fig. 5.56). It may be difficult to distinguish the result from intramedullary tumor. Later, atrophy supervenes.

DEMYELINATION

Any part of the neural axis may be involved with multiple sclerosis. The spinal cord is a frequently affected site. Plaques of demyelination occur most often in the periventricular white matter and in the subpial regions of the brain stem and spinal cord. Multiple sclerosis plaques are zones of selective demyelination with axonal sparing. There is subsequent gliosis. The patient with spinal cord multiple sclerosis presents with a vari-

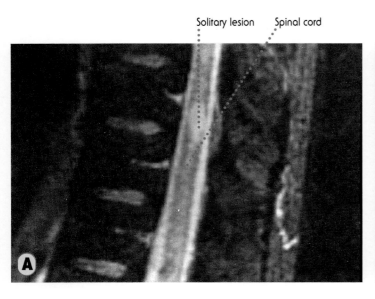

Solitary lesion   Spinal cord

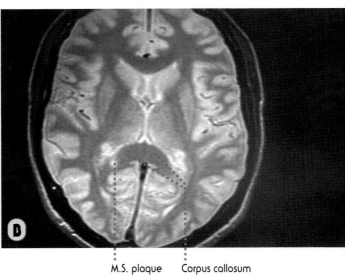

M.S. plaque   Corpus callosum

Fig. 5.57 MULTIPLE SCLEROSIS (A) T2-weighted sagittal image. There is a small solitary lesion in the thoracic spinal cord without mass effect. **(B)** T2-weighted axial image. Because of a strong clinical suspicion of multiple sclerosis (hyperreflexia, positive oligoclonal bands), a supplementary MRI of the brain was performed. This shows a second lesion in the splenium, further supporting the diagnosis of multiple sclerosis.

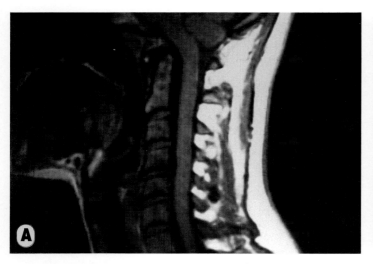

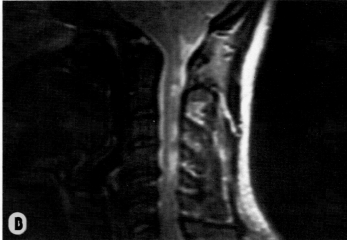

Fig. 5.58 MULTIPLE SCLEROSIS (A) T1-weighted sagittal image. The cervical spinal cord is mildly enlarged without a focal mass. **(B)** T2-weighted sagittal image. There are several high-intensity plaques in the cervical spinal cord. T2-weighted images are essential to demonstrate such small, intrinsic lesions of the spinal cord.

ety of symptoms most frequently related to spasticity due to demyelination of the cortical-spinal tract.

The edema associated with areas of demyelination is best visualized on T2-weighted images. The appearance is of a hyperintense region with or without cord expansion. If only a solitary lesion is seen, the appearance is relatively nonspecific and a T2-weighted examination of the head should be performed to search for other evidence of the disease (Fig. 5.57). Frequently these patients have asymptomatic intracranial lesions. Multiple, geographically separated lesions in the spinal cord should be considered diagnostic of multiple sclerosis until proven otherwise (Fig. 5.58).

OTHER MYELOPATHIES

An acute, disseminated encephalomyelopathy may occur after exanthomatous viral disease of childhood, upper respiratory tract infections, or vaccinations. Spinal cord involvement may be diffuse or localized. Sagittal T1-weighted images demonstrate the cord enlargement that may in time resolve (Fig. 5.59). T2-weighted images may show a more localized area of cord edema (transverse myelitis).

Vacuolar degeneration of the spinal cord has been described in many patients with acquired immunodeficiency syndrome. Pathologically, the myelopathy

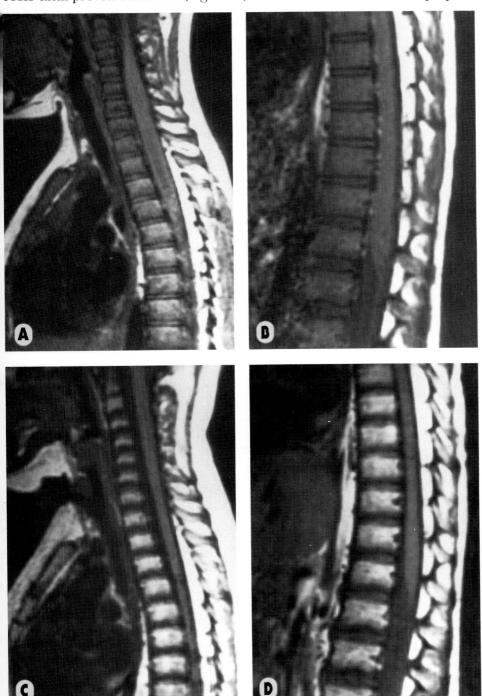

Fig. 5.59 IDIOPATHIC MYELITIS (A) and **(B)** T1-weighted sagittal images. The entire spinal cord is diffusely enlarged. The central portion of the spinal cord is hypointense, presumably due to edema. **(C)** and **(D)** T1-weighted sagittal images. Follow-up examination after four months demonstrates that the spinal cord has returned to a normal size.

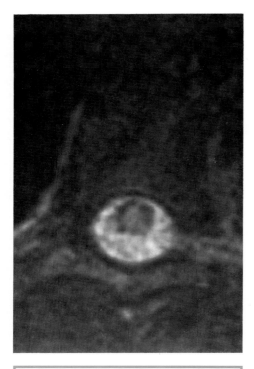

Fig. 5.60 VACUOLAR DEGENERA-TION OF AIDS T2-weighted axial image. The high intensity of the spinal cord edema is demonstrated centrally in the spinal cord.

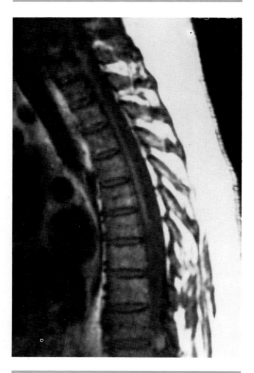

Fig. 5.61 THORACIC SPINAL CORD ATROPHY T1-weighted sagittal image. The thoracic spinal cord is diffusely atrophic. The cause could not be determined.

most resembles that of subacute combined degeneration of vitamin B_{12} deficiency. The degeneration primarily involves the lateral and posterior columns. Patients present with ataxia and paresis. T2-weighted images may show cord edema (Fig. 5.60).

SPINAL CORD ENLARGEMENT AND SPINAL CORD ATROPHY

Magnetic resonance examination, on occasion, demonstrates either a localized area of cord swelling or diffuse spinal cord enlargement. A specific etiology for the cord pathology may be difficult to determine. Spinal tumors—low grade gliomas, in particular—may enlarge the spinal cord without a recognizable mass. There may be no discernible border or edge to the tumor. It may diffusely involve the spinal cord or a more localized segment. Infarction, radiation myelitis, vasculopathy, infective and postinfective myelopathy, and demyelination may all have similar appearances. They all tend to be hypointense on T1-weighted images and hyperintense on T2-weighted images. The administration of a contrast agent may characterize the lesion by showing localized neoplasm enhancement.

Cord atrophy is a frequent secondary phenomena following demyelination, infarction, trauma, prolonged compression, and other insults. It represents the end stage of these varied disease processes. The atrophy is best assessed on a combination of sagittal and axial T1-weighted images (Fig. 5.61).

TRAUMA

Pathological changes in experimental spinal cord injury have shown that immediately following trauma, hemorrhage occurs in the subpial gray matter and spreads through the white matter within minutes. Capillary damage allows extravasation of blood. Within hours, there is diffuse axonal damage and extensive tissue necrosis. Although complex fractures of the vertebrae are best demonstrated with polytomography and/or CT, MRI demonstrates this spinal cord injury to best advantage.

Sagittal images are best for localizing the level of involvement and for displaying the abnormal anatomy (Fig. 5.62). An area of hypointensity on T1-weighted images and hyperintensity on T2-weighted images are characteristic of a spinal cord contusion (Fig. 5.63). Significant hemorrhage may appear as areas of hyperintensity on T1- and T2-weighted studies of patients in the subacute phase of the injury; but this finding is infrequent on MRI, even though it is consistently seen pathologically.

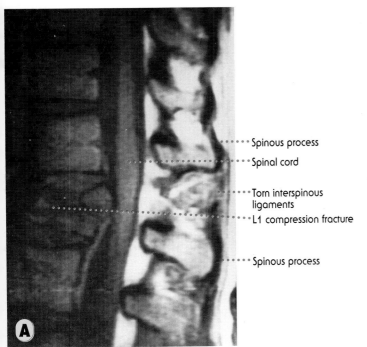

Spinous process

Spinal cord

Torn interspinous ligaments

L1 compression fracture

Spinous process

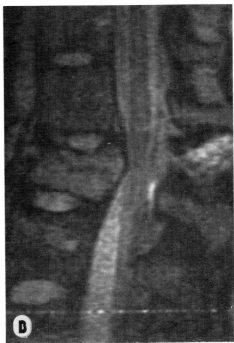

Fig. 5.62 LUMBAR COMPRESSION FRACTURE (A) T1-weighted sagittal image. The L1 vertebral body is compressed. The spinal cord is deviated posteriorly but does not appear compressed. **(B)** T2-weighted sagittal image. Subacute hemorrhage and edema into the torn interspinous ligaments are clearly visible. There is no evidence of a spinal cord contusion.

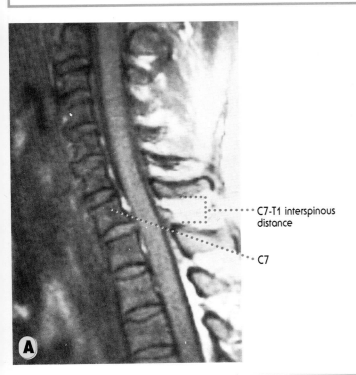

C7-T1 interspinous distance

C7

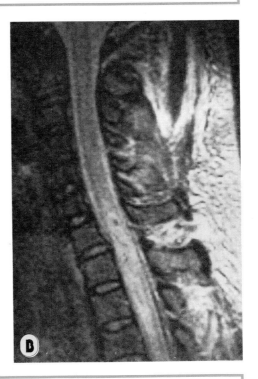

Fig. 5.63 CORD CONTUSION AND RUPTURE OF INTERSPINOUS LIGAMENT (A) T1-weighted sagittal image. This young woman suffered a hyperflexion injury. There is slight anterior subluxation of C7 on T1, minor prolapse of the disc at that level, and widening of the spinal cord from the top of C7 to T2. The C7-T1 interspinous distance is increased. **(B)** T2-weighted sagittal image. The contused cord is edematous, seen as the hyperintense lesion within the substance of the cord. Similarly, edema in the C7-T1 interspinous ligament is hyperintense.

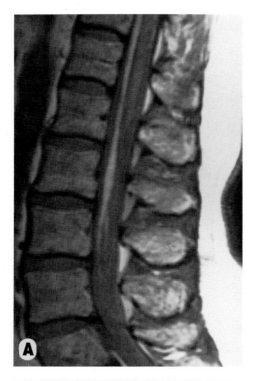

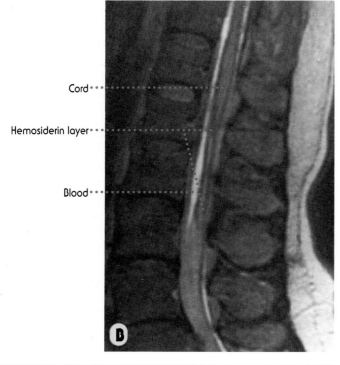

Cord ···

Hemosiderin layer ···

Blood ···

Fig. 5.64 SUBARACHNOID HEMORRHAGE **(A)** T1-weighted sagittal image. The hyperintense subarachnoid blood is anterior to the spinal cord. **(B)** T2-weighted sagittal image. The blood remains hyperintense on the T2-weighted image. Note that the epidural and subcutaneous fat are considerably less intense. There is a band of reduced signal on the surface of the cord and nerve roots due to the presence of hemosiderin.

HEMORRHAGE

Magnetic resonance imaging is excellent for the evaluation of subacute and chronic subarachnoid hemorrhage within the spinal canal. Acute subarachnoid hemorrhage is not frequently identified by MRI. Shortening of the T1-relaxation time, due to the formation of methemoglobin, allows for visualization of subarachnoid hemorrhage as high signal intensity on T1- and T2-weighted images (Fig. 5.64). Later hemosiderin staining of the surface of the spinal cord may be evidenced as a surface band of reduced signal on T2-weighted images.

DEGENERATIVE DISEASE

DISC DISEASE AND SPONDYLOSIS

Intervertebral discs form an amphiarthrotic joint that unites two adjacent vertebral bodies. They consist of two cartilaginous end-plates, the nucleus pulposus, and the anulus fibrosus. The cartilaginous end-plates are hyaline cartilage, which covers the central portion of the superior and inferior vertebral surfaces. The anulus fibrosus is a ring of cartilaginous fibers that surrounds the nucleus pulposus. It is attached superiorly and inferiorly to the vertebral body by Sharpey's fibers. The nucleus pulposus is comprised of a gelatinous matrix of collagen and proteoglycans. Increasingly fibrous components along its periphery blend the nucleus pulposus with the anulus. The vertebral end-plates and adjacent cortical bone have low signal intensity on both T1- and T2-weighted images. They frame the vertebral body with a fine line of low signal intensity. On T1-weighted images, the nucleus has slightly decreased signal intensity, as compared with the anulus. Sharpey's fibers are of very low signal intensity. On T1-weighted images, the inner anulus is of intermediate signal intensity, and the peripheral anulus fibrosus is of decreased intensity (Fig. 5.65).

Progressive chemical and structural alterations in the nucleus pulposus occur with aging. The semifluid nucleus pulposus contains 85% to 90% water bound to hydrophilic mucopolysaccharides. Dehydration occurs as a primary feature of disc degeneration. The degeneration results in decreased signal of the nucleus and anulus particularly on T2-weighted images. This change in MRI appearance has been shown to correlate with the changes of disc degeneration relative to discography. Degenerative changes in the anulus may lead to concentric and radial tears and cause protrusion of the nucleus pulposus. This event is reflected in the MRI appearance of decreased signal intensity on the T2-weighted images due to the dehydration, as well as in the loss of the definition between nucleus and anulus due to fissuring (Fig. 5.66).

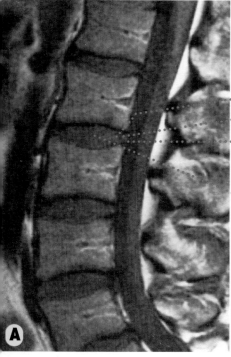

Inner fibers of anulus
Outer fibers of anulus
Posterior longitudinal ligament
Nucleus pulposus

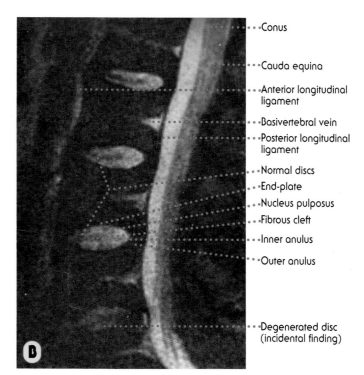

Conus
Cauda equina
Anterior longitudinal ligament
Basivertebral vein
Posterior longitudinal ligament
Normal discs
End-plate
Nucleus pulposus
Fibrous cleft
Inner anulus
Outer anulus
Degenerated disc (incidental finding)

Fig. 5.65 NORMAL L2-L3 AND L3-L4 INTERVERTEBRAL DISCS **(A)** T1-weighted sagittal image. The nucleus pulposus is slightly hypointense relative to the inner anulus. The peripheral anulus is dark, blending with the posterior longitudinal ligament. (An incidental finding was broad-based bulges of the L4-L5 and L5-S1 discs.) **(B)** T2-weighted sagittal image. The intensity of the nucleus is much higher than that of the inner anulus. The outer anulus remains dark. The dark horizontal band in the disc is a common finding in the normal adult. It represents a fibrous cleft in the nucleus.

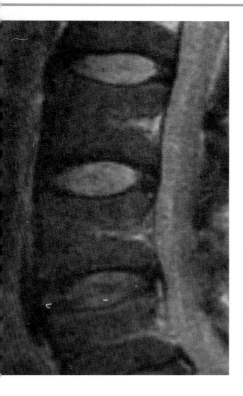

Fig. 5.66 DEGENERATIVE INTERVERTEBRAL DISC: ASYMPTOMATIC VOLUNTEER T2-weighted image. The L2-L3, L3-L4, and L4-L5 discs are shown. The L4-L5 disc is of reduced height and signal intensity, reflecting degeneration and desiccation. This is an extremely common finding even in asymptomatic volunteers. As an isolated finding, "degenerated disc" is of questionable diagnostic value.

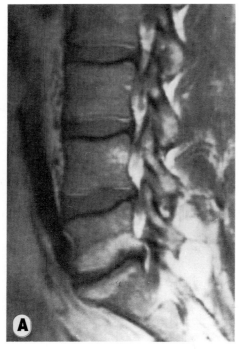

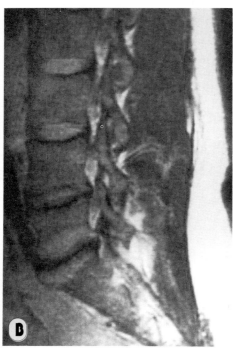

Associated with the primary changes in the disc there are secondary degenerative changes in the end-plates and the adjacent bone marrow. In acute disc degeneration, there is fissuring of the cartilaginous end-plates and vascularized fibrous replacement of the marrow adjacent to the end-plate. These changes result in decreased signal intensity on T1-weighted and increased signal intensity on T2-weighted images of the marrow adjacent to the end-plate. Further end-plate disruption and replacement of hematopoietic bone marrow by fatty marrow results in bands of increased signal intensity on the T1-weighted images (Fig. 5.67). Further disc narrowing and degeneration with subsequent sclerosis of the adjacent vertebra results in replacement of the bone marrow with thickened trabeculae. This causes decreased signal intensity on both T1- and T2-weighted images adjacent to the disc space. This decrease in intensity corresponds to the plain film appearance of sclerosis adjacent to the narrowed disc. Changes in the end-plate and adjacent marrow of decreased signal intensity on T1-weighted images and of increased signal intensity on T2-weighted images, have been described in infective discitis. Distinguishing features include the irregularity of end-plate destruction in discitis and the high signal intensity on T2-weighted images of the infected disc as compared with the characteristically decreased signal intensity of the degenerative disc.

Herniation of the nucleus pulposus may occur in a posterolateral direction through the anulus fibrosus where the restraining effect of the anulus is insufficient. Anular protrusion occurs as a result of disc narrowing due to the dehiscence of the nucleus and resulting disc space narrowing. Disc herniations variously manifest themselves as bulging, prolapsed, extruded, and sequestered discs. In a bulging disc there is degeneration of the nucleus with resulting narrowing of the disc space. The anulus remains intact but bulges posterior to the vertebral body (Fig. 5.68). Prolapsed disc signifies herniation of the nucleus through a radial tear in the anulus, which produces a focal prominence immediately beneath the most peripheral portion of the anulus (Fig. 5.69). If the disc protrusion extends beyond the peripheral portion of the anulus to lie beneath the posterior longitudinal ligament, it constitutes an extruded disc (Fig. 5.70). In practice, it may be impossible to determine the relationship of the disc material to the outer

Fig. 5.67 DEGENERATIVE END-PLATE CHANGES (A) T1-weighted image. The L5-S1 disc is reduced in height and in signal intensity, indicating degeneration. The hyperintense signal in the vertebral bodies of L5 and S1, adjacent to the end-plates of the L5-S1 disc, is the most common of the observed patterns of end-plate changes associated with degenerative disc disease. **(B)** T2-weighted image. The abnormality is less apparent on this sequence. This pattern of end-plate involvement is thought to be due to replacement of normal marrow by fatty marrow. It is also thought to prestage the sclerosis commonly observed on plain radiographs and CT.

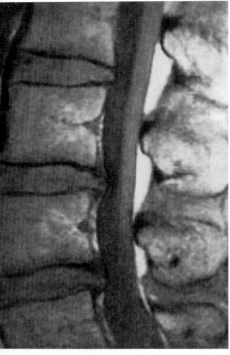

Fig. 5.68 BULGING DISC/ANULUS: ASYMPTOMATIC VOLUNTEER T1-weighted image. There is broad-based bulging of the disc and anulus at three levels: L2-L3, L3-L4, and L4-L5. It is increasingly more pronounced at the lower levels. The anulus is intact throughout. A disc bulge may be difficult to differentiate from a disc herniation. Axial sections are helpful—the bulge is broad-based, the herniation focal.

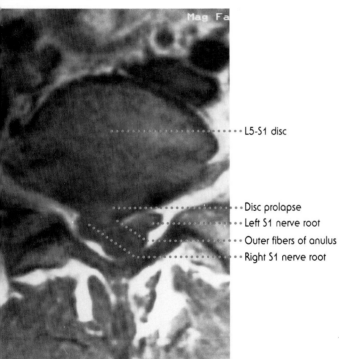

L5-S1 disc

Disc prolapse
Left S1 nerve root
Outer fibers of anulus
Right S1 nerve root

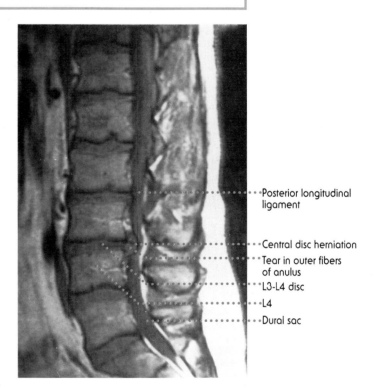

Posterior longitudinal ligament

Central disc herniation
Tear in outer fibers of anulus
L3-L4 disc
L4
Dural sac

Fig. 5.69 POSTEROLATERAL L5-S1 DISC HERNIATION T1-weighted axial image. The posterolateral disc prolapse encroaches on the right S1 root.

Fig. 5.70 L3-L4 DISC HERNIATION T1-weighted sagittal image. The herniated central L3-L4 disc pushes the posterior longitudinal ligament posteriorly, compressing the thecal sac.

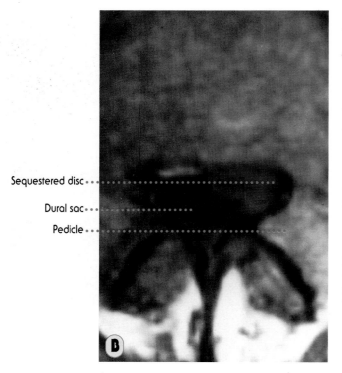

L2

Sequestered disc
fragment

L3

Normal epidural fat

L4

A

Sequestered disc

Dural sac

Pedicle

B

Fig. 5.71 SEQUESTERED DISC (A) T1-weighted sagittal image. The extruded disc has migrated behind the body of L3 and is no longer in continuity with the disc space. **(B)** T1-weighted axial image. The disc is clearly seen in the spinal canal at the level of the pedicles, remote from the disc space.

anular fibers and to distinguish, therefore, between prolapsed and extruded discs. The term herniated disc encompasses both of these entities and suffices for most purposes. An extruded disc remains in communication with the body of the nucleus through the radial tear in the anulus. In sequestered disc herniation, there is extrusion of material through the radial tear in the anulus, but it is no longer continuous with the remaining disc (Fig. 5.71). The isolated fragment is sequestered either anterior or posterior to the posterior longitudinal ligament.

CERVICAL SPINE Cervical degenerative disc disease and spondylosis are common and frequently asymptomatic. Disc herniations, posterolateral osteophyte formation, foraminal narrowing, and spinal cord compression may be seen without corresponding symptoms or signs. Careful clinical and radiological correlation is required to ensure that the demonstrated abnormality relates to the patient's symptoms. Myelography and CT-myelography are the traditional imaging modalities for a patient who presents with cervical radiculopathy. CT-myelography has proven more accurate than myelography alone in displaying the cause and location of nerve root compression, due to this modality's superior ability to distinguish between disc and osteophytes and to visualize lateral disc protrusions. Magnetic resonance imaging has many advantages over CT-myelography. It is noninvasive, while at the same time allowing for images in multiple planes and assessments of changes in the spinal cord itself. Although MRI is as sensitive as CT-myelography in identifying nerve root compression, differentiation between protruded disc material and posterolateral osteophytes is more difficult, because of the overlap in MRI appearance between these entities.

Disc herniations can be visualized by MRI in either the sagittal or axial plane as a protrusion of the nucleus into the spinal canal posterior to the normal disc margin (Figs. 5.72–5.74). It is often possible to distinguish between an extruded and a sequestered disc by demonstrating the continuity of the herniated fragment with the intervertebral disc in the latter entity. Most herniated disc material is hypointense or isointense relative to the adjacent anulus on T1-weighted sequences.

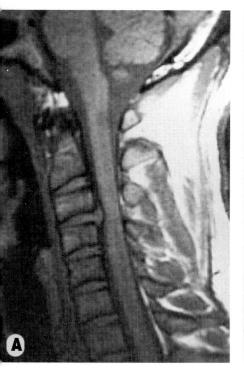

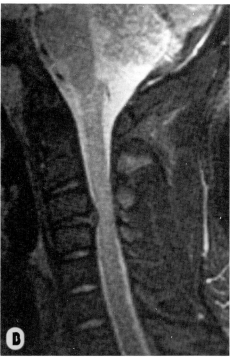

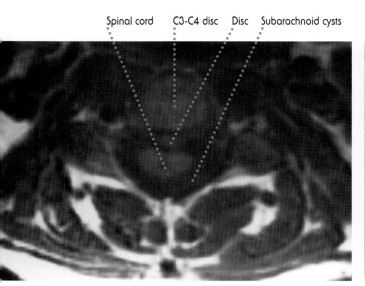

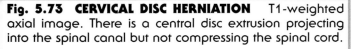

Spinal cord   C3-C4 disc   Disc   Subarachnoid cysts

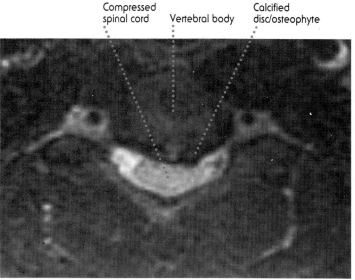

Compressed spinal cord   Vertebral body   Calcified disc/osteophyte

Fig. 5.73 CERVICAL DISC HERNIATION T1-weighted
axial image. There is a central disc extrusion projecting
into the spinal canal but not compressing the spinal cord.

Fig. 5.74 CERVICAL DISC HERNIATION T2-weighted
axial image. This image demonstrates the difficulty in
distinguishing between extruded discs and osteophytes.
A portion of the extruded disc is isointense with the
nucleus. The calcified portion is hypointense and indistinguishable from osteophytosis.

Posterolateral osteophytes are of variable intensity on T1-weighted images. They are often markedly hypointense, similar to cortical bone. If there is partial marrow replacement within the osteophyte, the signal intensity is higher (Fig. 5.75).

THORACIC SPINE   Symptomatic thoracic disc herniation is distinctly uncommon. Patients may present with sudden onset of paraparesis, but radiculopathy is infrequent. In most cases, thoracic disc herniations are pathologically identical to those seen in the cervical spine (Fig. 5.76), except that the former are frequently calcified and, therefore, are of low signal intensity on T1- and T2-weighted images.

LUMBAR SPINE   Disc herniations are most common in the lumbar region. The L4-L5 and L5-S1 discs are the most frequent sites. Symptoms of low back pain with radiation in a dermatome distribution is typical. Lumbar disc herniation is a leading cause of functional disability and has major socioeconomic consequences. Because of the greater thickness of the lumbar disc, it is easier to distinguish between disc protrusions, extrusions, and sequestrations in the lumbar spine. Most disc protrusions and extrusions are isointense or hypointense relative to the adjacent anulus on both T1- and T2-weighted images (see Figs. 5.69 to 5.71). Sequestered disc herniations are frequently hyperintense relative to the adjacent disc on T2-weighted images. Most disc herniations are in the posterolateral direction. However, central and lateral herniations are not at all uncommon. Lateral discs can be easily overlooked, unless the foramina are closely scrutinized on axial and parasagittal sections (Fig. 5.77).

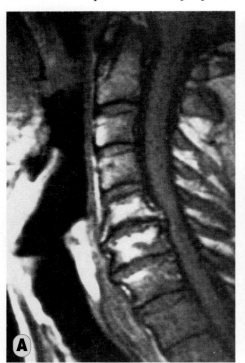
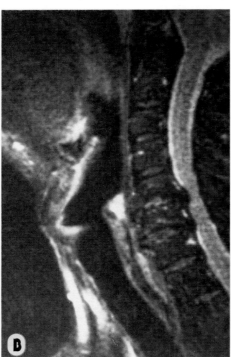
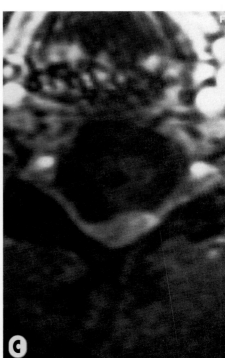

Fig. 5.75 CERVICAL OSTEOPHYTE   (A) T1-weighted sagittal image. Large posterior and anterior osteophytes arise at the C5-C6 interspace. Hyperintense fatty marrow replacement is seen adjacent to the involved disc. This marrow extends into the posterior osteophyte of the inferior C5 end-plate. The osteophyte arising from the superior end-plate of C6 is hypointense cortical bone. **(B)** T2-weighted sagittal image. The subarachnoid space is obliterated, and the spinal cord is compressed at the C5-C6 interspace by the posterior osteophyte. **(C)** Axial gradient recalled echo image. The posterior osteophyte deforms the left side of the spinal cord. The subarachnoid space is narrowed.

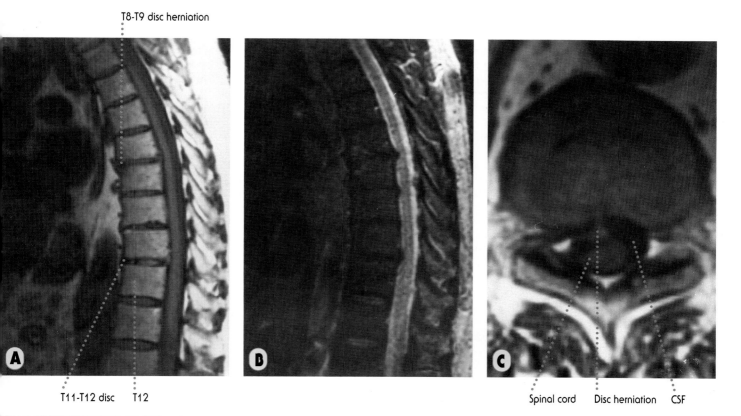

T8-T9 disc herniation

T11-T12 disc   T12

Spinal cord   Disc herniation   CSF

Fig. 5.76 THORACIC DISC HERNIATION **(A)** T1-weighted sagittal image. Disc herniation is present at T8-T9 and T11-T12. **(B)** T2-weighted sagittal image. The extent to which the disc protrudes into the subarachnoid space is more apparent on T2-weighted images. **(C)** T1-weighted axial image. The T11-T12 disc herniation lies to the right of the midline and deforms the anterior surface of the spinal cord.

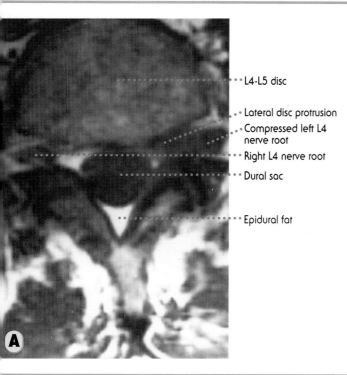

L4-L5 disc

Lateral disc protrusion

Compressed left L4 nerve root

Right L4 nerve root

Dural sac

Epidural fat

Epidural veins

L3 nerve root

L3-L4

L4 pedicle

Lateral disc protrusion

Fig. 5.77 LATERAL L4-L5 DISC PROTRUSION **(A)** T1-weighted axial image. A left lateral disc protrusion compresses the left L4 nerve root in its foramen. **(B)** T1-weighted sagittal image. This image through the level of the left pedicles demonstrates the lateral disc protrusion compressing the L4 nerve root.

SPINAL STENOSIS

Spinal stenosis may be divided into primary and degenerative types. Primary spinal stenosis is related to congenitally thick vertebral laminae, short pedicles, and a secondarily narrow spinal canal. Degenerative spinal stenosis is secondary to a variety of factors, of which disc degeneration appears likely to be the initiating factor. Disc degeneration and resultant loss of disc height cause a chain of events that ultimately leads to spinal stenosis. The loss of disc height causes diffuse anular bulging or protrusion of the disc, which compromises the anterior aspect of the dural sac. The loss of disc height also causes malalignment of the posterior facet joint, which increases mechanical stress and ultimately results in secondary arthritic changes. The resultant instability causes reactive ligament hypertrophy and osteophytosis. The instability also results in anterior, posterior, or lateral subluxations that further compromise the spinal canal; a combination of bony and soft tissue spinal canal narrowing severely compresses the lumbar nerve roots. Disc degeneration and loss of height resulting in such instability causes increased stress to the attachment of Sharpey's fibers. This results in anterolateral osteophyte formation and spondylosis. Typical large, horizontally oriented osteophytes develop.

CERVICAL SPINE   Cervical spondylosis and spinal stenosis are a frequent cause of cervical myelopathy. Affected patients present with symptoms of progressive spasticity in their lower limbs. There may or may not be associated radiculopathy. T2-weighted sagittal images best demonstrate the cord compression (Fig. 5.78). Areas of increased signal intensity in the spinal cord are frequently seen on the T2-weighted images (Fig. 5.79). These areas of hyperintensity probably relate to myelomalacia from longstanding compression.

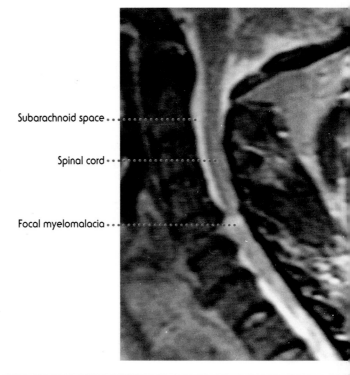

Subarachnoid space

Spinal cord

Focal myelomalacia

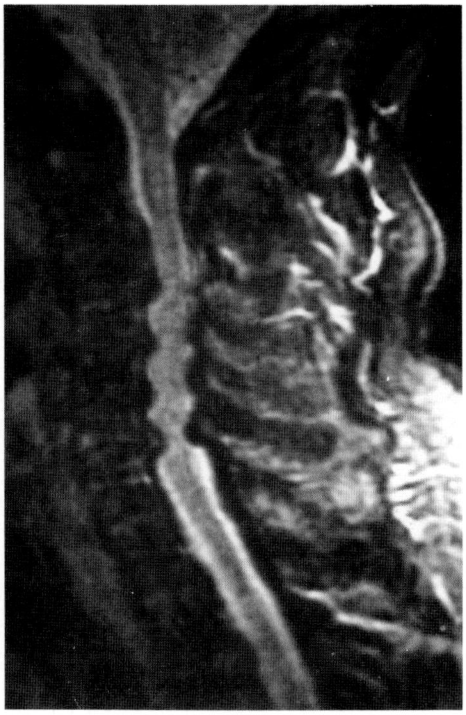

Fig. 5.78 CERVICAL SPONDYLOSIS T2-weighted sagittal image. The spinal cord is compressed anteriorly by osteophytes and posteriorly by hypertrophic facets at multiple levels.

Fig. 5.79 MYELOMALACIA T2-weighted sagittal image. There is multilevel spondylosis. There is a focal hyperintense lesion in the spinal cord at C5. This is presumed to be an area of cord softening (myelomalacia) secondary to longstanding compression.

LUMBAR SPINE Spinal stenosis causes compression of the lumbar nerve roots. Patients so affected present with low back and leg pain. The classical history is of spinal pseudoclaudication, in which the patients' symptoms become maximal on walking and are relieved at rest. Bladder control, and less frequently, bowel control may be limited or lost. The patients are older than those studied for disc herniations and usually present in their sixth decade. In primary spinal stenosis, the presentation may be earlier. Magnetic resonance imaging demonstrates the narrowing of the spinal canal and displacement of the epidural fat (Fig. 5.80). Associated bone changes are better assessed by CT.

POSTOPERATIVE SPINE Assessment of the postoperative back remains difficult. Failure to adequately relieve the patient's symptoms following back surgery is a frequent clinical problem. Recurrent disc hernia-tion (or residual herniated disc material) and epidural fibrosis are the common causes. It is clinically important to distinguish between these two entities, as recurrent disc herniations are treatable by repeat surgery and epidural fibrosis is not. Differentiation on the basis of signal intensity alone is not possible. They are best distinguished on the basis of morphology, location, and mass effect, and, secondarily, on signal characteristics and pattern of contrast enhancement.

Epidural fibrosis is a process of fibrous scarring often extending from the laminotomy site anteriorly to surround the nerve root sheath. It is poorly defined and tends not to have significant mass effect. It manifests itself by the replacement of the epidural fat and thickening of the adjacent dura rather than its displacement (Fig. 5.81). Disc herniations do tend to have mass effect, and their relationship to the adjacent disc can often be determined.

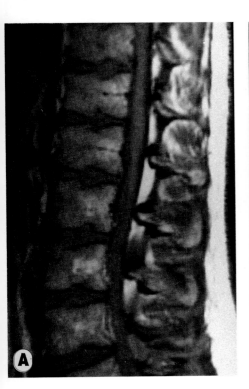
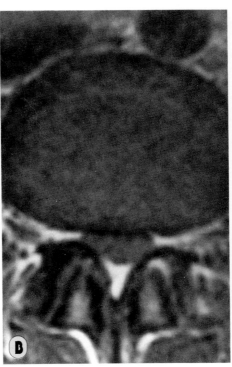
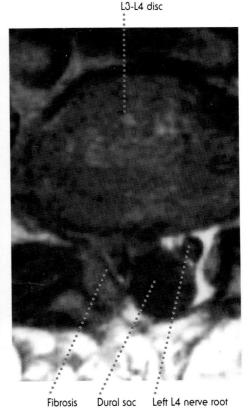

L3-L4 disc

Fibrosis   Dural sac   Left L4 nerve root

Fig. 5.80 CONGENITAL SPINAL STENOSIS (A) T1-weighted sagittal image. The entire lumbosacral spinal canal is narrow in the anteroposterior dimension. **(B)** T1-weighted axial image. The stenosis exists because of congenitally short pedicles, resulting in narrowing of the canal and thecal sac. It is characterized by a trefoil shape to the canal, whereas normally it is triangular.

Fig. 5.81 EPIDURAL FIBROSIS T1-weighted axial image. There has been a previous laminotomy for disc herniation. Epidural fibrosis encases the right L4 nerve root. There is little mass effect; the dural sac and nerve root are not displaced.

Although the appearance is variable, epidural fibrosis is usually hypointense or isointense on T1-weighted images and mildly hyperintense on T2-weighted images. Whereas protruded and extruded discs are most often isointense or hypointense on both sequences, free fragments or sequestrations often are hyperintense on T2-weighted images and, therefore, cannot be distinguished from the fibrosis. Enhancement of epidural fibrosis with paramagnetic contrast agents, a helpful diagnostic aid, is similar to the contrast enhancement demonstrated on infused CT examinations. It has been shown, however, that the margin of a herniated disc can also enhance (Fig. 5.82).

Following anterior cervical discectomy, a bone plug may be inserted at the disc level (Cloward proce-dure). A well-defined hypointense plug on the T1-weighted images is typical and should not be con-fused with other pathology (Fig. 5.83).

POSTERIOR LONGITUDINAL LIGAMENT CALCIFI-CATION   Extensive calcification of a thickened posterior longitudinal ligament in the cervical spine, may cause cervical cord compression and symptoms similar to cervical spondylosis. A densely calcified and thickened posterior longi-tudinal ligament is obvious anterior to the spinal cord on radiographs and CT. Magnetic resonance images demonstrate a thick linear mass of low signal intensity anterior to the spinal cord (Fig. 5.84).

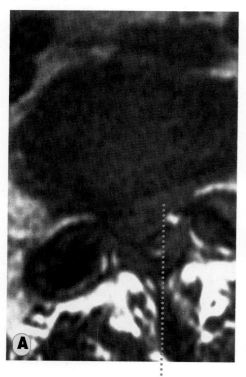
Soft tissue lesion

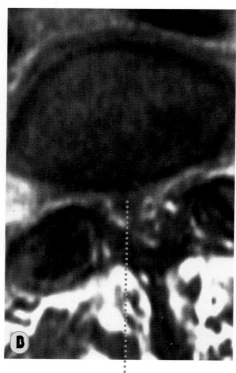
Lesion

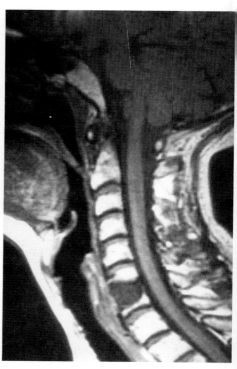

Fig. 5.82 HERNIATED DISC (A) T1-weighted axial image. There is an indistinct soft tissue lesion on the left side of the spinal canal, anterolateral to the thecal sac. **(B)** Post-gadolini-um-DTPA. The lesion enhances mod-erately, predominantly along its pos-terior margin. Enhancement is more typical of epidural scar; but as this case demonstrates, it is not uncom-mon to see it along the margin of a herniated disc. (Courtesy of Dr. G. Sze, Department of Radiology, Yale University, New Haven, CT)

Fig. 5.83 POSTOPERATIVE SPINE: CLOWARD PROCEDURE   T1-weighted sagittal image. A Cloward procedure has been per-formed at C6-C7. The bone plug used following the anterior discec-tomy is of low intensity relative to the adjacent normal marrow.

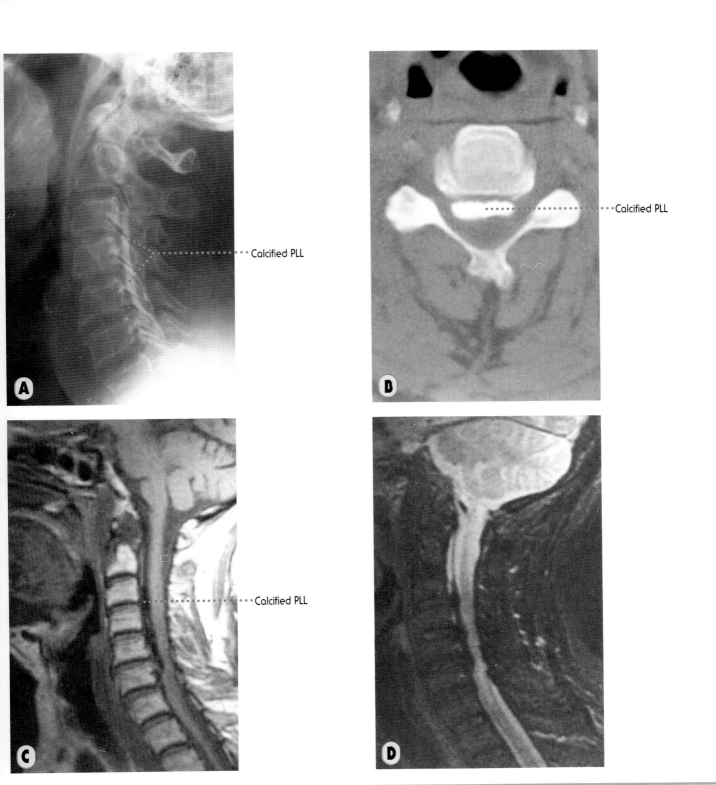

Calcified PLL

Calcified PLL

Calcified PLL

Fig. 5.84 POSTERIOR LONGITUDINAL LIGAMENT CALCIFICATION **(A)** Lateral cervical spine radiograph. The densely calcified and thickened posterior longitudinal ligament (PLL) is visible behind the cervical vertebra. **(B)** Computed tomography axial image. CT further demonstrates the extent of the PLL calcification. The spinal canal is narrowed by the densely calcified mass. **(C)** and **(D)** Sagittal T1- and T2-weighted images. The calcified PLL is clearly visible as a band of marked hypointensity, identical to cortical bone.

BIBLIOGRAPHY

BOOKS

Burger PC, Vogel SF. *Surgical pathology of the nervous system and its coverings*, 2nd ed. New York: John Wiley, 1982.

Modic MT, Masaryk TJ, Ross JS. *Magnetic resonance imaging of the spine*. Chicago: Year Book, 1989.

Okazaki, Harus. *Fundamentals of neuropathology*. New York/Tokyo: Igaku-Shoin, 1983.

JOURNAL ARTICLES AND BOOK CHAPTERS

Aisen AM, Martel W, Ellis JH, et al. Cervical spine involvement in rheumatoid arthritis: MR imaging. *Radiology* 1987;165:159–163.

Bronskill MJ, McVeigh ER, Kucharczyk W, et al. Syrinx-like artifacts on MR images of the spinal cord. *Radiology* 1988;166:485–488.

deRoos A, Kressel H, Spritzer C, et al. MR imaging of marrow changes adjacent to end plates in degenerative lumbar disc disease. *AJR* 1987;149:531–534.

Enzmann DR, Rubin JB. Cervical spine: MR imaging with a partial flip angle, gradient-refocused pulse sequence. I: General considerations and disc disease. *Radiology* 1988:166;467–472.

Flannigan BD, Lufkin RB, McGlade C, et al. MR imaging of the cervical spine: neurovascular anatomy. *AJR* 1987;148:785–790.

Hackney DB, Asato R, Joseph PM, et al. Hemorrhage and edema in acute spinal cord compression: demonstration by MR imaging. *Radiology* 1986;161:387–390.

Han JS, Benson JE, Kaufman B, et al. Demonstration of diastematomyelia and associated abnormalities with MR imaging. *AJNR* 1985;6:215–229.

Kubarik MA, Edwards MK, Grossman CB. Magnetic resonance evaluation of pediatric spinal dysraphism. *Pediatr Neurosci* 1986;12:213–218.

Kulkarni MV, McArdie CB, Kopanicky D, et al. Acute spinal cord injury, MR imaging at 1.5 T. *Radiology* 1987;164:837–843.

Lee BCP, Zimmerman RD, Manning JJ, et al. MR imaging of syringomyelia and hydromyelia. *AJNR* 1985;6:221–228.

Ludwig H, Tscholakoff D, Neuhold A, et al. Magnetic resonance imaging of the spine in multiple myeloma. *Lancet* 1987;ii:364–366.

Masaryk TJ, Ross JS, Modie MT, et al. Radiculomeningeal vascular malformations of the spine: MR imaging. *Radiology* 1987;164:845–849.

Minami S, Suzoh TS, Nishimura K, et al. Spinal arteriovenous malformation: MR imaging. *Radiology* 1988;169:109–115.

Mirvis SE, Geisler FH, Jelinek JJ, et al. Acute cervical spine trauma: evaluation with 1.5 T MR imaging. *Radiology* 1988;166:807–816.

Modic MT, Masaryk TJ, Mulopulos GP, et al. Cervical radiculopathy: prospective evaluation with surface coil MR imaging, CT with metrizamide, and metrizamide myelography. *Radiology* 1986;161:753–759.

Ross JS, Masaryk TJ, Modic MT, et al. Vertebral hemangiomas: MR imaging. *Radiology* 1987;165:165–169.

Rubin JB, Enzmann DR. Optimizing conventional MR imaging of the spine. *Radiology* 1987;163:777–783.

Sarpel S, Sarpel G, Yu E, et al. Early diagnosis of spinal-epidural metastasis by magnetic resonance imaging. *Cancer* 1987;59:1112–1116.

Schneidernan G, Flannigan B, Kingston S, et al. Magnetic resonance imaging in the diagnosis of disc degeneration: correlation with discography. *Spine* 1987;12.

Yu S, Haughton UM, Ho PSP, et al. Progressive and regressive changes of the nucleus pulposus. Part II: The adult. *Radiology* 1988;169:93–97.

Yu S, Sether LA, Haughton UM. Facet joint menisci of the cervical spine: correlative MR imaging and cryomicrotome study. *Radiology* 1987;164:79–82.

INDEX